Professor Margaret Alston OAM

Professor Margaret Alston, B. Soc. Stud (Syd), Dip. Comp. Applic. (RMIHE), M. Litt (UNE), PhD (UNSW), assumed duties as Head of Department of Social Work at Monash University in 2008. She established the Gender, Leadership and Social Sustainability (GLASS) research unit at Monash, has published widely in the fields of rural gender and rural social issues, and has been a keynote speaker at a number of national and international conferences over the last several years. She is currently researching the gendered impacts of climate change in Australia and the Asia–Pacific region. Margaret received her Medal of the Order of Australia in 2010 for services to social work and the advancement of women, particularly in rural areas.

Associate Professor Wendy Bowles PhD

Wendy Bowles is a social worker with a practice grounding in the disability field. She is Associate Professor of Social Work and Human Services and Sub-Dean Workplace Learning in Faculty of Arts at Charles Sturt University. Wendy has co-authored *Ethical Practice in Social Work* and *Research for Social Workers: An introduction to methods,* as well as publishing chapters and articles on rural social work practice, social work ethics, fieldwork education and disability issues. Wendy is an active member of various boards, advisory groups and committees as well as her professional association: the Australian Association of Social Workers for which she chairs the National Field Education Sub-Committee.

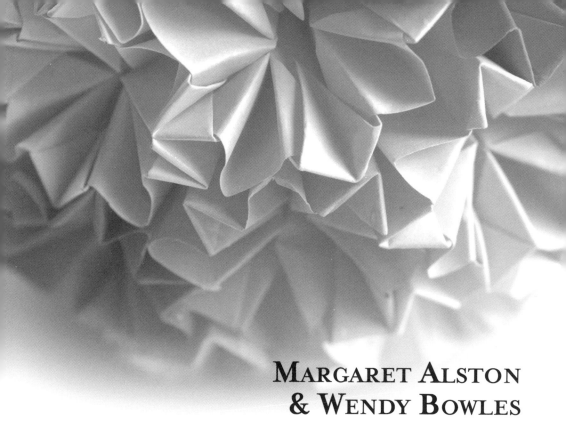

Margaret Alston & Wendy Bowles

3RD EDITION

Research for Social Workers

An introduction to methods

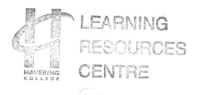

LEARNING
RESOURCES
CENTRE
HAVERING
COLLEGE

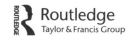

Routledge
Taylor & Francis Group

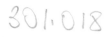
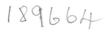

First edition published 1998
by Allen & Unwin

Second edition published 2003
by Routledge

This edition published 2013
by Routledge
2 Park Square, Milton Park, Abingdon, Oxon, OX14 4RN

Simultaneously published in the USA and Canada
by Routledge
711 Third Avenue, New York, NY 10017

and in Australia and New Zealand
by Allen and Unwin Pty Ltd
83 Alexander Street, Crows Nest, NSW 2065, Australia

Routledge is an imprint of the Taylor & Francis Group, an informa business

© 2013 Margaret Alston and Wendy Bowles

Index by Sue Jarvis
Set in 11.5/14 pt Minion by Midland Typesetters, Australia
Printed in China at Everbest Printing Co

British Library Cataloguing in Publication Data
A catalogue record for this book is available from the British Library

Library of Congress Cataloging-in-Publication Data
A catalog record has been requested for this book

ISBN13: 978-0-415-50677-9 (hbk)
ISBN13: 978-0-415-50681-6 (pbk)
ISBN13: 978-0-203-08414-4 (ebk)

Contents

Tables

Figures

Acknowledgements

We would especially like to thank our publisher, Lizzy Walton, for her assistance and support in bringing out the third edition of this book. Jenny Coopes' cartoons flavour the chapters with just the right spice. We particularly wish to thank our partners for their ongoing support, and our friends and family who make it all possible.

Introduction

We are delighted to bring you the third edition of *Research for Social Workers*. Since the first edition was published, social work research has developed in new and exciting ways, and this edition reflects many of these changes. There are new chapters on 'Systematic Reviews' and 'Research in Post-disaster Recovery and Other Crisis Situations', and 'Statistics for Social Workers' is now covered in two chapters. All chapters have been updated, with most incorporating new material.

Our initial aims remain the same:

- To make research methods accessible to students and social work practitioners with plain English explanations of research concepts and principles.
- To enable social work students and practitioners to undertake their own research by providing a step-by-step guide.
- To encourage the social work community to become critical consumers of research.
- To assist with the development of a social work research culture, or research-mindedness amongst social workers (Humphries 2008; Dominelli 2005), which extends our understanding of social work knowledge and practice across the world.

One defining change scholars may notice is that we are encompassing research examples from across the world. It is our aim to make this textbook accessible to social workers everywhere, and thus we have set out to ensure that the book captures some of the realities of social work in global settings.

As social work practice has grown increasingly sophisticated, and more diverse in its range of fields and settings, the place of research in social work has become more critical. Today, research is relevant to just about every area of social work practice: from the initial stages of an intervention—determining the needs of an individual, group or community; through to testing new ideas and deciding which course of action to take; and finally, to evaluating practice and justifying social work's existence. Social work has become central to new areas of global concern such as post-disaster recovery and human trafficking, and it is our intention to give our social work colleagues some direction on the ways in which we might use research to enhance our work in critical situations. Springing from the research traditions of sociology and psychology, social work is now developing its own research orientation and knowledge base, grounded in human rights and social justice, providing fertile ground for social work theory and practice to flourish. However, many social workers still do not recognise the potential of research, nor its value for them as practitioners.

This book introduces research concepts and skills for social workers. It is a valuable resource for social work students as well as social work graduates who wish to hone their research skills. Readers will gain not only an understanding of the principles and approaches that are most relevant to social work practice, but also have access to a step-by-step approach to undertaking research in their work. *Research for Social Workers* deals with research issues from a social work perspective, using social work examples and incorporating social-work-based methods. It has been written as a guide for beginners in appropriately non-technical language, but it will allow readers to move into a research program with confidence and ability. As academics, researchers and social workers ourselves, we are committed to enabling social workers to include research as an essential—indeed fundamental—part of their professional toolkits. This means becoming critical consumers of research, as well as confidently being able to incorporate research into everyday practice.

Today, social work research reflects the many differences in approach, politics and theory that exist in social work practice. Hence it is important that social workers understand the variety of research approaches available, and are aware of the different theories and epistemologies on which they are based, so that their personal approaches to research are more informed and explicit. Thus the book begins with a brief exploration of what constitutes the spectrum of social work research and how theories influence all aspects of research—from choosing the general topic area and the overall approach to defining the problem and selecting methodologies.

Because this is an introductory text for beginning researchers, the various approaches are presented as ideal types to highlight the differences and the debates that surround them. However, we do not view the research process as consisting of mutually exclusive, dichotomous approaches (for example, inductive/deductive or qualitative/quantitative). In our own research, we tend to use multi-method approaches and the examples chosen in the book reflect this. Nonetheless, for an introductory text we feel it is important to set out the different approaches separately, so that beginning researchers can clarify the differences and identify the different orientations in existing research as they develop their own conceptual approach to research practice.

In Chapter 1 we sketch an outline of different approaches to social research, concluding with a discussion of the politics and ethics of research. In these times when many social issues have become laden with political ideology, it is particularly important to be aware of the various ideological and political agendas of the different stakeholders in the research process, and the policy and practice implications of the research we undertake. In Chapters 2 and 3, we cover the issues involved in choosing your topic area and defining the problem. Steps in the research process are summarised in Chapter 4, and sampling procedures are covered in Chapter 5. Research methods that are most relevant to social workers— surveys, interviews, needs analyses, evaluation, action research, methods of establishing best practice and other methods—are discussed in Chapters 6 to 11. This includes a new chapter about an emerging field of social work research, systematic reviews. Chapter 12 also introduces a new topic: research in post-disaster recovery situations. The information from this chapter is applicable to other crisis events, and provides strategies and techniques that will assist workers to use research effectively in order to inform and build good practice in this emerging area of practice. Chapters 14 and 15 present different ways of analysing data and producing results, with reference to the various computer software packages available. Chapters 16 and 17 introduce statistical concepts and techniques. The book concludes with a discussion of how to ensure that research leads to action, and an exploration of some of the most effective ways of influencing policy and practice (Chapter 18). Finally, Chapter 19 provides a detailed guide to writing your research proposal, including how to produce a budget.

As the aims outlined at the beginning of this Introduction are achieved, so will social work's voice strengthen, and with it social work's ability to achieve its mission of advancing the pursuit of social justice for disadvantaged groups, fostering human rights, overcoming oppression and working to improve well-being for all people.

PART I

Beginning social work research

I *Social work research*

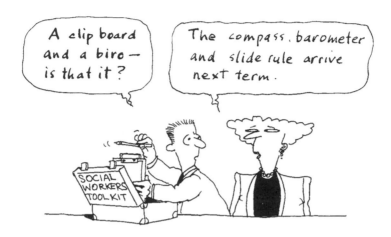

This chapter introduces you to social work research. As social work is an evolving, dynamic profession, it requires a solid research base to advance and develop responsive and sustainable practice. However, before we introduce you to a rich understanding of social work research, we want to provide you with some reassurance. Research is *not* all about numbers. If you are one of those social workers or students who have had unhappy experiences with mathematics, do not despair! Social research is more about critical awareness, careful thinking and the ability to view situations from new perspectives rather than it is about numbers. In the twenty-first century, a whole range of approaches to research exist—some involving more mathematics than others. With the advent of computer software packages, it is more important to understand the thinking or logic behind the mathematics, and the theoretical perspectives behind the thinking, than to be able to calculate the numbers themselves.

In this chapter, we examine some of the different forms of research and the power of the underlying beliefs that shape them. Quantitative, qualitative, emancipatory, feminist and postmodern influences on research methods are discussed. Each of these offers a range of possibilities for creative and exciting research for social workers. All these approaches can be used by social work researchers and all are important for you to understand, not only because you may use them in your work, but also in order to understand the research undertaken by others. As you will see, these methods are not necessarily mutually exclusive. Indeed, much research today involves a mixture of methods—that is, researchers use a 'multi-method' approach, selecting aspects of different approaches that best suit their purposes. As this is a text for beginning researchers, we present the approaches separately so that you can see how they have evolved, and so we can introduce some of the debates that surround them.

We also consider some of the important political and ethical issues that surround research, before moving on in later chapters to the 'how to' of different research approaches. First we discuss what social research is and why, as social workers, we should study research.

Why study research?

Research provides us with evidence about the effectiveness of our practice; it can enhance our understanding of effective policies and practice, and it can advance socially just issues and socially inclusive practices (Smith 2009). As with other professions, we are being encouraged to develop 'research-mindedness' or the ability to inform our practice with research findings and to conduct our own research (Humphries 2008).

Whether we realise it or not, most social workers are constantly doing research or research-like activities. Consider the following:

- A social worker wonders which counselling methods used by different workers in her team are most helpful to the young offenders they see on a regular basis.
- A community worker in a new job at a council has a brief to find out what the local community thinks of a planned development to build an industrial complex in some bushland containing a disused quarry.
- A worker in a church-based agency holds a regular group for homeless youth and suspects that many group members are facing similar issues and problems in their lives.
- A social welfare worker wants to know what effects the new respite care service is having on families who are under stress.
- A worker in the disability field who has been asked to establish a new service for young adults wonders what life is like from the perspective of the young people, and what kind of services—if any—they would like his agency to provide.

- A worker sent to a crisis situation wants to evaluate where the greatest need might be and how each of the services and organisations in the field is responding.

All these situations require research skills if social workers are to systematically and effectively address the questions and issues they face. The bottom line is that if you are to make informed decisions or undertake carefully thought through actions/interventions, you need research skills. More specifically, consider the following reasons for studying research.

Becoming an informed research consumer

Social workers are often confronted with government or interdepartmental reports in which research and statistics are quoted. If this is a familiar situation for you, you are probably uncomfortably aware that you may have taken such reports at face value and, because of a lack of research understanding, you may not have the ability to critique such reports. As Dudley (2011, p. 10) reminds us, we need to be 'effective in consuming research studies that are pertinent to [our] professional work'. You should heed Smith's (2009, p. 29) suggestion that we assess research findings by asking the following questions:

- Was the method used appropriate to this particular research question and research environment?
- Was the research carried out to an acceptable standard, according to the requirements of the chosen method?

Research studies can be biased or flawed for a lot of different reasons, and you might not be able to detect these reasons without a basic understanding of research methodology and the confidence required to assess these studies.

All social research has a political imperative. Some reports may take liberties in the way research is presented in order to achieve or to bolster a certain perspective. Some departments—for example, those keen to downsize—may disregard or under-report the success of certain programs. Some statistics may be used inappropriately or out of context to enhance an unsupported position. Likewise, some research reports might enhance positive findings in order to ensure continued funding. It is naive to think otherwise in an economic climate where large cuts have been made to welfare spending.

Consider also that when outside consultants are used by an agency or department to assess the organisation's functions, you should be in a position to critically analyse their work and examine whether or not they have given you a fair appraisal. It is imperative that you become an informed practitioner, capable of dissecting the information on which decisions are being made about policies that affect your department or your programs.

Evidence-based practice

A second and equally important reason why you should have competent research skills is to allow you to justify your practice interventions in an informed way, based on research evidence. It is not enough to rely on your intuition—intuition is susceptible to bias, and may reflect your own values rather than client benefits. Increased accountability to funding bodies and to the people for whom the services are established requires workers to assess adequately what the people we are working with want and need, how our interventions are affecting people's lives, and how our programs and approaches can be improved. Increasingly around the world, social workers are being expected to work in an evidence-based culture—that is, to know whether or not what they are doing is working.

There are a number of ways in which practice effectiveness may be assessed. For instance, as a practitioner you may be called on to examine the effect of certain interventions on a group of clients. You might also be required to justify your agency's effectiveness by providing an evaluation of the use of its services and the effects of the services on the client group.

Again, you might be called on to show you are meeting the needs of a particular target group (needs analysis). Often practitioners keen to continue a new program are expected to evaluate the program in order that its effectiveness can be demonstrated—that it is meeting its objectives, that it is developing as intended and that it is producing desired outcomes (program evaluation). The future development of the program may depend on well-constructed evaluation research. As well, maintaining—and indeed increasing—your funding level may depend on your analysis of research conducted to justify a service (cost–benefit analysis).

It is also vital that you have the confidence and competence to act as a contributing partner in research projects. There are often occasions when your agency or department will conduct or contribute to a research project. Having an understanding of research methods will allow you to ensure that a social work perspective is part of the project.

Participating in the policy process

Increasing our research-mindedness also enables us to assess the impact of government social policies and to assist in constructing such policies. It is social work's role as a profession to take a lead in the formulation of policy that affects the most vulnerable members of our community, and to criticise or support government policies. In the past, social workers have not been known for applying pressure effectively—at any level of government—to change or modify policies. As an example, cuts in welfare programs in many countries have not been matched by rich social work research assessing the consequences of a loss of services for vulnerable people.

With improved research skills, you will be on firmer ground in joining in the policy process—in commenting on current policies or evaluations of policy and developing a case for new or different policies.

Undertaking postgraduate education

One important outcome of studying research at undergraduate level is that it will facilitate your entry into Masters and doctoral programs. This reason should not be discounted, as it is our experience that students may be reluctant to pursue postgraduate study because of their lack of knowledge about research and their fear of attempting a major research project. Yet we need such students to build a strong theoretical and research base in order to upgrade the standing of our discipline. Of course, you must also be aware that studying research at undergraduate level is a requirement of professional social work associations around the world, and so is a basic requirement for those of you wishing to attain a social work degree.

Developing social work knowledge and theory

A very important reason for studying research is to aid in the development of social work knowledge and theory. Having studied, or being currently involved in studying, social work, you would be aware that the development of social work theories and knowledge rests on the shoulders of practitioners who are able to test and evaluate their usefulness. We need these developments to come from social workers themselves, rather than from other disciplinary areas. For all these reasons and more, you will benefit from the study of research methods.

Practising in an ethically responsible manner

Social work codes of ethics around the world support ethical research practice. For example, the ethical codes of the British, US and Australian social work associations all contain detailed sections on how to undertake ethical research. We discuss this in more detail later in the chapter.

What is social research?

From the above discussion, it can be seen that many different types of research are used in the welfare field. Which approaches you choose will depend on the purpose of the research, your background and beliefs, the agenda of the organisation funding the research and, increasingly, the perspectives of the people and/or programs being researched.

Examples of the variety of social research used in the welfare field

- Needs analysis
- Action research
- Outcome evaluation
- Cost–benefit analysis
- Secondary analysis
- Content analysis
- Client satisfaction surveys
- Qualitative in-depth interviewing

Nearly all forms of research involve the search for patterns or themes—ways of simplifying a mass of information into meaningful stories or relationships. Good research helps us to make links, gain insight into apparent contradictions, explore new territory and raise difficult questions. In the process of searching for patterns or themes, all types of research involve some form of measurement. In Chapters 2 and 3, we will explore the different types of measurement used in the process of translating broad research issues into researchable questions.

In the welfare field, almost all types of research are undertaken in order to make a decision or to take some action. If we went to the trouble and expense of undertaking a research project, it would be most disappointing if the finished report sat on a shelf gathering dust. It is often said that research is a means of putting off tough or expensive decisions. Instead of being the end of the process, your report should be the first step in changing a policy, deciding on an intervention strategy or setting up a new service.

Taking these considerations into account, the definition of research (below) describes the way the terms 'social research' and 'social work research' are understood throughout this book. The research literature contains as many definitions of research as there are forms; this definition captures the broad elements that are generally agreed upon as being shared by most research that is undertaken in the social welfare field.

Definition of social research

Social research is the systematic observation and/or collection of information to find or impose a pattern, in order to make a decision or take some action.

Definition of social work research

Social work research implies action, pursues social justice and collects systematic information in order to make a difference to people's lives.

Drawing on several writers who are now articulating what it is to be a social work researcher (e.g. see Smith 2009; Hardwick and Worsley 2011), we agree that social work research differs from other forms of social research in that it is action-oriented, has a clear relationship between research and practice, incorporates an understanding of the social, political and economic context, is embedded in social work values, may enable the participation of those researched and is designed to make a difference.

The power of research as a tool for social change is fundamental to our understanding of the place of research in social work. Just as the goals of social work involve not just understanding the world, but actively intervening to change things in some way, so too does social work research involve action, decisions and change.

Types of research

The ways in which researchers find or impose patterns from or on the mass of information available in order to make decisions or take action depend very much on the beliefs and theories from which they operate. Before we decide what type of research to do, it is important to understand the assumptions and perspectives that underlie the major approaches to research, so that we are not 'blinkered' by our methodology or unaware of its limitations.

The different research approaches used today are best understood in the context of their history and how they developed in relation to each other. We will discuss five of the major research approaches, in order to demonstrate the variety that exists:

- quantitative research
- qualitative research

- the emancipatory approach
- feminist research
- postmodern research.

These research approaches are summarised as ideal 'types' rather than actual descriptions of research as it happens in the 'real world'. The descriptions highlight the major differences between the approaches to allow you to distinguish between the different types and to think about which research methods would be most appropriate in different situations. In fact, many researchers use a variety of methods—the multi-method approach— and the different approaches themselves can have considerable overlap. We begin with what was until recently the dominant and orthodox form of research.

Quantitative research

Quantitative research is the oldest form of social research. It grew out of the natural science paradigm of the eighteenth and nineteenth centuries and the intellectual tradition known as 'positivist' or 'realist' (Humphries 2008). This type of research is based on the idea that there is an objective 'reality' that can be measured accurately, and that operates according to natural laws, which can be 'discovered' by rigorous, objective research (Sarantakos 2005). Just as a natural scientist in the nineteenth century might examine a rock and test its properties, so it is assumed that a social scientist can 'objectively' study a group or social system, or study reality from the outside (Sarantakos 2005; Morris 2006).

It is also assumed that the effect of the researcher's own presence is minimal or non-existent, so that 'pure' reality can be studied. In other words, it is assumed that whatever the researcher is told, or observes, would actually be happening whether they were present to observe it or not. Similarly, it is assumed that any other researcher who studies the same social phenomenon would come up with the same findings because the research has been done in a structured and measurable way (Hardwick and Worsley 2011).

Originally, the people who were being studied using this approach were not included in the decision-making processes about the research (they were 'objects' for study rather than 'subjects' involved in the process). Indeed, often the only concessions made to them being people rather than the inanimate objects researched in the physical sciences were precautions taken to protect privacy, anonymity and safety.

Traditionally, researchers in the quantitative positivist tradition begin with ideas or theories about the world, which they then go out and test empirically. Thus they carefully design the structure of their research and the concepts they are researching *before* they go out into the field. Going from the general to the specific, or beginning with the theory and testing ideas empirically, is known as the 'deductive' approach to research (Hardwick and Worsley 2011; de Vaus 2002). We will discuss how these ideas or theories are turned into researchable questions in Chapter 3.

At the most extreme end of the quantitative spectrum of research methods lies experimental design. In recent times, this method has experienced a revival in some areas of social work research, particularly in the United States and some parts of the United Kingdom (Humphries 2008; Morris 2006). Experimental designs involve strict conditions, including random assignment of subjects (people) to experimental groups (the group being given the intervention) and control groups (the group that does not have the intervention). The researcher manipulates the independent or treatment variable systematically to determine what effects treatment (intervention) has on the experimental group. Because people are placed randomly in the control and experimental groups, it is assumed that all the other factors (variables) that could influence or interfere in the effect of the treatment variable are balanced out between the two groups. Thus any change measured in the experimental group can be assumed to be due to the treatment variable. Proponents of experimental design in social work argue that this is the only 'true' way of rigorously testing the effectiveness of interventions.

While experimental designs—also known as 'randomised control trials', or RCTs (Humphries 2008)—may be possible in some social work situations where a single intervention is being offered, such as correctional or prison settings, it is not always possible or desirable to randomly allocate people to experimental or control groups, because those in the control group will not receive the intervention—presenting an ethical dilemma. In addition, critics of this approach argue that social reality cannot be reduced to simplistic manipulations of one variable at a time—life is much more complex than this. Rather than being 'objective', this approach is based on a world-view that assumes humans act in ordered, rational ways. Critics of positivism and its offshoots maintain that these assumptions are not universal truths, but a particular theoretical perspective (for example, feminist critics argue that this reflects a largely white, male, middle-class view of the world).

Due to these and other considerations, a whole range of quantitative measures have been developed that 'compromise' one or more of the conditions of classic experimental research design. For example, there are quasi-experimental single-case designs in which practitioners can evaluate the effects of their interventions with a single person, and non-experimental surveys and group designs where inclusion in the sample is not based on random allocation.

Quantitative researchers typically use techniques such as surveys, questionnaires and structured observations. Using statistics, they analyse the information they have collected to see whether their ideas about patterns or relationships are supported by 'the facts' as revealed in their research. Because they are interested in 'truth' and discovering natural 'laws' of society, quantitative researchers place great importance on whether the people they study are representative of a whole population, and whether their results can be applied to this larger group. Various sampling and statistical techniques are used in attempts to ensure that conclusions can be 'generalised' (applied) to all the people in the population, and not just to those who were included in a particular study.

Examples of quantitative research

- The Census
- Large opinion polls
- Some forms of evaluation—for example, outcome evaluations, cost–benefit analyses
- Research that aims to establish whether there is a relationship between two or more variables—for example: Is there a relationship between income and religion?

Although quantitative research has provided many useful insights into the social world, some of its most basic assumptions have attracted stringent criticism. These have led to alternative research approaches. A general term for a variety of research methodologies that has arisen from critiques of quantitative approaches is 'qualitative research'.

Qualitative research

Instead of beginning with theories of patterns or relationships and testing them in the 'real world', qualitative researchers prefer to start the other way around and begin with their experiences or specific observations. They begin their research with no preconceived ideas, and allow the patterns or themes to emerge from their experiences. From careful observations, immersion in the world of the 'researched', in-depth interviews and a range of other techniques, qualitative researchers build their theories from the patterns they observe in their data (sometimes called 'grounded theory'—e.g. see Corbin and Strauss 2008). Thus their approach is inductive: it moves from specific observations or interactions to general ideas and theories. This is in direct contrast to deductive quantitative researchers, who begin with general theories and move to specific situations. Whereas quantitative researchers aim to 'discover' universal social 'laws', and test theories that explain causal relationships, qualitative researchers are more interested in understanding how others experience life, in interpreting meaning and social phenomena, and in exploring new concepts and developing new theories.

In contrast to quantitative researchers who emphasise the importance of 'objectivity', and of research being 'value free', many qualitative researchers reject the whole notion of objectivity, arguing that research can never be value free. Rather than assuming that there is an 'objective reality' that exists independently of people and can be measured, qualitative researchers believe that 'reality' depends on how people experience and interpret life. From this point of view, reality is 'socially constructed', and so cannot be separated from experience or measured from the outside. Instead, the challenge is to understand reality from the 'inside'—from other people's perspectives.

A crucial part of such understanding is the way the researcher interacts with the researched, and how the two parties affect each other during the research process. This is another major difference between qualitative and quantitative research. Quantitative researchers believe that the researcher should remain separate from those being researched, and that the researcher has minimal or no effect on what is being researched. Qualitative researchers maintain that this is impossible—instead, the researcher should acknowledge their own values, biases and position in relation to the researched. They advocate a research process that is a two-way interaction between the researcher and the researched, in which the parties are on a more equal level—sometimes 'co-evolving' the research structure as they go. Thus a qualitative researcher might conduct very flexible, open interviews so that the conversation can cover topics, perspectives and meanings that are important to the people being researched. Qualitative researchers reject structured surveys and interviews, arguing that these structures reflect the values, assumptions and 'social constructions' of the researcher rather than the perspective of the people being researched. According to qualitative researchers, quantitative methods distort reality because they only measure those aspects of it that are 'quantifiable'. Much of social life, qualitative researchers maintain, can only be understood in the context in which it is experienced, and can never be captured in artificially structured questionnaires, which impose a particular view of reality upon the people being researched.

Similarly, qualitative researchers—unlike quantitative researchers—do not emphasise statistical procedures or the importance of representativeness. Instead, they generalise their results using theory, logic, and further exploration and discussion of themes with the people with whom they are researching. Statistics can be used for limited purposes in qualitative research, such as summarising or describing what many people felt. However, most purist researchers in this tradition would not see any point in 'imposing' advanced statistical procedures on the information they have collected.

Examples of qualitative research

- A researcher spends several months 'hanging around' with a gang of 'street kids' to investigate their lifestyle and the issues that are important to them (participant observation).
- In-depth interviews are conducted with rural women and workers from relevant human service agencies to explore attitudes to domestic violence in the country.
- Observations of council meetings and interviews with local councillors are conducted to examine how they perceive 'grassroots democracy'.
- Meetings are held with groups of elderly residents in an inner-city suburb to understand their concerns and priorities, and to find out what they would like from the local neighbourhood centre.
- Focus groups are held with women and men in small coastal villages affected by cyclones to determine what safety and early warning systems are needed.

Unlike quantitative research, which has its roots in positivism and theoretical disciplines closely related to it (for example, you might come across terms such as 'logical positivism' and 'postpositivism'), there are many different theories underpinning qualitative research that emphasise different aspects of it, and that arise from different critiques of positivism. Some of the theories on which various types of qualitative research methods are based include ethnography, symbolic interactionism, constructivism, hermeneutics and critical theory. Many textbooks on qualitative research methods (e.g. Morris 2006) contain descriptions of these different theories, which you will need to understand in more detail if you are going to attempt some of the qualitative techniques.

Qualitative research has experienced its share of controversy. One of the major criticisms of these methodologies is that they ignore the larger social structures and forces that influence existence by concentrating only on the microcosm of human experience. In this way, accusations of being 'apolitical' have been levelled at some qualitative researchers. Ethical questions have also been raised about some forms of qualitative research, such as 'participant observation', where the researcher joins a group or community 'in disguise' and then publishes the results of their observations without the knowledge or consent of the people themselves. Still others have questioned the uses to which both quantitative and qualitative research has been put. From our discussion so far, it might seem that qualitative and quantitative research are incompatible opposites— and indeed, up until the 1960s, this was how the two schools were viewed (Pyke and Agnew 1991; Rothery 1993; Taylor 1993). However, purist qualitative or quantitative researchers are rare. More commonly, research- ers combine aspects of qualitative and quantitative methodologies to accomplish their purposes. Instead of viewing qualitative and quantitative approaches (or inductive and deductive thinking) as diametrically opposed, many theorists see them as different phases of a cyclical process of devel- oping knowledge (Humphries 2008; de Vaus 2002). For example, de Vaus (2002) describes research as a cycle of theory-building and theory-testing that incorporates inductive and deductive approaches. Thus researchers may begin with an idea that they explore in a qualitative fashion before testing more developed hypotheses using quantitative methods. The two approaches can be used in a cyclical, logical fashion designed to develop and refine theorising.

Many researchers use both qualitative and quantitative questions to explore different aspects of the same issue in a questionnaire. Once you have understood the differences between qualitative and quantitative approaches, it is best to see them both as being useful and necessary skills for good researchers to have in their repertoire.

The third type of research that we discuss in this chapter—which has largely arisen as a result of critiques of purist forms of qualitative and quantitative research—is emancipatory or critical research, sometimes called 'anti-discriminatory research' (Humphries and Truman 1994) or, more recently, 'anti-oppressive' research (Strier 2007). Critical theorists have an ideological commitment to address oppression or the misuse of power. This research thus encompasses feminist theory, anti-oppressive theory and neo-Marxism, for example. Morris (2006) puts this best when she argues that researchers operating from this paradigm take an ideological stance and use their research to actively address oppression. Some critical theory researchers combine qualitative and quantitative approaches to achieve their goals, while others may use more qualitative or more quantitative methods, depending on their purpose. What distinguishes this research is not its methodology, but its goals. Feminist research has become such a large and influential form of critical theory research that it is now acknowledged as a form of research in its own right. We begin our review of these types of research with a brief introduction to emancipatory research, followed by a closer look at feminist research.

Emancipatory or anti-oppressive research

During the twentieth century, it became increasingly clear that research, together with the knowledge it brings, is not essentially 'good' in itself, nor does it necessarily contribute to universal betterment, as was originally believed in the eighteenth and nineteenth centuries. The use of the atomic bomb in World War II is seen by many as the end of the age of innocence for research. Even before this time, however, anthropologists had been disillusioned by the way the results of their research had been used for political and military ends in Africa during World War I.

At the same time as it was being realised that research can be used for various political ends, many social scientists were coming to see that research has largely been an instrument of the powerful, used against the powerless. Traditionally, researchers have studied 'downwards': there are far more studies of indigenous people's culture than that of the colonists; of the working class than the aristocracy; of patients' behaviour than that of doctors; of consumer behaviour than that of corporations. There have also been several published accounts of the difficulties of studying 'upwards'—for example, studying white-collar crime or the culture of sociologists. Hardwick and Worsley (2011, p. 55, quoting Oliver 1992) note that those who are researched tend to be the less powerful:

> People who are poor, unemployed, mentally ill, women, black people, disabled people and children are all frequently studied. In comparison research has uncovered little about the lives and activities of psychiatrists, bank managers, policemen, politicians, policy makers, political terrorists, captains of industry or even researchers themselves.

As these realisations were being reached, challenges were being mounted from within the ranks of 'the researched' regarding the value of research for them, and their right to be part of decision-making about how research would be done. With the rise of consumer rights movements and liberation movements worldwide, people who traditionally had been seen as passive 'objects' of research began demanding that research should have some benefits for them as well as for the researchers and those who sponsored the research. The disability lobby has been particularly effective at taking back control of the research agenda. Indigenous peoples now insist on having control of research that is carried out in traditional communities, and on being part of the decision-making process about the aims, methods, results and recommendations of that research. Developing countries negotiate agreements, including the possibility that indigenous researchers will be trained as part of major international research projects on their soil, in return for allowing the research to proceed.

At the same time, people from groups who previously have been excluded from conducting research but are more usually the researched—women, people from races and cultures other than white Anglo-European/American, people with disabilities—are now entering the professions, including the research area. They are exposing discriminatory assumptions in much of what has been previously accepted as 'objective' research knowledge and methodology. They are also demanding that researchers be accountable to the people they research, not just to the people who pay for the research.

Principles have been developed for anti-oppressive research (Morris 2006, p. 135, drawing on Potts and Brown 2005):

- Anti-oppressive research is social justice and resistance in process and outcome.
- Anti-oppressive research recognises that all knowledge is socially constructed and political.
- The anti-oppressive research process is all about power and relationships.

As with qualitative research, the theoretical traditions of emancipatory research come from a variety of areas, including Marxism, feminism, critical and conflict sociology, as well as educative consciousness-raising theories such as those of Paulo Freire (1970). However, in contrast to both quantitative and qualitative approaches, emancipatory researchers argue that the point of research is not merely to study the world, but also to change it (Strier 2007). For too long, such researchers argue, research has been in the hands of the powerful, where it has been furthering the interests of the power elite at the expense of the powerless. The job of the emancipatory researcher is to uncover the myths, beliefs and social constructions that contribute to the continuation of the status quo, in order to reveal how power relations are really operating to control the powerless. In the process, emancipatory researchers aim to liberate, enlighten or empower those people who are subjugated.

Emancipatory researchers take for granted that research is never value free. What is important is whose side you are on. Emancipatory researchers deliberately 'take sides' with the people who are oppressed or struggling against their oppression. Thus, they are overtly political.

Emancipatory researchers sit somewhere between the purist quantitative and qualitative positions in terms of their views of 'reality' and 'objectivity'. They view society as being full of contradictions and tensions between dominant and oppressed groups, between those who impose their reality on others and those who are the 'other'. In this view, people are shaped by external forces operating in the interests of the powerful (similar to the assumptions of universal objective laws of quantitative researchers), but may also be aware of their oppression and attempt to resist the dominant group's version of 'reality' (similar to the beliefs about the importance of subjectivity of qualitative researchers).

With its growing body of literature, and contributions to many debates about the nature of research and knowledge, feminist research has become an important area of emancipatory research in its own right (e.g. Morris 2006).

Feminist research

Like other forms of emancipatory research, feminist research is characterised by its goals rather than its methods. During the last 20 years, this form of research has made an immense impact on society in general, and especially on the position and role of women (Ackerly and True 2010; Morris 2006; Reinharz 1992). As an approach to research, it has undergone a lively evolution and is still evolving.

Feminist researchers study women as *gendered* subjects (Sands 2004). In their quest to study women, their lives and work, feminist researchers apply academic and research techniques to expose the sexism inherent in male-dominated social sciences and research (sometimes referred to as 'malestream research'). For example, early second wave feminist researchers highlighted the 'gender-blindness' of official statistics, which made it impossible to determine the status and condition of women separately from the male 'head of the house' (e.g. see Oakley 1985; Roberts 1981).

Thus feminist researchers showed how traditional ways of measuring the world have ignored or silenced women's viewpoints and position because the researchers literally cannot 'see' them.

'Feminist research' traditionally has been defined as a focus *on* women, in research carried out *by* women who were feminist, *for* other women (Stanley and Wise 1990, p. 21) and, from its beginnings, feminist research has been committed to changing women's lives. More recently, there has been a greater emphasis on gender equality research, as women's subordination is viewed as relational and therefore contextualised in relationships between women and men. Nonetheless, the vexing issue of women's status across the globe occupies the time of many feminist researchers committed to making a difference to women's lives and circumstances.

During the earlier phases of feminist research, there was a distinction made by feminists between quantitative methods, which were seen as being 'male', and qualitative ones, viewed as 'female'. Feminist researchers favoured qualitative research not only because it seemed a better way of capturing the complexities of women's lives but also because it brought forward women's stories. Feminists also felt that qualitative methods were less hierarchical and placed the researcher and researched on an equal footing. Since then, a plurality of approaches has developed: feminist researchers now use a variety of methods, including quantitative research, and have introduced some innovative techniques of their own in their task to study and improve women's lives. These include consciousness-raising groups, textual analysis and collaborative strategies such as keeping group diaries and discussing the meaning of results or presenting results back to respondents for interpretation with the researcher. Many writers emphasise that the ongoing debate within this plurality of multiple approaches is itself an important part of feminist research. They maintain that it is crucial for different approaches to be respected, and that no single approach gain dominance as *the* form of feminist research.

Feminist researchers often criticise the 'artificial dichotomies' that exist in mainstream research—for example, the deductive/inductive split or the theory/method divide. They argue that instead of being separate or opposites, such concepts are inextricably linked to each other. For example, two early writers on feminist methodology, Stanley and Wise (1990), have said of the traditional inductive/deductive split:

> Researchers cannot have 'empty heads' in the way that inductivism proposes; nor is it possible that theory is untainted by material experiences in the heads of theoreticians in the way that deductionism proposes (1990, p. 22).

Another of the critical, and perhaps one of the most respected, early writers on feminist methodology, Reinharz (1992), defines feminist methodology as the sum of feminist research methods. In her definition, feminist research is research that is done by researchers who claim to be feminist, or that is published in explicitly feminist journals and books, or that receives awards from organisations that give awards for feminist research.

Like emancipatory researchers, feminist researchers come from a variety of theoretical backgrounds, including socialist feminism, radical feminism, liberal feminism, Marxist feminism, critical, poststructural and postmodern perspectives.

Ten themes of feminist research methodology identified by Reinharz

- Feminism is a perspective, not a research method.
- Feminists use a multiplicity of research methods.
- Feminist research involves ongoing criticism of non-feminist scholarship.
- Feminist research is guided by feminist theory.
- Feminist research may be transdisciplinary.
- Feminist research aims to create social change.
- Feminist research strives to represent human diversity.
- Feminist research frequently includes the researcher as a person.
- Feminist research frequently attempts to develop special relations with the people studied (in interactive research).
- Feminist research frequently defines a special relation with the reader.

Source: Reinharz (1992), reproduced in Morris (2006).

Early writers on the feminist method, Stanley and Wise (1990, p. 38) proposed a set of four basic assumptions about the world, based on the work of Margrit Eichler, with which they expect all feminist researchers would agree. These four points (see box) echo many of the themes discussed in relation to emancipatory research in the previous section.

Four assumptions of feminist research

- All knowledge is socially constructed.
- The dominant ideology is that of the ruling group.

- There is no such thing as value-free science, and so far the social sciences have served and reflected men's interests.
- The perspectives of men and women differ because people's perspectives vary systematically with their position in society.

Like many qualitative researchers, feminist researchers often ensure that they are included as an essential part of the research process, and are explicit about their beliefs and background, how they became involved in the topic and their relationship with the people with whom they are researching. In their quest for empowerment of women and understanding women's perspectives, feminist researchers may also develop close relationships with the people they involve in their research.

Examples of feminist research
- A researcher holds conversations with rural women over several months to discuss and write up their experiences of farming and their attitudes towards these experiences.
- A women's support group collects statistics and evidence about how domestic violence is dealt with in its region compared with other types of violence, in order to raise community awareness and to lobby for a women's refuge.
- A social welfare worker involves her colleagues in a study of their daily work practices to analyse the similarities between social work and traditional 'women's work'.
- Beginning with her own experience, a researcher explores the meaning of mastectomy in Western culture through an analysis of works of fiction, poetry and women's magazines.
- A social worker conducts focus groups with women in crisis shelters to determine whether disaster-recovery responses take account of women's health, welfare and safety issues.

As is the case with quantitative and qualitative forms of research, feminist research has its critics. There was some criticism of feminist research in its early days for not including the voices of women from marginalised groups. However, more recent work incorporating the notion of intersectionality, or the intersection of multiple identities, has enabled a much richer engagement of feminism with diversity (Davis 2008; Gunnarsson 2011). Terming much of the broad range of feminist research methodologies discussed above as 'standpoint/critical' feminist research, feminist social work researchers who support postmodern approaches, such as Clark (2005) and Campbell and Fonow (2009), have criticised what has now become known as traditional feminist research. Campbell and Fonow (2009), for example, argue that we must examine our own understanding of what we view as real, becoming much more self-reflective about the taken-for-granted 'truths' we observe. They argue that we must get lost and found and lost again with our participants as we explore and analyse our work. Tellingly, they alert us to the dangers of an uncritical view, which may exclude other equally valid perceptions and gloss over differences in women's original accounts. Our review of the major approaches to social work research concludes with a brief brush with postmodernist research to illustrate just how wide the spectrum of research available to social workers has become.

Postmodern research

Much of the social work research discussed so far—both quantitative and qualitative—comes from a modernist perspective, which ultimately falls back on a belief in a knowable, 'real' world, the truth of which can be discovered through rational processes (e.g. Howe 1994). However, the postmodern world in which social work and social research now finds itself challenges all this.

Instead of certainties and 'realities' which can be explored scientifically, postmodernism asserts that 'truth' or knowledge is created through language and meanings, and is different for different people, depending on their experiences. Thus, instead of a single, knowable reality, postmodernist researchers speak of a plurality of voices, each with its own locally constructed reality. No single reality is more valid than another—indeed, diversity and difference should be celebrated. Instead of focusing on structural disadvantage or the study of fixed notions of 'men' and 'women', for example, postmodernist researchers turn their analysis to language itself (often termed 'discourse'), and 'to examining what voices women (and men) are using within the context of unequal gender and other social relations' (Trinder 2000, p. 51).

With its emphasis on language as the site for the complexities of how power is mediated through discourse and relationships, and its insistence that there is no single reality, postmodernism poses some fundamental challenges to social work that will keep theorists and researchers busy for some time (not least in trying to untangle the sometimes inaccessible language postmodernists use!).

Proponents of a postmodern feminist approach to social work research argue that postmodern research retheorises the individual as an effect of the social, thus overcoming the problem of artificially distinguishing between the person and their environment (e.g. see Denzin and Lincoln 2005; Haene 2010). Rossiter argues that this opens the way for a new view of social work's traditional claim to work with the 'person in environment', which offers an opportunity to 'unify social work as a democratic project' (Rossiter 2000, p. 29). Taking this thinking one step further, Haene (2010) argues that there is a convergence between postmodern research and thera-peutic approaches, suggesting that the role of practitioners is very similar in purpose and design to that of researchers. Rowntree (2010, p. 450) also argues that 'narrativism', or the capacity for people to understand their lives through stories, provides social work researchers with the ability to use interviews to understand cultural stories—or to make sense of people's experiences within their cultural context. Thus it could be argued that some social work methods transfer readily to social work research.

Regardless of how far we proceed with this argument, there is little doubt that postmodernism offers the prospect of a more complex under-standing of the way power operates between social workers and their clients, and of the way our work can provide the basis for critical reflection.

Initially, critics of postmodernism argued that it might threaten the very existence of social work because, with no fundamental reality or 'truth', how can one know whether one is working towards social justice or injustice? Gray (1995), for example, warned of the dangers of relativism and subjec-tivism undermining the notion of ethical practice in social work. However, there is now greater consensus regarding postmodern approaches, and acknowledgement that these offer social work the opportunity to become more reflective and inclusive, as well as the capacity to more closely link theory with practice.

Conclusion and summary

In this brief review of some of the major approaches to research, we have attempted to show how important it is to understand the underly-ing assumptions, beliefs and goals of each approach, and how these shape the ways in which research is done. We have also argued that while some approaches are incompatible (for example, experimental design and postmodern analysis), many other approaches are not mutually exclusive. Some types of quantitative and qualitative research can be integrated to produce richer results than will be achieved by simply using one method-ology or another. Research in the real world is messy, and often cannot be limited to a particular 'ideal type'. Instead, researchers tend to use techniques and methods from a variety of approaches, depending on their purpose, as shown in the discussion on emancipatory and feminist research.

The important point to take with you from this discussion is that it is imperative that you are explicit about the theoretical and value framework within which you conduct your research. Similarly, an important aspect of being an informed consumer of research is that you can identify what theory or approach underlies the research you are reading about. We conclude this chapter with a summary of the political and ethical issues that arise whenever a person becomes involved in research.

The politics of research

We now know that research is not a value-free endeavour that inevitably produces knowledge for the good of all people. Instead, we must accept that research is an activity laden with ethical and political consequences. Several fundamental and related political questions must be addressed before any research is begun (Morris 2006). These are:

- Who is the research for? (Whose interests does it serve?)
- What is the purpose of the research? (How will the results be used?)
- Who decides topic areas and how are these choices made?
- Who defines the critical concepts embedded in the research?
- What secondary data are available, how were they collected and for what purpose?
- Who funds the research and why?
- How will the research be disseminated and for what purpose?

While we cannot always be sure how our research will be used in the long term, it is important to be as clear as possible from the beginning about the purposes of the research and whose interests it will serve.

Key players in the research process

One way to address these questions is to be clear about the key players who must be taken into account in the planning of your research.

Key players in the research process

- The researcher or researchers
- The people who are researched
- Sponsors who pay for the research

- People who will benefit from the research
- People who are targeted to be convinced by the research (e.g. policy-makers)

From the discussion in this chapter, it should be clear that the research process is rarely straightforward, but rather is the outcome of negotiations or bargains between each of these groups of people, who may have conflicting interests. Sometimes these categories will overlap—for example, if an organisation run by people with disabilities hires a researcher to investigate the housing needs and preferences of its members, then at least three of the above categories will be the same. The fact that people share categories does not necessarily make the negotiations any simpler, however. Still, when planning a piece of research, it can prevent many problems later if we can distinguish between who the key stakeholders are and what our own attitudes and position are in relation to them.

Who owns the research?

Another important question that needs to be sorted out before research begins relates to who owns the research. In the early days of social research, it was assumed that the knowledge generated by research was somehow universally owned. Nowadays, research knowledge is more often treated as a kind of private property, which is owned by the people who sponsor (pay for) it. If the people who commission the research do not approve of the results, they may refuse to publish them, and the researcher may have no legal redress about this. To prevent as many difficulties as possible in this area, it is important to have a clear contract with the sponsor of the research, to specify who owns, and who is responsible for, the research data and outcomes.

Aspects to include in a research contract
- Who owns the data?
- Who owns the research instrument?
- Who owns the findings?
- Who owns the report?
- Who is responsible for the recommendations?
- Who owns the intellectual property rights?
- Who can publish what and where?

The ethics of research

Just as research is never value free, ethics is a vital part of every research project. These days it is generally accepted that social research must meet five ethical criteria in order to be considered ethically acceptable. As we have discussed, these principles have been accepted not only because most researchers wish to conduct ethical research, but also because of the demands for a 'fair go' from the people being researched.

Ethical criteria for research

- Autonomy/self-determination (includes informed consent and confidentiality)
- Non-maleficence (not doing harm)
- Beneficence (doing good)
- Justice (are the purposes just?)

Source: Hardwick and Worsley (2011).

The principle of autonomy involves issues such as respect for people and their right to decide whether or not they will be involved in research. When asking people to be involved in your research, it is important that you can demonstrate that they have given their *informed* consent to participate and that their *right to privacy* is protected. This means that they understand the nature of the research and its purpose, the risks for them and what will be asked of them.

Other ethical aspects of the principle of autonomy include the right to *privacy*, including the right to withdraw from the process at any stage and to refuse to answer certain questions if they wish, the right to *anonymity* and the right to *confidentiality*. Confidentiality means that the information given to the researcher will not be divulged to others, except in reporting research results as agreed, and also that the information will not be used for any purpose other than the research. We also need to ensure that our research does not disrupt people's lives, that we do not use deception and that our research is based on principles of social justice (Humphries 2008).

Researchers are also required not to harm their subjects in any way and, conversely, to do some good, or to be of benefit, to the people who are being researched. Often in proposals to ethics committees you will be asked to document the risks your research might pose to the participants, and what measures you will take to minimise these.

Principles of justice or fairness are also ethical issues which, as we have seen, can be viewed differently depending on your perspective. Research is often a complex issue involving ethical dilemmas in which you may have to choose between undesirable alternatives.

Three questions that might help you to decide on the ethical value of your research project are:

- Would the participants be willing to do further research of this kind?
- Would I be happy for my own family to participate?
- What are the benefits for the people being researched?

We add a final principle: making a positive contribution to knowledge—a task that involves issues of professional standards. You must ensure that your purpose is worthwhile, that your data are gathered carefully and that you have chosen appropriate methods of research design, data collection and data analysis. Results must be reported honestly, and this should include any problems, errors or distortions of which you are aware. You cannot publish data that you did not collect, and you must not falsify data.

In relation to other researchers, it is imperative that you give credit and refer to others who have contributed to your work. Plagiarism, or using other people's work without acknowledgement, is a serious offence in research and scholarship generally.

Social work codes of ethics

Many national social work codes of ethics are explicit in including research within their practice standards. For example, the National Association of Social Workers' (NASW) Code of Ethics in the United States devotes section 5.02, 'Evaluation and Research', to sixteen ethical responsibilities that social workers have in relation to research and evaluation (NASW 2008).

Similarly, the Australian Social Work Code of Ethics (AASW 2010) includes a section (5.5.2 'Research', AASW 2010, pp. 36–8) containing several clauses relating to (1) the general approach to research; (2) respect, consent, privacy and review; and (3) publicity and distribution of research findings, all of which apply the ethical principles discussed in this chapter to social work research. In addition, references to research appear throughout the general parts of the AASW Code. For example, social workers are to 'set and enforce explicit professional boundaries (with research participants) to minimize risk of conflict, harm, exploitation' (clause 5.1.6 (j)) and 'Social workers will ensure clients anonymity and remove identifying details when permitted to use confidential information for purposes such as ... research' (clause 5.2.4 (j)). In addition to these clauses, which also relate to other people with whom social workers relate, most social work codes of ethics from across the globe will note the requirement for social workers to promote the general ethical principles and standards of the code when conducting research.

The British Code of Ethics for social work, adopted in April 2002, goes even further in its stipulations about how social workers should do research. In addition to the requirements listed in the other two codes, this code emphasises the anti-oppressive or empowerment focus of social work, and reminds social workers to work together with disempowered groups, individuals and communities in devising and achieving research agendas (BASW 2002).

Having research included in social work codes of ethics in this way means that social workers who ignore or violate ethical principles when undertaking research face serious penalties imposed by their profession, which may affect their whole career.

The role of ethics committees

Most universities and major welfare and research institutions, such as large hospitals, government departments and research councils, have ethics committees that review research proposals before researchers can begin their work. Some organisations also have their own research codes of ethics. When planning your research, you must find out the requirements for your particular situation. Usually you will have to document the ethical implications of your research for the committee before it can be approved. Often the questions on the form address the ethical principles outlined above. Filling out an ethics form will also help you to be clearer about the nature of your research.

Ethics committees play an important role in protecting the public from unethical research. They are part of ensuring that we are accountable for our actions, and universities and research institutions impose severe penalties if the procedures agreed to are not followed.

Summary

In this chapter, we have defined social research and introduced some of the major types of research. Principles of quantitative, qualitative, emancipatory and postmodern research are described in order to demonstrate the variety of research approaches that are possible, and the ways in which different approaches are shaped by their underlying beliefs about the world. We have noted the different theories on which the approaches are based, the different types of methods and techniques used, and how each form of research views the role of the researcher differently. All of these approaches are used by social workers doing research. Although for simplicity we have presented 'ideal types', in reality social work researchers may use a mixture of some of these approaches, depending on their purposes. It is important to understand a variety of approaches if you are to have the flexibility to research different social work issues in the most appropriate way. It is also important that you are able to identify the underlying approaches of your own and others' research. Finally, we have discussed some of the political and ethical implications that researchers must consider before they begin their research.

Discussion questions

1.1   What are the differences between quantitative, qualitative and emancipatory, or anti-oppressive, research?
1.2   What challenges does postmodern research pose?
1.3   What are the main tenets of feminist research?
1.4   With which forms of research do you feel most comfortable?
1.5   Why are politics and ethics so important in planning your research?
1.6   List some key ethical issues to consider in any research proposal.

Exercises

Find an example of one piece of quantitative, qualitative and feminist research. (Use your local library—try journals or books that are collections of research.) Answer these questions about each of the articles:

1.1   For whom was the research conducted?
1.2   What was the purpose of the research?
1.3   Are you told how the results were used? What actions or decisions were taken as a result?
1.4   Identify the people in the following categories:
   • the researcher/s
   • the participants or people being researched
   • those who benefited from the research

- those who sponsored the research
- those who were targeted to be convinced by the research.

1.5   Can you identify any conflicts of interest between these groups?

1.6   What were the theories underlying the research?

1.7   How was the information gathered?

1.8   How were the patterns or themes determined (how were the data analysed)?

1.9   What conclusions were drawn?

1.10 How is the role of the researcher discussed in the article?

1.11 What role did the people who were researched play in the process of the research?

1.12 What risks existed for the people who were researched? For the researcher?

1.13 Were there benefits for those who were researched? What were they?

1.14 Do you think the participants would be willing to undertake further research with this researcher?

1.15 Would you have been happy to participate in this research?

Further reading

Babbie, E. 2010, *The Practice of Social Research*, 12th edn, Wadsworth, Boston. Chapters 1, 2 and 3 contain a good discussion of the foundations of social scientific inquiry and the different theories and paradigms that underlie research, as well as an introduction to ethical issues.

Grinnell, Richard M. and Unrau, Yvonne A. (eds) 2010, *Social Work Research and Evaluation*, 9th edn, Oxford University Press, New York. Part 2 considers ethics and culturally competent research.

Hardwick, Louise and Worsley, Aidan 2011, *Doing Social Work Research*, Sage, London. This book provides a refreshing analysis of what makes social work research unique, and provides a useful discussion of ethics in social work research.

Humphries, B. 2008, *Social Work Research for Social Justice*, Palgrave Macmillan, Basingstoke. Chapter 1 introduces the notion of research as contentious and Chapter 2 discusses ethics for social work research.

Reinharz, S. 1992, *Feminist Methods in Social Research*, Oxford University Press, New York. This book remains a classic for feminist researchers, and provides a very good discussion of feminist methods.

Sarantakos, S. 2005, *Social Research*, 3rd edn, Macmillan, Sydney. This book provides an in-depth discussion of the differences between qualitative and quantitative research paradigms, as well as ethics.

Yegidis, B.L. and Weinbach, R.W. 2009, *Research Methods for Social Workers*, 6th edn, Allyn & Bacon, Boston. Part 1 examines the link between social work research and practice, including a detailed chapter on ethics.

2 Choosing your topic area

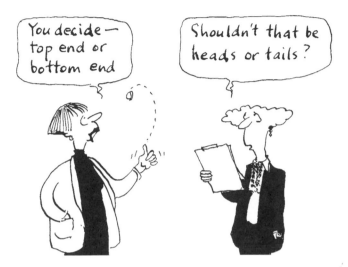

In this chapter and the next, we will explore choosing your research topic, and then examine how to transform the issue, problem or area in which you are interested into researchable questions. We will look at how both quantitative and qualitative researchers go about this process.

Sometimes this first step—choosing your research topic or problem, and developing research questions—is also the step that brings the project to a halt before it has even started. Some beginning researchers are so overwhelmed by all the possibilities and the enormity of the task that they never get on to the research itself. Kaufmann (1973) was the first to coin the phrase 'decidophobia' to account for the paralysing inability to make a decision. We suggest that this concept can aptly be applied to beginning researchers who find the whole notion of undertaking research particularly anxiety-provoking.

One of the main elements of 'decidophobia' is wanting to do too much at once. You cannot possibly solve all the problems, or even answer all the questions you have, in one research project. The first lesson in defining your research problem, then, is to accept that you will only ever be able to research a small part of the issue in which you are interested. This is often a disappointment to the beginning researcher. Be warned, and warn those with whom you are researching: you will always have to narrow down your research topic and address only *some* of the issues that interest you. Defining the research topic is a crucial step in this process. It can be a big help in overcoming 'decidophobia', and in enabling you to get on with your research.

The first step in defining the issue or problem to be researched is to determine the general area. This first step is crucial, and should be framed as a problem statement rather than as a question (Yegidis and Weinbach 2009). As we saw in Chapter 1, often a research area presents itself during the course of your work, or from personal experience. Alternatively, you might answer an advertisement for funding for a research topic, or be approached by someone from your organisation about a project. However the research topic presents itself, before you leap into planning the project or even narrowing down the topic area, it is important that you are aware of your own values and preferred theoretical perspectives, and how these will influence the way you conceptualise the project.

Theory, values and your research topic: The importance of a conceptual framework

Inevitably, the theories from which you operate, your beliefs about the world and the values you hold—whether you are conscious of them or not—will influence the research topic you choose and the way you go about researching it. For example, if you are asked to evaluate a residential facility for people with disabilities, the way you approach this will depend on how you see the problem. If you hold a largely functionalist view of the world, you may assume that staff and residents are working together to achieve the program's goals, so you may only interview staff, or perhaps staff and residents together, as part of your evaluation. If, however, you are coming from a more critical tradition, you may assume that the staff and residents will have different—even opposing—views, so you will design a project that seeks those views separately. Perhaps you may choose only to interview staff, or only to interview residents—indeed, if you operate from certain perspectives it may not occur to you to interview the other group. In addition, a feminist researcher would want to ensure that the results for men and women—whether staff or residents—could be analysed separately. A postmodern feminist might be inclined to assess language and power relations within the institution with a particular focus on how these issues affect women.

Similarly, a person immersed in symbolic interactionism might be most interested in how the facility is experienced by the residents themselves, and spend considerable time understanding their perspective about how the institution is run. This researcher may analyse the interactions between staff and residents in terms of how meanings are developed and shared. Another researcher, operating from a critical perspective, may be more interested in uncovering the power differentials between staff and residents in decision-making, and how the structures within the facility affect these relationships. They may also be interested in wider political and social structures and how these affect life in the facility.

Again, a postmodern researcher might be interested in how people develop meanings and relationships, and how they co-construct terms such as 'staff' and 'resident'. They might wish to analyse how the discourse of 'residential setting' mediates relationships. Rather than assuming that power lies in social structures and roles within the organisation, they would assume that power is more fluid, and a feature of relationships, meanings and language. Their methods of observation and the focus of conversations would be quite different from those of other researchers from different approaches.

Every aspect of research is influenced by our theories and values. The important point being made here is that researchers must be aware of what our underlying theories and values are, as well as how they influence our choice of, and general approach to, the topic, and incorporate this understanding into our thinking as we develop our conceptual framework or plan for the research.

Part of deciding on the topic area involves developing a conceptual plan for how you will undertake the whole project. Usually this is not a straightforward and linear process, but rather a cyclical one. As you read more, talk to different people and discover more about the topic, so your conceptual framework develops. This will include the underlying purpose of the research, the topic area, the particular questions or focus in which you are most interested, the methods you intend to use, the steps in the research process and the means by which you will analyse the data, as well as what you hope will happen as a consequence of the research. At the same time as you are working out the topic of your research, you will be formulating this conceptual plan for how you intend to investigate it. If you can be explicit about the values and theories which underlie your approach, you will be much clearer about your purpose and alert to any conflicts of interest that may occur with other players in the process.

Often funding bodies or academic institutions require a research proposal before they give their approval to a research project. Completing a research proposal can be a good start to setting out the conceptual framework for your research. Even if such a proposal is not required, it is imperative that you write down a plan of the way you are conceptualising your topic and the process by which you will research it before you begin the research itself. Having a clearly defined plan will save you much time and energy later. As you begin to think about your research topic and to develop your conceptual plan, there are several people whose opinions you should take into account.

Who decides on the topic area?

Whatever the path by which you become involved, it is critical that *you* are interested in the topic. Research requires much time and effort. Unless you are curious and interested in the area you are about to research, there is little point devoting your valuable time and energy (and those of other people) to it. Questions that might help you decide whether you really are interested include: What is my interest in this issue? What can I learn from it? How will it contribute to my own or others' work? What do I hope to achieve by my involvement? Will I have the time, considering my other commitments, to complete the research?

In Chapter 1 we saw that there are four other types of key players, in addition to yourself, who must be taken into account when you are formulating the topic you wish to research. The first group is the *people being researched*. Who are they? What are their attitudes to the issue you are interested in? Will you be able to get access to them, and if so will they want to be involved? What is in it for them?

Second, you must consider the *organisation* paying for or sponsoring the research. Often this will be the agency where you already work. You will need to explore questions such as: What are the organisation's aims for the project? Do these conflict with the aims of the people being researched? Do they conflict with your own interest in the problem? How can you resolve such issues so that the project can go ahead? Will the organisation provide adequate resources? If not, are there other avenues of funding for the project? Will the organisation permit you the time for the project? All these issues have to be negotiated carefully as part of refining the research topic.

The third group we identified in Chapter 1 was the *people who will benefit from the research*. Who are they? Will the people you are researching receive some benefits? Will your agency? Will you? Finally, you need to consider the *people who the research is aimed at convincing*. How can they be involved in the topic so that they become committed to taking the decisions or action to which your research results point?

Selecting an advisory group

One way of addressing many of these issues is to meet with members from each of these groups, in order to assess their interest and involvement and how they see the problem. A useful mechanism is a steering committee or advisory group consisting of representatives from each of the groups of key players. This group can be the 'sounding board' against which you try out your ideas, negotiate the purpose of the research, and work out the questions you wish to ask and the general approaches you will take. Such a group, with the different perspectives of its members, can help you avoid many political and ethical pitfalls in the research process, and ensure that your project meets the needs of the key players. It can also be a great help throughout the life of the project, not just at the problem-formulation stage.

Of course, forming this advisory group will not be without its challenges. All members must feel that they have sufficient respect and influence that they are not intimidated into silence. A representative from the group who is being researched should be someone who is used to being on committees and working with welfare professionals, or at least someone who is not afraid to offer their opinion in such a group. Having a 'token' member on an advisory group who feels unable to speak up is pointless, and sometimes destructive. It can give the impression that there is support from the group being researched when this is not the case at all. Even if it is not possible to form a group such as this, it is most important that you identify the key players and consult with people from each of the four categories about how they see the topic, as part of the process of defining the problem you will be researching.

Criteria for defining the research topic

At least four criteria must be met before you finalise your research topic. Most social work research textbooks have at least one chapter on ethics guiding research. We have drawn from these the criteria we view as critical for guiding social work research projects. Together, these criteria address many of the questions raised in this introductory discussion.

> **Criteria for choosing the research problem**
> - Is it relevant?
> - Is it researchable?
> - Is it feasible?
> - Is it ethical?

Unless the problem you choose is *relevant* to the social welfare industry—that is, unless it will lead to 'making a decision or taking some action', as we have specified in our definition of research in Chapter 1, there is no point in proceeding. Research topics can be either 'pure' or 'applied', although these terms are really ideal types at each end of a continuum. *Applied research* is directly related to organisational or program goals, and is often seen as being immediately 'useful'—for example, evaluating the effect of a living skills program on residents' quality of life. *Pure research* topics, on the other hand, involve theoretical development, or exploring more general issues that affect social welfare—for example, the factors that contribute most to good quality of life. While not as immediately useful as the first 'applied' topic, this more 'pure' topic is still relevant, since many services aim to improve quality of life. Whether your topic is at the applied or pure end of the research continuum, it must be relevant or the interest and resources will not be available.

Some problem areas are simply not amenable to methods of social research. Ethical questions, which are extremely relevant to welfare policies and people working in social welfare, may not be *researchable*. For example, the topic 'Should homosexual and lesbian couples be allowed to foster children?' is not researchable using methods of social research. This question is a problem of values or ethics rather than one of systematically finding 'patterns' in the social world, as specified in our definition in the Introduction. On the other hand, the topic 'Are there different outcomes for children fostered by homosexual and lesbian couples compared with children fostered by heterosexual couples?' is theoretically researchable because it involves a search for patterns and the systematic collection of information.

Once you have established that your problem area is both *relevant* and *researchable*, you need to ensure that it is also *feasible*. Feasibility is about whether it is possible for you to actually *do* the research. Your topic needs to be manageable and possible within the resources you have. In the example above, if agency policies have only recently included homosexual and lesbian couples as foster parents, it will be impossible to study the long-term outcomes for children, no matter how relevant and researchable the issue. Similarly, if your topic is too broad, it will not be feasible. Even if homosexual and lesbian couples have been fostering children for some time, few researchers would be able to examine a large topic such as comparing all the issues affecting foster children's quality of life and how these relate to whether their foster parents were in homosexual, lesbian or heterosexual relationships. However, researchers might be able to investigate smaller, more manageable questions such as the length of time the foster placements lasted, children's ability to form friends at school, academic performance and emotional security.

Narrowing the topic even further from these four issues to just one (for example, emotional security) may transform your study into a feasible project within the resource limitations you and your organisation have. When considering feasibility, you must also consider the time and costs involved. A research project will not be feasible unless it is affordable. It is very easy to under-estimate costs. Ex-foster children and parents may have scattered widely. How long will it take to locate them? How much will phone calls, postage, printing and travel to interviews cost? Another aspect of feasibility is making sure that you are collecting information in a form that you, or someone you can afford to pay, can analyse. Thus expertise, and access to expertise, constitute another important part of feasibility.

Feasibility involves questions of ethics as well as of resources. For example, if you wanted to research children's previous experiences of being fostered by homosexual and lesbian couples as compared with heterosexual couples, it is highly unlikely that the relevant organisation would allow you to interview the children. Similarly, schools, counselling agencies and other organisations involved with foster children will have policies which prevent researchers gaining access to their clients, especially about sensitive issues, in order to protect privacy and confidentiality and to prevent harm. Before you decide on your topic, it is crucial that you make sure that your topic and methods meet the ethical guidelines of the agency(ies) through which you want to contact the people you are researching, and that you will be able to collect the data you need in order to address the question.

Sometimes a topic can be made feasible by changing the focus of the question. In the example above, if the researchers amend their topic to an investigation of long-term outcomes for children who had been fostered by homosexual, lesbian and heterosexual couples five to ten years ago, they may be permitted to review case histories from client records, with proper safeguards in place to protect privacy and confidentiality. In some circumstances, the agency may also be willing to approach ex-clients and foster parents on behalf of the researchers, to gain permission for the researchers to contact them to discuss becoming involved in the research.

The fourth criterion that must be met before your topic is finalised is that it must meet general *ethical criteria* for research. In Chapter 1 we reviewed the major summarising principles that must be followed in order to conduct ethically acceptable research, as well as the sorts of guidelines for ethical research set down in social work codes around the world. It is most important to check that your topic meets these criteria. Ask yourself the three questions that were also listed to help you further think through the ethical implications of your topic area. In most instances you will have to submit your research proposal to an ethics committee, as we discussed in the previous chapter, so it is important to think through these issues as part of formulating your research topic.

Purpose of research and your topic

The purpose of your research also affects how you view your topic. There are three broad types of research purpose.

The three main purposes of research
- Exploring social phenomena or theories (exploratory research)
- Describing various aspects of the social world (descriptive research)
- Explaining social phenomena (explanatory research)

The three purposes of research are part of a continuum. D'Cruz and Jones (2004, p. 19) refer to this continuum as having a 'tight' end (explanatory) and a 'loose' end (exploratory), depending on the specificity of the research question. We would argue that most studies contain elements of all three phases of the continuum because we tend to explore, describe and attempt to explain our research situation. For example, the first part of a study may begin with a concern to describe a particular phenomenon such as juvenile delinquency, including a description of who juvenile offenders are most likely to be, what their backgrounds are and what sort of offences they commit (descriptive research). The study may also include a goal of examining various causes of juvenile delinquency (explanatory research).

Exploratory research is undertaken when little is known about an area. Often exploratory research is the prelude to a more detailed study, but it is also an important form of research in its own right. Imagine that youth violence has been the source of newspaper headlines in a major regional city recently. Gangs of unemployed youths are being blamed in the media for all sorts of crimes, from a recent outbreak of robberies of small businesses to attacks on old-age pensioners, break-and-enters into private dwellings and an increase in assaults on public transport. The local council employs you as a researcher to find out more about youth violence. Let us assume that the purpose of your research is exploratory. You may interview a wide range of people to gain an understanding of how violence, and especially youth violence, is perceived in that city. You may talk to professionals such as teachers, police, court officials, health centre and hospital personnel, local counsellors, juvenile justice workers, youth workers, refuge workers and ministers. You may also talk to members of local youth groups and clubs, churches, publicans, high schools, centres for unemployed youth or security officers who patrol the city at night. If you have the trust of health workers or victims' groups, you may be able to interview or meet people or groups of people who have been identified as having experienced youth violence. In this way, the researcher gathers information and gains insights into how youth violence is perceived (or not perceived) in the city by the different groups. Usually exploratory studies identify the general terrain of a topic or problem area, and the important themes and issues that arise within this area.

If, on the other hand, the purpose of the study into youth violence is *descriptive*, the researcher usually already knows, or has found out, much of the information that an exploratory study provides. In descriptive research, the researcher's aim would be to describe more specific details and patterns of youth violence. The researcher may be finding out the types of violence that have been recorded by the various agencies, the number of assaults reported the categories of people who have been assaulted and the ages of people who have been identified as perpetrators. If she finds that youth violence is indeed a problem for the city discussed above, the researcher may look for descriptions of the patterns of events leading up to and following incidents of this violence, for the 'typical' story of what occurs, how it is reported and what happens after violence has been reported. With the right methodology, she may also be able to investigate the types of violence that are not reported, and the stories surrounding such events. Thus descriptive research aims to find out in more precise detail than exploratory research the *what* of social phenomena.

In contrast to descriptive and exploratory research, the purpose of *explanatory research* is to investigate the *why* of social phenomena—that is, to answer questions about their causes. Thus an explanatory study stemming from newspaper articles on youth violence in the city may endeavour to explain why youth violence occurs in this particular city, or particular areas of this city, or what factors are associated with its increase. It may attempt to explain what causes young people rather than other age groups to become violent. If the method used is quantitative, hypotheses about what causes youth violence and its increase in this setting may be developed and then statistically tested. If the methodology is qualitative, hypotheses about the causes of youth violence and its increase will be developed during the course of the study, as data are collected and the literature searched for theoretical explanations.

As you can see from these brief examples, research with exploratory, descriptive and explanatory purposes can use either quantitative or qualitative approaches or a multi-method mixture of both. Whatever approach you use, it is most important that you are clear about the purpose or purposes of your research, and what you hope to achieve from your study of the topic.

Summary

As you begin to formulate your research topic, you will also begin to develop a conceptual framework or plan for the research, which includes the purpose of the research, specific questions, methodologies, structure for carrying out the research and data analysis. As far as possible, you need to clarify your own and others' theoretical/value positions, as an important prelude to establishing the broad purpose of the study. Generally, research projects have exploratory, descriptive or explanatory purposes. It is essential that your research questions and methodologies reflect these purposes. Several issues arise when you are choosing your research topic, even before you have defined your research problems or questions—all of which require clear and careful thought. Having established the general territory of the problem, it is important to identify who the key players are, what they want to achieve and whether the problem itself is relevant, researchable, feasible and ethical.

Discussion questions

2.1   What is 'decidophobia' and how might it be overcome?
2.2   Whose views should be considered when you are developing your research topic?

2.3 What are the four criteria for choosing a research topic?

2.4 'Under what conditions do women have the right to choose abortions?' Is this a researchable topic?

2.5 An article appears in the local paper debating whether discipline in schools is declining. Give some examples of the different sorts of questions that might be generated by research with exploratory, descriptive and explanatory purposes.

Exercises

You are a university student on placement at the local council in a small rural town. You have been given the following newspaper article about domestic violence and are asked to research it.

DOMESTIC VIOLENCE COMMITTEE

_____ newly formed Domestic Violence Committee will meet for the first time today following the issue of a record number of domestic violence orders following Monday's _____ Local Court sitting.

Fourteen domestic violence restraining orders were issued after Monday's court.

It was the largest number ever issued here.

A committee to formulate effective response systems to the problem, and to follow up progress in individual cases, has been formed.

2.1 Who would be the key players from each of the four groups whom you could consult about this topic?

2.2 What might be the underlying theories and values that would influence this research topic?

2.3 What exploratory questions could you ask about this topic?

2.4 What descriptive research questions could you ask about this topic?

2.5 What explanatory research questions could you ask about this topic?

2.6 Is this topic:

   (a) relevant?
   (b) feasible?
   (c) researchable?
   (d) ethical?

Further reading

Grinnell, Richard M. and Unrau, Yvonne A. (eds) 2010, *Social Work Research and Evaluation*, 9th edn, Oxford University Press, New York. This edited collection provides a useful section on approaches to knowledge.

Smith, Roger 2009, *Doing Social Work Research*, Open University Press, Maidenhead. Chapters 1, 2 and 3 give a good overview of social work research. Chapter 3 is devoted to a discussion of critical perspectives.

Wadsworth, Yoland 2011, *Do It Yourself Social Research: The Bestselling Practical Guide to Doing Social Research Projects*, 3rd edn, Allen & Unwin, Sydney. This best-selling guide to doing social research outlines in plain language the process of doing social research—in particular the why and how.

Yegidis, B.L. and Weinbach, Robert W. 2009, *Research Methods for Social Workers*, 6th edn, Allyn & Bacon, Boston. Part 2 of this book outlines the planning stages of the research process and gives advice on how to plan for the project.

3 Developing research questions

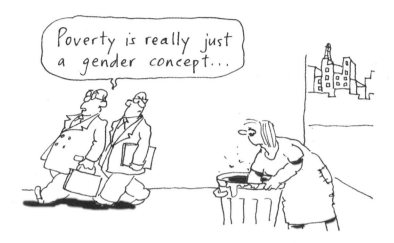

In Chapter 2 we discussed some of the issues involved in choosing your research topic. In this chapter, we go into more detail about how to transform your general research topic into researchable questions. Qualitative and quantitative approaches do this in different ways, and from different directions.

Developing quantitative research questions

In Chapter 1 we discussed how the quantitative approach begins with theories and questions which are examined in carefully designed studies. Researchers using this approach must determine how they are going to test their ideas in the social world. Developing your research questions is important in quantitative research, because the types of questions asked heavily influence the whole design of your study and the sorts of data analysis you will be able to perform. Many social work textbooks concentrate on qualitative research approaches. What we provide here is a useful conceptual understanding of the process of turning a research question into a measurable or quantifiable analysis. For more detailed discussion of quantitative research, you should read widely in social research and look at texts on other methods.

The process of thinking through research questions from the level of ideas or theory to measurable indicators (called variables) that can be used in social research is called 'operationalisation'. This process has been described as a 'descending level of abstraction' (Saks and Allsop 2007, p. 194) because researchers transform a problem or topic area that is in their heads into something that they can see or touch or measure out in the 'real world'.

The ladder of abstraction has several 'rungs' that must be negotiated on your way to transforming your ideas into measurable variables. In fact, you will find that, rather than being a ladder, the structure you are descending is actually more like a playground 'pyramid'. In quantitative research, you begin at the top, the narrowest point of the pyramid (the initial concepts), and climb down, instead of standing on the ground and climbing upwards. As you descend, each layer becomes wider and wider so that there are increasingly more choices and pathways you could take, the closer you get to the ground.

While there are many possible rungs (levels of abstraction) in the pyramid, we will discuss just four, to demonstrate how the initial topic or problem area can be transformed into researchable questions as you descend the pyramid to the 'ground' of actually doing the research. The four rungs we will discuss are: *concepts, dimensions* (or constructs), *indicators* and *variables*.

Concepts

The top rung of our pyramid is the concept. Concepts are just the ideas or theories with which you begin; they are terms that usually summarise clusters of related elements. For example, most people understand and use the concept 'poverty' in daily conversation. When discussing whether or not someone is 'poor', however, we may or may not be referring to the same things. First, this is because the idea of 'poverty' could have many quite varied aspects, depending on the cultural, social and historical context. Second, people have different views about what is important in constructing or dissecting the notion of 'poverty'. For example, some people may emphasise the amount of income a person has, while others will temper this with intervening variables such as the size of the family dependent on that income. Others may see poverty as a much more complex mix of lack of access to income, services and supports, and therefore a lack of ability to participate in society—more commonly termed social exclusion. The way 'poverty' is defined is therefore significant for further analysis related to policy development—for example, in the ways we might address poverty alleviation. Our understanding of poverty, and hence poverty alleviation, may encompass access not only to income, but also to assets such as clean water and food supplies, employment and health, welfare, transport and communications services. Thus how we define such a concept significantly impacts on the research that follows.

In researching the issue of 'poverty', one's theoretical perspective will also influence the type of research question that will shape the research. For example, critical theorists may be interested in the way the wage system and welfare provisions create power differentials between groups in society. Thus they may see structural elements as influential in determining the research question. Feminist theorists may be more interested in how the experience of 'poverty' (however defined) might differ for women. Seccombe (2011, p. 39) notes that there are several theoretical perspectives that give insights into poverty, including the *individual* perspective, which places responsibility for life chances on the individual; the *social structural* perspective, which takes note of inequalities inherent in the labour market, institutions and government that affect people's economic position; and the *culture of poverty* approach, which uses both individual and structural elements to explain poverty. She further notes these are not gender neutral, and represent a male perspective as the dominant position. What you should note from this brief discussion is that the theoretical lens we are using to understand our research question will shape how we determine what it is we are measuring.

Thus, concepts are 'summary ideas' that may mean different things to different people. It is important to define concepts clearly so that those reading our research know what we mean by the concepts we use, even if they do not agree with our definitions.

Usually there are at least two major concepts in each research topic, and most often these are expressed as a question about how the concepts are related. For example, let's take the question 'How does gender influence poverty?'

There are two major concepts involved in these questions. The first is the concept or idea of 'gender', which can readily be defined as the way that women's and men's lives might differ depending on social and cultural constructions of what it is to be male or female in a given situation. There is also the concept of 'poverty'. At first glance, the 'gender' concept is relatively simple, while 'poverty' is more complex. Because it is more abstract, the concept of 'poverty' is actually higher on the pyramid of abstraction than the concept of 'gender'. To discuss both these concepts in more detail, we need to descend to the next rung of our pyramid: the level of dimensions.

Dimensions

The elements or aspects that go together to make up concepts are called 'dimensions'. There may be differing numbers of dimensions in each concept, although there would seem to be only one dimension to the concept of 'gender'—whether one is male or female. However, gender is a complex concept if one includes transgender elements. For the sake of simple illustration, here we will stay with the notion of gender as being a dichotomous notion of being male or being female.

In contrast, there are many possible dimensions to the concept of 'poverty'. We listed some of these dimensions in our discussion of what could be involved in the concept of poverty. Defining the variable and being clear in your definition allows you to descend the ladder of abstraction. In her study of poverty and welfare dependence, Seccombe (2011) uses dimensions of welfare dependency, stigma, lack of employment opportunities and the importance of social supports to analyse the impact of poverty on welfare recipients. She notes that key influencers of poverty include lack of employment; lack of child care; minimal child support from children's other parent; inadequate transport infrastructure; racism and sexism; and a welfare system that penalises initiative.

For our purposes, the dimensions of poverty might include:

- income
- number of dependants
- employment opportunities
- accessible services, including health and transport
- child care
- child support
- welfare system support/penalty
- social supports.

Already we can see how the pyramid broadens as we descend each rung to make our definitions of the problem clearer and more specific. From one concept (poverty), we now have at least eight dimensions—and you may think of others that could have been selected. However, at least for this study, we are beginning to have an understanding of the way we might approach a study of how poverty might be differentially experienced by women and men.

Indicators

Indicators are measurable aspects of dimensions, usually expressed in observable or behavioural terms. Defining dimensions in this way, makes clear exactly what is being measured and how concepts are being defined. By describing indicators in behavioural or measurable terms, quantitative researchers also hope to enable others to measure the same phenomena, perhaps under different circumstances, in order to expand knowledge in the particular area of interest. Thus, in our example, by defining what we mean by 'gender' and 'poverty' we allow other researchers the possibility of replicating our study and expanding or commenting on our findings, in other situations. For example, if we were to undertake our study in Australia, other researchers may wish to study poverty in different countries or cultures, or among different age groups.

Just as there can be many dimensions to a single concept, so there can be many indicators created to measure one dimension. (Remember, as we descend the pyramid the layers become ever broader.) Many quantitative researchers advocate using a range of indicators to measure a single dimension, especially if the dimension is complex. How might we operationalise the dimension of 'poverty' into measurable indicators?

In our study, there are a number of indicators that we might use to measure the experience of 'poverty'. These might include more obvious quantifiable measures of income, number of dependants, distance to services, accessibility of services and supports (that is, how easy is it for people to get to services), employment opportunities in the local region, availability of child care, child-support payments, welfare-support payments and the level of social supports people might have in their community. We might also include more intangible indicators of poverty, such as levels of social participation, feelings of well-being, levels of anxiety and experiences of hopelessness, violence, freedom and choice. These indicators can be measured by asking respondents to rate each indicator on a scale. How these scales are measured, and what information they could provide, is discussed on our next rung of the pyramid, 'variables'.

Before discussing variables, let us consider how the relatively simple dimension, 'gender', is defined. This seems relatively straightforward and can be assessed by simply asking whether a person is male or female. However, it might also be useful to include additional questions such as age, ethnicity and location to add complexity to the analysis of gendered experiences over time and place.

Assessing the complexities within a given research question raises an important issue which must be considered when we are operationalising research questions: the *unit of analysis*.

Units of analysis

The unit of analysis is the unit we study, or the unit from which we gather the information we need—it is the measurable dimension at the bottom of the ladder of abstraction. In social work research, the unit of analysis is usually an individual, a group or a social event. In our study, the major unit of analysis is the individual rather than the family or household. It is important to note that even within the same household poverty may be experienced differentially by women and men. In a number of research projects conducted in various Asia-Pacific countries during the 2000s, Margaret Alston found that women and men were differentially affected by climate events and experienced different levels of hardship and hence poverty. Thus it is important to look at the individual in a study such as this to determine how individuals rather than households are affected.

From this example, it can be seen that even apparently simple concepts require careful thought and definition if they are to be transformed into measurable indicators for quantitative social research. Defining the unit of analysis is an important part of this process.

Variables

The bottom rung of the 'pyramid of abstraction'—the level before we reach the 'ground' and start actually doing the research—is specifying just how we will measure our indicators and what 'level of measurement' we will use. Variables are indicators expressed in measurable terms, with the form of measurement made explicit. Variables must vary—that is, they must have more than one value. For example, in the case of gender we have one variable— being female or male. For the indicators making up the dimension 'poverty', we can use ordinal levels of measurement for our tangible dimensions— for example, asking people to tick the level of their income from a small number of groupings such as less than $5000, $5000—less than $10 000, and so on. We can also assess accessibility of services by asking similar questions, such as 'the distance to my nearest health service is: less than a kilometre, 1 kilometre to less than 5 kilometres, and so on. For the more intangible variables, such as levels of anxiety or sense of well-being, we can use five-point scales, with (5) being 'very high' or 'very satisfied' and (1) being 'very low' or 'very dissatisfied', to create variables. These scales are commonly called Likert scales and are widely used in questionnaire or survey research. It allows qualitative data to be given a quantitative dimension to enable statistical testing. We can then discuss the level of poverty in terms of the individual indicators within this dimension, or in summary form, by putting each person's scores on all the variables together into one single 'poverty' score.

Dependent and independent variables

In explanatory research, researchers explore questions about how one variable affects another, or about the causes behind some social phenomenon. The terms 'dependent' and 'independent' are used to describe pairs of variables that are in a relationship with each other. The *dependent variable*, symbolised by a Y in research texts, is the one that researchers are most interested in understanding or explaining why it varies. An independent variable, on the other hand (symbolised by an X) is one that the researcher believes may produce at least some of the variation in the dependent variable. Another way of expressing this is that the value of Y is dependent, to some extent at least, on the value of X.

In our study, there are many dependent variables developed to measure the concept of 'poverty', which we wish to understand. Gender is the independent variable—that is, we want to know whether the experience of poverty is affected by gender.

There are other kinds of variables as well as dependent and independent variables. We will discuss these in greater detail in Chapter 7.

Hypotheses

Once variables have been defined, many quantitative researchers go on to develop hypotheses about their variables. Hypotheses are *statements about variables* and the relationships between them. They are derived from the research questions about concepts that began the process of operationalisation. Hypotheses are important in quantitative research because they clarify and guide the research process, including how the data will be analysed. There are many forms of hypotheses: they may be descriptive ('poverty is increasing in the twenty-first century'), relational ('poverty is related to gender'), directional ('poverty is higher amongst women') or non-directional ('there is a relationship between poverty and gender').

In social research, we can never actually *prove* that there is a relationship between two variables. The closest we can get is to *disprove* the hypothesis that there is no relationship. The hypothesis that states that there is no relationship between two variables is called the *null hypothesis*. Most statistical tests aim to reject the null hypothesis. If we can be fairly sure that there is evidence of a relationship, then we reject the null hypothesis and accept the alternative or research hypothesis. These days, null hypotheses are rarely stated in research reports. However, it is important to know that 'rejecting the null hypothesis' is the basis of most statistical tests that provide support for the existence of a relationship.

Hypotheses may be explicit or implicit. In our study of how gender affects experiences of poverty, there are several implied hypotheses—for example, 'women are more likely to experience poverty' and 'there is a relationship between poverty and a lack of employment opportunities'. We will discuss how qualitative researchers develop hypotheses after discussing levels of measurement and their importance. For now, it is a useful exercise for beginning researchers using quantitative approaches to try to formulate hypotheses using the variables they have operationalised, as a way of clarifying exactly what they are researching.

In summary, as quantitative researchers descend the 'pyramid of abstraction', they transform general research questions about concepts into specific hypotheses about variables.

Example of descending the pyramid of abstraction

Research question

Does gender influence an individual's experience of poverty?

Concepts

Gender
Poverty

Dimensions

Gender
Poverty

- Income
- Number of dependents
- Distance to services
- Access to services
- Employment opportunities
- Child care
- Child support
- Welfare support
- Social supports

Example of indicators

Gender
- Sex
Experience of poverty
- Level of participation, feelings of well-being, levels of anxiety, experiences of hopelessness, violence, freedom and choice

---

Examples of variables

Gender

• Male/female

Experience of poverty

• Five-point self-rating scale: Very high (5), High (4), Neutral (3), Low (2), Very low (1)

Example of hypothesis

There is a relationship between experience of poverty as self-rated on a five-point scale and gender.

Levels of measurement

An important aspect of specifying variables is determining the level of measurement they will have. This in turn affects the kinds of statistical procedures that can be performed (see Chapter 16 and 17). There are four levels at which variables may be measured. Each level provides different kinds of information.

Nominal level

The nominal level is the simplest level of measurement. It sorts variables into categories. For example, the categories for the variable 'gender' are 'male' and 'female'. These are usually assigned numbers, so that they can be coded for analysis. However, the numbers do not imply order or magnitude. If 'female' is coded '1' and 'male' is coded '2', we are not assigning females more value, or a higher score, than males. We are simply differentiating them.

Ordinal level

The ordinal level of measurement is the next level of measurement above nominal. As well as being able to divide a variable into categories, at the ordinal level we can rank the categories from high to low, or from best to worst. In our study, the five-point scale measuring experience of poverty is an example of an ordinal level variable. Note that while we know that a score of (5) means that someone has a very high level of, for example, anxiety than someone who has scored (4), we do not know how much more anxious the first person is, or whether there would be the same amount of difference between two people who scored (3) and (4) as between two people who rated their experience at (4) and (5).

Interval level

In addition to the properties of nominal and ordinal level measurement, interval level measurement is distinguished by there being equal intervals between the ranks or ordered categories. This means that we can add and subtract—a useful function for summarising large amounts of information. An example of an interval measurement is the IQ scale. While the difference between an IQ of 80 and 90 is supposed to be the same as the difference between an IQ of 160 and 170, it is not possible to claim that someone with an IQ of 160 has twice the IQ of someone with an IQ of 80.

Ratio level of measurement

The ratio level of measurement is the closest level to numbers or mathematics. Not only do measurements at this level include all the properties of the previous three levels, but at this level there is also an absolute zero point. This permits us to multiply and divide results—another very useful property for summarising large amounts of information to give us a typical 'picture' of the issue we are studying. Examples of variables at ratio levels of measurement include age, height and timespan in years or in minutes. In practice, many interval level measurements are also at the ratio level, but it is important to understand the difference between the two.

There are four rules that must be followed in all measurement of variables. First, variables must have at least two categories (they must *vary*). Second, categories must be distinct (that is, different). Third, categories must be mutually exclusive (the same person should not be able to fit into two categories of the one variable). Finally, categories must be exhaustive (all the people being studied must fit into one of the categories; even if the category is 'other', every person should be assigned to a category).

Checking the effectiveness of measurement: Reliability and validity

Having operationalised our research questions down to measurable hypotheses involving variables, including specifying the level of measurement of each of our variables, we must consider how effective our variables actually are. There are two main ways of evaluating the usefulness of our variables: checking their validity and reliability. Reliability and validity are treated differently in quantitative and qualitative research. We will discuss both in this section, as a prelude to examining how research questions are formulated in each.

Validity in quantitative research

The first important test of whether variables are effective in quantitative research is whether they are actually measuring what the researcher wants to measure—or, as Dudley (2011, p. 91) puts it, 'How good are the measures we are using?' This is termed *validity*. Ultimately, the validity of a variable depends on how we have defined the concept it is intended to measure, and how accurately the measure reflects the concept we are measuring.

Different texts deal with quantitative validity in slightly different ways. We refer you to some of these different discussions at the end of this chapter. Basically, there are four main ways to assess validity in quantitative research, and each method assesses a different aspect of validity. No one method is perfect. The method you choose will depend on the purpose of your measurement and what sort of evidence of validity is most important.

Face validity

Face validity is a term sometimes used interchangeably with content validity, which means the degree to which a measurement appears, on the face of it, to measure what it is supposed to measure (Babbie 2010). In other words, does it appear to reflect the concept you are measuring?

Content validity

Content validity refers to the extent to which variables cover the whole content, or all the major dimensions, of the concept being measured. For example, do the indicators we have chosen to examine experiences of poverty really capture the full extent of this experience, or has something crucial been omitted? Of course, it is never possible to cover all the meanings of a concept, but variables can be more or less successful in covering the content of a concept.

Criterion validity

Criterion validity means the measure is valid if scores correlate with other measures of the same concept (Dudley 2011). To establish criterion validity, you would compare the results from your measuring instrument with results from some outside criteria, or 'gold standard'—such as other well-accepted methods of measurement. For example, do individuals who score highly on our measures of poverty also score highly on other tests of poverty? There are several kinds of criterion validity, including *concurrent validity* (for example, the ability to predict accurately a person's current experience of poverty) and *predictive validity* (for example, the ability to predict how a person's experience of poverty will be two years from now).

Construct validity

Construct validity is concerned with how well a measure conforms to theoretical expectations, or how well it measures a theoretical construct. It does this by assessing how the variable relates to other measurable variables (Dudley 2011). Suppose, for example, that there was a well-accepted theory that said poverty was related to levels of violence experienced by women. If we measured levels of violence as well as experiences of poverty, and found that our measure of violence increased with increasing poverty, we could say that our measure of poverty had construct validity.

Remember that there is no ideal way to establish validity. The method you choose will depend on your purpose and what is available. A leading authority in this area, de Vaus (2002), recommends that if a good external criterion exists, use this; if the definition of the concept is well accepted, use content validity; and if there are well-accepted theories that utilise your concept, use construct validity.

Validity in qualitative research

Qualitative researchers view validity differently from quantitative researchers. Rather than beginning by making sure that their variables are accurately operationalised, qualitative researchers ensure validity through their methods of data collection and analysis. One way of ensuring validity of findings in qualitative research is to recheck findings with respondents to make sure the researcher 'got it right'. Qualitative researchers argue that qualitative research has its own validity because researchers are out in the field in the real world of their participants, and the researcher does not artificially shape the way data emerges. Qualitative researchers are also constantly checking and rechecking their data through ongoing and prolonged engagement with the research field and participant observation over time.

Possibly the most important way that qualitative researchers ensure their findings are valid is through the process of 'triangulation'. Triangulation is the use of a variety of methods and also sometimes researchers, theories, data-collection technologies or a combination of these to collect similar data (Rubin and Babbie 2011).

In fact, many qualitative researchers claim that because their methods and data-collection procedures are closer to reality and more flexible than those used in quantitative research, because they communicate about the nature of their research and its findings with the people involved, and because they have the opportunity of going back or expanding their research if their findings are found not to be valid in the first place, they have better ways of ensuring validity than quantitative researchers.

Reliability in quantitative research

Testing for reliability is the other way that researchers have of evaluating whether their variables and findings are effective. Reliability is about consistency. A variable is reliable if someone else who uses it gets very similar results to the original researcher, or if the original researcher uses the measure at a later time or with a similar group of people, and similar results appear (Rubin and Babbie 2011).

There are several types of reliability in quantitative research, as well as different ways of assessing whether research results are consistent. Reliability can refer to results being consistent over time, with groups of different respondents or across different variables.

The most common method of testing reliability is to use the same instrument on several occasions with the same group of people (called the *test–retest* method). This has many problems, in that differences in measurement could indicate real differences in the way the people feel over time or reflect some 'interference' effect of the previous test, which may have raised awareness of the issue in the people being researched. However, it is the major method of testing reliability that can be applied to single questions, as well as to scales.

Another method is the *split-half* method, whereby the variables or scales in an instrument are divided into two halves and administered separately. If the scores are similar, the instrument is considered to be reliable. There are several other methods of testing reliability, most of which also apply to scales.

Reliability in qualitative research

Qualitative researchers do not use the methods of controlling variables and manipulating the environment described above for quantitative researchers, and in fact are quite critical of these approaches. Instead, qualitative researchers try to ensure reliability or consistency by trying to find exceptions to their results, or to consciously list all possible sources of error.

Whereas qualitative research has paid detailed attention to questions of validity, it has tended to ignore issues of reliability. More recent accounts of qualitative research set out methods of ensuring reliability, such as using extra questions that are worded slightly differently, using a systematic and consistent line of questions with different interviewees, and carefully setting out how data were collected so that the research can be replicated.

Validity and reliability

Validity and reliability are different but related concepts. In quantitative research, reliability is a necessary but not sufficient precondition for validity. It is possible for research questions to be quite reliable but not valid. For example, the everyday question, 'How are you?' is likely to reliably get the reply, 'Well thanks', but the response does not necessarily indicate how a person is really feeling. Thus it is reliable but not valid. On the other hand, quantitative research questions that are valid are necessarily reliable because accuracy is an essential part of validity in this approach.

Having briefly noted how quantitative and qualitative researchers try to ensure that the variables they develop are effective by being concerned about validity and reliability, we conclude this chapter with an examination of how qualitative researchers develop research questions.

Developing qualitative questions

Whereas quantitative research begins at the top of the pyramid of abstraction and involves careful thinking through of research questions before the research commences, qualitative research begins as close to the ground as possible, and gradually works upwards through the rungs of the pyramid, developing questions and hypotheses as it goes. Some qualitative researchers claim to actually start on the 'ground' with no initial ideas at all, but we have seen that it is really impossible for researchers to begin with 'empty heads'. Rather, we tend to begin our research with theoretical baggage but limited understanding of the issue we are researching.

When thinking through their general topic, researchers from both qualitative and quantitative perspectives must take into account the issues that we discussed in the first half of this chapter. However, having decided on their general topic area, researchers using predominantly qualitative methods try not to define their concepts too clearly before they have talked to or observed the people with whom they are researching. Qualitative research will involve the research subjects in the process of defining the topic to a greater or lesser extent depending on the researcher's theoretical approach, and concepts will be loosely defined—if at all.

To illustrate this approach more clearly, it is helpful to use an example. Lee Purches (social worker) and Frances Jaeger (nurse) are two rural health workers who wanted to evaluate some support groups for women that Frances had set up in several small townships in a rural region. The support groups initially had been formed because workers at the local family care cottage had noticed that a large number of mothers with babies and small children were being referred to them with symptoms of postnatal depression. About a year after the groups were formed, the workers felt it was time to evaluate them.

With an egalitarian, feminist rationale, the groups had been set up as independent self-help units in several different small towns in the region, with each group developing its own aims, objectives and methodology. In line with this basic philosophy, the evaluators decided to involve the women in developing the approach to be taken to the evaluation, the aims of the evaluation and the questions that would be asked. Thus they went into the planning stages of the evaluation with an explicitly feminist approach, whereby the research would be *for* the women, not just *about* women.

First, the evaluators met with members from the original postnatal depression group from the family care cottage to discuss the aims of the evaluation, and to invite the women's participation. They then consulted with leaders from the various groups to discuss what questions and approaches the women would find most useful. The leaders in turn consulted with their groups and reported back to the researchers.

To the evaluators' surprise (and initial dismay), the women wanted a much broader approach to the research than the evaluators' original idea. Instead of just an evaluation, the women wanted a more general inquiry about postnatal depression and its impact on women's lives, and to explore issues of community awareness of the issue. Following further discussions with the women and local health workers, the topic of how living in a rural area affects the experience of postnatal depression was also included.

Throughout this discussion phase, research questions were being worked and reworked with the women and other interested people. The participants decided to design a questionnaire that would be posted to the members of the support groups in the various towns. A questionnaire was chosen rather than interviews or group discussion because of the distances involved, and also because it was hoped that the women would be able to be more honest if they could write their thoughts anonymously. Note that the questionnaire traditionally has been associated with quantitative research, yet in this case it was being used in a qualitative framework (with some quantitative questions being included as well).

The questionnaire turned out to be much longer than the evaluators would have liked, due to all the questions that the women wanted included. In addition, in the tradition of qualitative research, the researchers were then overwhelmed with an enormous amount of information in response to the questionnaire. Women wrote extra pages and described their thoughts and feelings in great detail in response to the open-ended qualitative questions that were asked. More detail on these sorts of questions will be provided in Chapter 7.

From this brief introduction to formulating research questions in qualitative research, you can see how the qualitative researcher begins at the opposite end of the pyramid of abstraction from the quantitative researcher. Rather than beginning at the top of the pyramid, qualitative researchers begin as close to the ground as possible, and then allow their questions and hypotheses to emerge from their observations, discussions or 'immersion in the field'.

In the example of the evaluation of the rural women's support groups, we have seen how the researchers circled between the bottom rungs of the pyramid, beginning with a general idea for the research (evaluation), which was slowly refined as the researchers gradually developed their questions, always returning to the 'ground' to check with the people they were researching that this was the approach that was wanted. By the end of this process, the research questions had significantly changed from the researchers' original ideas for a simple evaluation of a health care program for women to a study about postnatal depression in rural areas that included the evaluation. From the discussions with the group and the group leaders, a hypothesis about rural areas affecting the experience of postnatal depression also emerged. These three ideas (the group evaluation, experiences of postnatal depression and influence of rural lifestyle) were then further examined in a qualitative questionnaire.

Variables at different levels of measurement were used in this study. However, the emphasis was on qualitative, open-ended questions, and thus the major level of measurement was nominal.

Summary

In this chapter, we have discussed how general ideas or problem areas for research are transformed into researchable questions. From our discussion of the factors involved in choosing the general area for the research, we examined how quantitative and qualitative research questions are developed, beginning at different ends of the pyramid of abstraction. In both examples of research that were used to demonstrate this process, we have shown how research questions and designs are, in fact, often a mixture of qualitative and quantitative approaches. These days, quantitative researchers often begin with qualitative-type inquiries as they develop and test their concepts, dimensions, indicators and variables, to make sure that they are valid and relevant to the people who are being researched. We have also seen how qualitative researchers can use quantitative methods, such as questionnaires, to refine their questions with the people with whom they are researching.

The important lesson from this discussion is to understand that clear and careful thought about your research topic is an integral part of the research process, and not something that can be rushed through so that you can 'get on with asking people questions'. If you are doing quantitative research, it is vital that you operationalise your concepts and dimensions properly, because once these are set, you are committed to a particular course of action and it is difficult to correct mistakes. In qualitative research there is more flexibility, because qualitative researchers can alter their questions and directions as they go. However, qualitative researchers need to end up with results that are valid and reliable, and careful thinking about their research questions during the process of their research is just as important as it is for quantitative researchers at the beginning of theirs.

Discussion questions

3.1   A study appears comparing the average income between countries. What is the unit of analysis?

3.2   What is wrong with the following question? 'Please tick the box that indicates your weekly income:

$10–$20   ☐
$20–$50   ☐
$50–$300   ☐
$300–$1000'   ☐

3.3   What level of measurements are the following?
   (a)   Marital status:
       •   Single
       •   Married
       •   Living with partner, not married
       •   Divorced
       •   Widowed
       •   Separated
   (b)   Age expressed in years
   (c)   Number of children
   (d)   Satisfaction rating of a movie on a scale of 1–10 where 1 = not at all satisfied and 10 = very satisfied.

3.4   What is the difference between a hypothesis and a research question?

3.5   Read the following statements. Name the variables and their probable level of measurement. Indicate whether there are dependent or independent variables in each statement and if so, label them accordingly:
    (a) 'The price of wheat increases with the annual yearly rainfall.'
    (b) 'The longer the marriage, the more satisfied are the partners.'
    (c) 'Women have lower incomes than men.'
    (d) 'Increasing blood alcohol levels cause increasingly serious car accidents.'

3.6   A researcher into youth culture is repeatedly told during her time with a gang that they are not involved in hard drugs, only 'soft' drugs. Shortly after her research is written up, members of the gang are arrested for heroin trafficking. What could be said about the reliability and validity of her results?

3.7   The researcher from the previous question is beginning her research and has decided to use a qualitative approach. How might she go about defining her research questions?

Exercises

3.1   Operationalise the questions from the descriptive topic that you devised in the exercise in Chapter 2 into a researchable form for a quantitative researcher. List the concepts, dimensions, indicators and variables that could be involved, including more than one dimension for each concept, and more than one indicator for each dimension.

3.2   Specify the level of measurement of each of your variables.

3.3   Formulate a number of hypotheses from your variables.

3.4   What are the independent and dependent variables?

3.5   What is the unit of analysis for your study?

3.6   Is this topic relevant, feasible, researchable and ethical?

Further reading

Conceptualising and operationalising quantitative research, including measurement, validity and reliability

Babbie, E. 2010, *The Practice of Social Research*, 12th edn, Cengage, Boston. See Chapters 4 (on research design) and 5 (on conceptualisation, operationalisation and measurement).

Grinnell, Richard M. and Unrau, Yvonne A. (eds) 2010, *Social Work Research and Evaluation*, 9th edn, Oxford University Press, New York. See Chapter 11, 'Measurement'.

Yegidis, B.L., Weinbach, W.W. and Myers, L.L. 2012, *Research Methods for Social Workers*, 7th edn, Pearson, Englewood Cliffs, NJ. Chapter 10 covers the issues dealt with in this chapter in more detail.

Conceptualising and operationalising qualitative research and measurement issues

Merriam, S. 2009, *Qualitative Research*, Jossey-Bass, San Francisco. Chapter 9 deals with validity and reliability.

Padgett, D. 2008, *Qualitative Methods in Social Work Research*, 2nd edn, Sage, Thousand Oaks, CA. Chapters 1 and 2 provide insights into how to develop qualitative research questions.

4 Steps in the research process

Measuring Poverty.

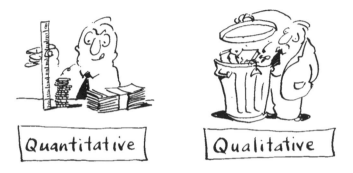

Quantitative   **Qualitative**

You have begun with a situation that perplexes, excites or alarms you. You must now decide about which aspect of the problem you wish to focus on and what it is you hope to achieve. You will have decided on the methodology or combination of methodologies that best suits your purposes. This chapter, which focuses on the steps you must now undertake to complete a piece of research, is designed to demystify the research process by breaking it into a series of comfortable stages that you can use as a model for future research projects. Your research plan will act as a blueprint, guiding you through the project. We have also included examples of research plans to familiarise you with the process of turning an idea into a recognisable research design. You should remember that the stages outlined here are not meant to be rigidly followed in each research project, but should act as a flexible guide to your work.

If you are conducting a study, you should always begin by making a flexible conceptual plan outlining the process you will follow. Your plan should include the stages shown in the box.

Research steps

1 Defining the problem
2 Choosing the methodology
3 Reviewing the literature
4 Preparation
5 Research design:
   - Sampling
   - Data collection
   - Administration
   - Data analysis
   - Reporting
6 Conducting the research
7 Disseminating the findings

Factors influencing the nature and success of your research

Research projects are not developed in a vacuum. A variety of factors will influence the content of your research design—its subject-matter, scope, methodology and so on. For social workers, these factors also include the agency in which you work, your professional background and your own limitations of time and expertise. It will also include your theoretical orientation, the political and cultural context of the work and your need to meet ethical requirements (Rubin and Babbie 2010). The prospects of your research attracting funding (its competitiveness) will also be influenced by a variety of factors, such as the currency of the issue. It is important that you understand these when preparing your research.

Agency context

As noted in Chapter 2, your agency will necessarily influence the type of research you are able to do, and hence the type of research proposal you are able to draft. Some agencies are more committed to research than others, and will influence your ability to act as researchers. Some agencies provide support and seed funding for small research projects which, while they may be small, are excellent sources of funds for 'learner' researchers. If funding is available for a small project, there may also be the opportunity within the agency to discuss your project with more experienced researchers. Take advantage of internal funding and support, and the possibility to learn all you can before entering the competitive, cut-throat world of external funding.

Where agencies do not provide research funding and support, you may need to convince your employers about the potential value of research. In the present tight economic environment, agencies may be happy to discuss an evaluation study, for example, which will show that they take seriously their responsibility to be accountable to external funding sources and to clientele. Shared projects between groups of agencies are also a possibility. Such projects provide excellent collegial experiences as well as allowing enhanced inter-agency cooperation. If you are daunted by the prospect of conducting your own research, seek collaboration with other workers in your region or in your specialist area.

You should also bear in mind that the agency for which you work will have a distinct philosophy that will influence the type of research you can undertake. Some private welfare agencies, which operate from a well-defined religious framework, will circumscribe the types of research that they will support. However, you should bear in mind that all agencies—public and private—operate from a framework that will influence the operations of their workers. What research is, and is not, possible will be influenced—sometimes powerfully and sometimes subtly—by the philosophy of the agency for which you work.

You should not ignore the organisational culture of your agency, a factor that will have a telling influence on potential research projects. How does the chain of management work? In other words, who has the power to endorse or influence your research proposal? How are decisions approved? What are the practices traditionally supported by your agency? Taking time to note the culture of your organisation may facilitate your research agenda.

Additionally, agency resources will have an impact on the scope of the research you may be able to undertake. The availability of advanced computer systems and administrative support staff will allow you to complete more detailed and complex research. The possibilities for research within your agency or within a group of agencies will also be influenced by the type of clientele, the size of the agency and the type of client files kept as ready sources of data. The availability of client files may negate the necessity for collecting new data. However, you and your agency must deal with ethical issues of confidentiality before you decide whether this is a viable alternative.

Agency influences on social work research

- Availability of seed funding
- Importance of proposed research to agency accountability
- Agency philosophy

- Organisational culture
- Agency resources
- Agency clientele

Theoretical and sociopolitical context

Your research project will be influenced by a number of very evident factors, such as the agency setting and the professional and practical issues that shape your work. Less evident will be the factors that implicitly influence the type of research you undertake and the way in which you carry it out. Chief among these is the theoretical background and orientation you bring to your work. Think about the way you practise social work. Do you operate from a psychotherapeutic framework? Maybe you favour systems theory or narrative therapy. In any case, you will no doubt be able to identify your practice orientation. In conducting research, you will have a similar distinct focus that shapes the way you 'practise' research—the way you identify a problem, the way you gather data about that problem and the way you interpret the data. For example, a feminist researcher examining the over-representation of children of single mothers in juvenile justice may seek to empower the women involved rather than categorise them, creating a quite different interpretation of a problem (see Chapter 2).

Another equally influential factor in the shaping of your research project is the socio-political context within which it takes place. What social issues are on the agenda? Think about the change in the welfare agenda already during the twenty-first century. Many Western countries have moved from a position where social justice and community responsibility for the vulnerable were fostered actively to a new era where the welfare state is in decline and individuals are often held responsible for their poverty. Think about the change of focus and note how this may affect the type of research conducted and the research agenda favoured by funding bodies. More recently there has been a great deal of research on the best ways to move people from welfare to work, but far less on the factors that create poverty traps. You should take time to be a 'conscientious consumer' in your reading of newspapers and analysis of government ministerial priorities. What are the trends and the 'hot topics'? How is the discourse of disadvantage being shaped and by whom? Is your research of advantage to the vulnerable? Be a reflective researcher (Hardwick and Worsley 2011, drawing on Fook 2002; Humphries 2008), consciously focusing on the context of your research practice rather than being uncritical or basing your work on habit (Thompson and Thompson 2008).

Theoretical, social and political context
- Your theoretical and practice position
- What are the 'hot' social issues?
- What is the political agenda of the funders?
- Who is shaping the agenda?
- Is your research empowering the disadvantaged?

Professional context

The social work industry, and its ethical position, will critically affect the type of research we might undertake. Specifically, there are some types of research that our profession will not sanction. These would include the possibility of inflicting harm on clients or withdrawing services in order to examine the consequences. We should also protect research subjects from any harm that may arise from the publication of results, obtain informed consent and ensure that insensitivity and bias are not part of our practice (e.g. see Rubin and Babbie 2010; Thompson and Thompson 2008). You should also note that research is often directed at assessing the most vulnerable. For example, we know far more about juvenile crime than we do about white-collar crime. Are vulnerable populations too easy a target and too powerless to direct the shape of research conducted around their circumstances? Our work requires a strong worker–client relationship, and we must not jeopardise this relationship by our research. The need for this confidential relationship may also prevent us from being able to observe other social workers at work for the purpose of collecting data.

Finally, your research proposals will be influenced by the emerging social work research culture, including evidence-based practice, as well as by your professional background, and your own values and ethical position.

Professional influences on social work research
- Professional code of ethics
- Protection from harm
- Confidentiality
- Informed consent
- Research focus
- Social/welfare work research culture
- Developing professionalisation

Personal context

Your research will be shaped not only by agency and professional concerns but also by the personal issues that affect you as a practitioner. These include your background, your workload and resources, and your track record.

Important issues you should consider are workload factors and the time you have available to conduct research. These issues may require you to undertake some negotiation with your employers. It is important that you, together with your agencies, recognise that research is 'real' work that can have a lasting impact on policy development, professional practice and agency resourcing. As such, it should be deemed to be part of your workload and not something you do in your spare time.

Your track record in research is important to the way your proposal to undertake research will be assessed. If you have experience as a researcher, this will improve your chances of success in a competitive round. You might ask, 'How does a beginning researcher achieve a track record?' The best way to gain experience is to be a junior partner in a research project with others who have the necessary skills to pass on valuable knowledge and insights. Don't be afraid to put up your hand and volunteer to help in a large project.

Personal influences on social work research

- Research background
- Workload and time pressures
- Track record

Practical issues

To be successful, research projects must be manageable. In defining the limits of your research, be aware that you cannot change the world with $10 000 (or whatever sum you are seeking), so do not try. Turning your research problem into a project that has a reasonable chance of success is a skill beginning researchers have a great deal of difficulty mastering. To do this properly, you must devote an adequate amount of time to developing your proposal.

Note that your proposal must be clear and concise. The problem must be explained so that the assessor of your proposal knows exactly what the problem entails, why it requires researching and how you as the researcher propose to do just that. In putting a proposal into a competitive environment, a potential researcher must be aware that they are competing for scarce funds. It is important that you do not waste your own time and that of the assessors with a poorly constructed proposal. The funding body or agency in which you work has to be convinced that this problem, which has excited you as a worker, is worth its time and investment. Consequently, research proposals should be developed with the same attention to detail and respect with which one would prepare a curriculum vitae. For a detailed summary of the items to include in a research proposal, see Chapter 19.

Practical issues affecting social work research
- Ensure the proposed research is manageable.
- Consult with colleagues and experts.
- Ensure the proposal is written clearly and concisely.
- Ensure it is properly costed.
- Ensure the proposal is well presented.
- Check for spelling errors and typos.

Having considered the factors that may influence your research, let's now turn to the important steps in the process of research.

Defining the problem

In Chapters 2 and 3, we learned how to turn a puzzling situation into a researchable question. In any research, you must define your problem, noting the dimensions of the issue, the target group affected, the political context and the anticipated outcomes. Decide whether your research is to be exploratory, descriptive or explanatory. Remember that your topic must be relevant, researchable, feasible and ethical.

There are several steps to follow when crafting and conceptualising the research problem. These might include:

- choosing the topic area
- critically evaluating why you are interested in this topic and what it is you wish to research
- choosing the particular focus for your research
- relating this to existing knowledge
- determining your specific research question or problem
- if quantitative, operationalising the concepts and variables.

Yegidis, Weinbach and Myers (2012) also note that context is important. You should decide where the research is to take place and when, what data you wish to collect, from whom, how you will collect the data, what variables you wish to measure, how you will analyse the data and how the findings will be disseminated.

This process is facilitated by carefully outlining your objectives and reasons for undertaking the study. While there are no limitations on the number of objectives, you should be careful not to take on more than you can handle comfortably. Beginning researchers have a tendency to try to solve the big-picture issues when they really only have the resources and expertise to concentrate on a small study. Limit your objectives on the basis of the constraints that bind you.

If your study is to be predominantly quantitative, you will need to define the research problem accurately, and this will involve operationalising the variables as outlined in Chapter 3. Qualitative-based research allows a much looser conceptual understanding of the research question at the beginning of the process.

Methodology

We discussed different methodological choices in Chapter 1. You will remember that these include quantitative and qualitative approaches. A quantitative methodology would be most useful where you have extensive knowledge of the environment or situation you wish to study and are looking to test hypotheses about relationships between variables and to make statistical inferences from your quantifiable data. Quantitative research is generally about testing theory.

A qualitative methodology enables you to further your knowledge of the situation when seeking to describe social reality. An emancipatory approach, using quantitative and/or qualitative methodologies, would be appropriate for research that centralises the concerns of marginalised or disempowered people.

You should be aware that you might choose a combination of approaches if this best suits your study. A combination of methods, also called triangulation, is useful for obtaining a wide range of information on an issue. Think carefully about your study, and determine what it is you wish to achieve from the research and then select an appropriate framework. Remember, it is not a political statement to choose one or other methodology, and in fact you would demonstrate naiveté if you were to declare, 'I am always and only a quantitative [or any other] researcher'. It is better to be pragmatic and to decide on the basis of the constraints you face. Decide carefully, because your research plan is determined by the choice you make.

Literature review

Conducting a literature review is a vital part of your research. If you have prepared a research proposal, you will already have read widely. A literature review allows you to discover what knowledge is available about the issue you wish to investigate, to determine how your study will differ from existing work and hence add to the existing knowledge in the area, and it enables you to frame your work conceptually. Some researchers find themselves overwhelmed by the amount of literature available on a given topic. If you find yourself in this situation, you should selectively choose works that:

- represent the argument of a larger body of works
- present opposing views
- reflect current debate, legislation and policy.

Older works are not necessarily inferior, and you should consider references that are classical representations of new ideas or groundbreaking developments. Essentially, your literature review should indicate that you are up to date with current thinking in the area of study.

A review of the literature is a far simpler proposition now than it was even five years ago. Online access to library resources and to the vast resources of the World Wide Web allow you to conduct keyword searches of large data banks. Books and journal articles are much more accessible than they have ever been, and most journals are now available online, allowing you access to complete articles. There are also very sophisticated websites available with a great deal of information to assist you. For example, many government departments have detailed websites containing policy documents, media statements and other useful material and links. If you have difficulty finding these resources, ask your librarian to help you scan the national and international literature and resources in your chosen area. If anything, you will find there is so much data that it is difficult to know where to begin.

You should read widely at first before narrowing down your reading as you define your topic. Read references carefully and critically analyse existing studies to determine what you can best do to extend your understanding of the issue. You might decide to research the issue in a new context, or with a previously unresearched group. For example, if your research topic is child protection, you might study the implications of established practices in a rural situation or with an ethnic population. Your literature review should be thorough so you are sure that what you propose to do is original research. As you further refine your topic, your reading will become more focused and specialised. It is a good idea to summarise the literature at this stage because this will form part of your final research report.

Preparation

Once you have defined your topic and analysed and reviewed the literature in your topic area, you need to undertake a number of tasks before you can launch into the research. Funding the project will be an issue for any piece of research. You should develop a research proposal for your agency or for a funding body, following the outline in Chapter 19. A further issue that must be dealt with during this preparatory stage is seeking ethics approval from the ethics committee at your agency, your university or the funding body. You should also spend some time discussing the proposed research with experienced researchers, colleagues and friends in order to help you to develop a suitable design and to gain the benefit of others' experience.

Research design

Having defined your problem, chosen your methodology, reviewed the literature and completed the preparatory stages, you must now develop an appropriate research design. A research design indicates how your data will be collected, analysed and reported, and includes the types of sampling, as well as the methods of data collection and analysis to be used. Your design is a plan of action that indicates how you propose to research the defined problem and is necessarily shaped by the problem and the methodology. For instance, if your study is qualitative and largely exploratory, you will have a more flexible design. During the course of the study, the questions are refined and clarified, and the researcher chooses the sample subjects as the research progresses. A quantitative study, on the other hand, will be far more precise, with a definite plan of action at the beginning of the study.

Sampling

Both qualitative and quantitative researchers employ sampling techniques. However, quantitative researchers employ probability sampling and so claim representativeness. Qualitative researchers eschew representativeness, claiming that non-probability techniques are more useful for assessing the social reality in which they are interested. Types of sampling will be outlined in Chapter 5. What you must ask yourself is whether your sample is truly adequate for the problem being studied. If you are conducting quantitative research, is your sample representative of the target group or is it biased in some way? For example, if you propose to study attitudes to euthanasia, would it be appropriate to survey university students only? Students may be largely responding to such an issue in an impersonal and non-reflective way. A sample should include those directly involved in the problem being investigated—in this case, terminal patients, relatives, doctors and nurses.

A qualitative sample is usually chosen purposively to reflect the situation under review. For example, Ann Oakley, a feminist researcher, conducted a groundbreaking study of housework in the 1970s that fundamentally altered the notion that housework was not 'work' (Oakley 1985). It still surprises many to learn that she interviewed only 40 women for this study. However, her sample was chosen purposively to reflect women working full time in the home in working-class London; it was small and she was not claiming that it was representative of all women. Her work was so well crafted that she influenced a generation of feminist researchers. Choose your sample to reflect accurately the problem you wish to study or the area you wish to explore.

Data collection

The way you go about collecting your data is just as important as the way you draw up your sample. While data-collection methods will vary according to the type of information you are seeking, the research question and the resources at your disposal, there are no right or wrong methods for a given situation or a given methodology.

Methods are merely tools for the social scientist, and each method is used where and when it proves to be most suitable. We should, however, choose methods that are the best ways of obtaining the information required. For example, questionnaire data will tell us how people felt about a particular issue at a given point of time, but may not be consistent with how they actually behave when the situation in question arises. A good example might be a survey of a group of nurses in nursing homes that finds they are adamant that the elderly in their care deserve the best quality of life that can be provided. A study using observation methods may, however, have revealed that nursing homes are under-staffed and that patients may not always be fed and showered on time, and may be left sitting alone in their rooms for long periods of time. The nurses have not necessarily lied during their survey. The researcher has simply used an inadequate method to collect the data.

Methods employed in quantitative and qualitative research often overlap. For example, you might use interviews, surveys, unobtrusive methods or content analysis in either—we reiterate that the methods are merely the instruments used to elicit the desired information. What differs is the purpose for which they are used (or the theoretical perspective of the researcher) and the way they are used (or the implementation of the methods).

Quantitative methods are more precisely implemented. They are carefully developed and tested prior to the commencement of the study to determine the suitability of the chosen methods. For instance, if the instrument is to be a questionnaire aimed at determining the cause-and-effect links between variables, it must be tested carefully to determine whether the questions relate to the chosen variables. Qualitative methods are far more flexible, and allow the researcher to change and develop the methods employed. For example, survey methods may be unstructured or semi-structured, with topic areas specified and questions varying depending on the issues being explored. This allows the researcher to move into new areas of inquiry and to better understand the perspectives and priorities of the subject. Thus, while methods may be similar, the ways in which they are used by a quantitative or qualitative researcher may vary. As a researcher, you must be clear about your own perspective and what it is you are seeking to know. Based on this information, your plan will specify the method/s you have chosen.

Administration

Conducting any piece of research creates a significant amount of administrative work. Your plan should note the administrative arrangements that will be put in place to ensure the success of your method/s. If you have chosen to survey 1000 people, for example, what materials will you need? Will you need research assistants? How will they be recruited/paid? How will they be trained? Where will interviews take place and how will you set them up? What ethical clearances do you need to obtain prior to commencement? What will you do about non-response? Where will data be stored securely while awaiting processing? If you have chosen to do a qualitative study, you might have decided to use participant observation or unstructured interviewing as your method. How will you gain entry to the situation? Have you thought through the ethical issues? Have you the time and resources to spend a great deal of time in the research situation? For any method, there will be a multiplicity of administrative issues to be sorted out and documented in your plan.

Administrative tasks

- Materials organised
- Access to equipment arranged
- Assistants recruited and trained
- Interviews or access to the situation organised
- Travel and accommodation booked
- Data storage security arranged
- Ethical issues resolved

Data analysis

With extraordinary prescience, Richards and Richards (1990, p. 5) note that 'theories are not little lizards waiting under rocks to be uncovered; but webs of understanding constructed by the researcher, and used actively to make sense of the data'. The success or failure of any research endeavour lies in the researcher's ability to work with the data and to actively generate understandable theoretical arguments. (This will be discussed more fully in Chapters 14, 15, 16 and 17.) What have you discovered that you did not know before? How can you document these findings to clearly indicate the new information you have generated? This process is perhaps the most daunting one for new researchers, but it is also the most exciting because you have made discoveries and have created a new understanding of the research issue. Once you have undertaken this process of analysis, you will find that the research process is demystified, understandable and challenging.

The way your data are to be analysed is an integral stage of any research and should be planned carefully. If you have conducted a quantitative survey and have data requiring statistical analysis, you may need to employ an analyst or purchase appropriate computer software and seek relevant training. A qualitative research study produces vast amounts of new data—often unstructured—which must be coded, categorised and analysed. This can usefully be done by computer. Whatever means you choose, you must incorporate this into your plan and allow time and resources for training or employing others to do the analysis.

Reporting

The final section of your plan will detail how you propose to report your findings. What is the most appropriate medium to allow you to widely disseminate your findings so that they have maximum impact on the situation that led you to do the research in the first place? You might decide that this is an interdepartmental report, a conference paper, a journal article, a book or a newspaper article. You should see this stage as crucial to the resolution of the problem, and make resources available. You may need to contact agencies, editors or publishers before you commence your research so that no time is lost and your research findings do not become dated. Chapter 18 expands on this topic area.

Reporting your research
- Interdepartmental report
- Conference paper
- Journal article
- Book or book chapter
- Newspaper
- Pamphlet or flyer

Conducting the research

Your plan acts like a roadmap that indicates how your study will be conducted. It should be comprehensive so that no surprises emerge during the execution phase. When conducting the research, you should follow the plan you have developed, allowing some flexibility for the unforeseen issues that may arise. The execution phase takes a great deal of time, and represents the major commitment in terms of time, energy and focus. Do not be discouraged if your data do not support your position or if your research plan must be reassessed. Negative or non-significant findings are just as valuable as findings showing a significant relationship or positive effect. If people do not publicise such findings, the research community and the profession may be left with a distorted picture of the existing situation. The experience you gain is important, and your findings will contribute to the knowledge base of our profession regardless of whether or not they are earth-shattering revelations.

Disseminating the findings

Research should be viewed as having three equally important stages: the preparation phase, the execution phase and the dissemination stage. Your research findings may have the potential to completely change our thinking on a particular issue. However, unless you first communicate your findings effectively by writing them in a way that is clear and intelligible and, second, disseminate those findings widely, your research will merely gather dust on your bookshelf. Research reports should be written clearly and concisely in a way that interests the audience by avoiding jargon and masses of superfluous information. Take careful note of the points outlined in Chapter 18 when presenting your findings.

Research in action

To further your understanding of the differences between qualitative and quantitative methodologies, and the different types of research plans they generate, let us examine some examples. The article below appeared in an Australian rural newspaper.

DOMESTIC VIOLENCE COMMITTEE

_____ newly formed Domestic Violence Committee will meet for the first time today following the issue of a record number of domestic violence orders following Monday's _____ Local Court sitting.

Fourteen domestic violence restraining orders were issued after Monday's court.

It was the largest number ever issued here.

A committee to formulate effective response systems to the problem, and to follow up progress in individual cases, has been formed.

The article details a significant increase in the number of local women appearing before the local court seeking protection orders from their violent partners. It was sent to us by a colleague in the area. As researchers in the welfare field, we are alarmed by the social problems in the town that underlie these bald facts. You might ask yourself how, if you were a member of the newly formed Domestic Violence Committee, you would best go about finding out more about the situation in order to formulate an effective response.

The first issue is problem definition. What are your objectives? What is it we wish to find out? Are we interested in quantifying the problem or seeking to explore and understand the experiences of the women or the perpetrators in the town? Are we interested in how the police and legal systems are responding to the situation? What programs or actions have proved effective? Is this an historically isolated experience for this town, or is it a common feature of the gender dynamics in rural communities?

Is this town any different from other small rural towns, and how does it compare to coastal towns or cities? These questions illustrate how difficult it is to decide what you might fruitfully explore through your research.

To help define the problem, outline your objectives carefully. Do you want facts about the numbers of victims coming before the courts? Are you more interested in understanding the experiences of the women so that you can develop programs? Are you interested in the possible link between poverty/unemployment and violence? Your ultimate concern will no doubt be to influence programs and policy so that violence is no longer a feature of your town.

Let us examine some different approaches—one quantitative and one qualitative, with the qualitative example having a feminist orientation.

Quantitative study of violence experienced by women in rural areas

Definition of the problem

From the newspaper report, you have determined that violence is possibly an emerging and increasing problem in small towns. There are many aspects to this problem that might fruitfully be tested. However, your experience with this community is that you think it might be limited to rising unemployment levels. Therefore, you have decided to test this hypothesis and to determine whether there is a link with high unemployment levels. Your hypothesis acts like a guess or tentative answer to a perplexing problem. Your hypothesis is: 'Violence against women is increasing in small rural towns as unemployment levels increase'.

Note that you will need to operationally define certain terms in your hypothesis. Violence against women historically has been defined in various ways. However, there is now consensus that violence should be more broadly defined than just overt physical violence, and should include emotional, psychological and spiritual violence. More succinctly, it is also defined as violent or abusive behaviour used by a family member to control another family member (Domestic Violence Crisis Service 2011). This definition is comprehensive, but it is also difficult to research because many women do not report their experiences of violence. When they do, it is more likely that they will report physical rather than non-physical forms of violence. You might choose, then, to operationally define violence against women as 'cases reported to police and to social/welfare workers in local agencies'. Small rural towns might be operationally defined as towns with populations of 5000 or fewer. 'Unemployment levels' are operationally defined as government unemployment statistics for the areas studied.

Operationally defined, your hypothesis now reads: 'Violence against women, as evidenced by reports to police and social/welfare workers, is increasing in rural towns of 5000 or fewer people as official unemployment figures increase'. As a social worker, you are concerned to incorporate into your study an examination of treatment procedures and effective programs. Your study will have a further aim: to examine the responses of the helping professions in the towns surveyed.

Literature review

You must read widely to determine what studies have already been done in this area and to help you to further define your approach to your research. There is a great deal of literature conceptualising and contextualising violence, and you should read as much as you can so that you are aware of the theoretical work in the area you are researching. Many researchers are so keen to get into the field and begin collecting data that they may ignore the value of existing literature in helping to develop an efficient and sound study.

Preparation

Funding research is a constant problem for researchers and workers in the welfare field. You might seek funding from your agency, or from a combination of the services represented on the steering committee. Alternatively, the committee might choose to make a joint submission to an external funding body. In any case, cost your plan carefully so that you are not disadvantaged by a shortfall in funding.

In any research, particularly in an area as sensitive as violence, you should make sure you have ethical clearance from your own agency and/or the funding body's ethics committee. In this case, issues of confidentiality, privacy, access to counselling for interviewees and security for those taking part are all relevant ethical issues.

Research design

The best way to gather data that accurately reflects the defined problem is a skill that must be learned. To assist with this, a carefully developed research design is vital. Your design reflects the ideal sampling, data-collection and data-analysis methods chosen. You must draw up a careful plan to test your hypothesis, always bearing in mind that your plan will be limited by your funding and time constraints. Despite these, ensure that it retains its focus on the research problem. Let us assume that you have adequate funding and have permission to spend one day a week for six months on this study.

Sampling

The committee decides to restrict the study to ten rural towns with populations of fewer than 5000 in the state where you are working. Your sample of towns might be chosen randomly, or be determined by distance constraints so that the ten closest to your home form the basis of your study, or you might look at towns across a number of regions, including coastal and inland areas. Within the ten towns, the committee decides to survey a representative sample of local police and social/welfare workers. Your first task is to seek the names and addresses of these service providers so that your sample is complete.

Data collection

Your methods must be chosen well to gather the required data and adequately test your hypothesis. In this case, you are seeking reported cases of violence as well as unemployment figures and information on response mechanisms. Because you are looking for a link between the two variables, your data must span a specified period (say, two to five years) to determine fluctuations. Collecting data on employment figures will be relatively easy, as these can be obtained through the government employment services. These data will be broken down by local areas and will allow you to note fluctuations.

Collecting data on reported cases of violence will be more difficult, as you will need to survey a number of people to gather the required information. You might choose to draw up a questionnaire or interview schedule for the police and service providers in the selected towns. With a sensitive issue such as this, face-to-face interviews, although time consuming, will allow you to gather the information more successfully than mailed questionnaires. Your interview should cover issues dealing with historical trends in the reporting of violence, but should also examine a number of other issues that might affect reporting in order that you may determine whether any factors not related to unemployment are affecting the results. Issues such as changes in legislation, new services that make it easier for women to seek help, community education and community changes in attitude will have an impact on the reporting of violence, and may have a greater effect on results than unemployment. You will also include questions about types of service responses and effective programs.

Before entering the field, you should test your questionnaire by pre-testing questions and by conducting a pilot test in a town not in your sample. Piloting allows you to refine your questions to ensure that they are not ambiguous and are focused on the issue in question. With a quantitative study, your interviews will be standardised so that each person is asked the same series of questions.

Administration

The administration issues involved with this study will depend on the funds available. If you have sufficient funds to employ a research assistant who can conduct the interviews for you, you will need to allow time to draft the questions, to train the assistant, to conduct the interviews and to analyse the responses. You may also need to allocate funds for travel and accommodation in the various towns to be visited. Most importantly, you need to be sure your interview appointments have been made well in advance.

Data analysis

Once the interviews are completed, your analysis of the collected data will necessarily take a great deal of time. This is where you determine whether the evidence supports your hypothesis, or whether other variables have had a greater influence on reported violence. There are several quantitative data analysis computer programs available that will assist you at this stage of your research; these will be discussed further in Chapter 15.

Reporting results

Your results may indicate that increasing reports of violence are linked to increasing unemployment figures. They may also indicate a number of other issues that influence violence in the community. You may also have a great deal of valuable information on effective programs. Whatever the case, you should not lose sight of the original reason for conducting the study—your alarm at the numbers of women reporting violence in the newspaper story. Your report of the study should illuminate this issue and carefully present your findings. If your results are being published in a newspaper, there is little need to do more than report the issues. If you are writing a report, an article, a conference paper or a book, you should write about any additions to the conceptual understanding of the problem that you are able to make. Your work is useful regardless of how conclusive your findings are because it adds knowledge and informs others about your methodology and the application of methods to achieve the stated results.

Qualitative study of violence experienced by women

Because qualitative researchers are concerned to understand the lived reality of people's experience, such a study will necessarily be different to a quantitative study. In this case, the committee may decide that a qualitative study is essential to understand what is happening in the town. Qualitative research does not need a well-defined research hypothesis, but it does require you to clearly state the research problem. The committee may decide that the problem is essentially to find out more about violence in the town, what strategies women employ to deal with the situation, whether current responses are seen as acceptable, and what changes might be made to deal more effectively with violence. In this case, the plan is more flexible and will be shaped by the emerging data. Regardless of the methodology employed, a literature review remains an essential element of any piece of research. Your reading should help to shape your thinking and alert you to the issues that should be incorporated into the study.

Research design

Sampling

In qualitative studies, there is no claim that the sample is representative of the whole population, and little attempt to claim that findings are generalisable beyond the study population. Qualitative researchers are less interested in recognising patterns of behaviour, attitudes or other phenomena than they are in *understanding* social reality; therefore the sampling technique employed will be non-probability based, or purposive, because subjects will be chosen for a *purpose*. In this case, the committee decides to seek permission to speak with women who are seeking protection orders to find out what is happening to them, where they are seeking help, whether this is effective and what can be done to prevent violence. The committee also decides to speak with service providers in the town to find an effective response, to coordinate community education activities, to maximise protection for women and to undertake preventive measures against violence. Thus the sample might comprise women who have sought protection orders during the past two years and all service providers in the town.

Preparation

To undertake such a study the committee must clarify where funds will be obtained, who is to do the work and how the committee will oversee the project. Most importantly, the committee must address the ethical issues involved in the proposed study. How will victims of violence be approached to participate in the study, and what strategies will be put in place to ensure confidentiality is maintained? Clearance must be sought from relevant ethics committees so that those participants approached are not compromised. In this case, the local police officer and the magistrate are part of the newly formed committee. One of these officials might be asked to contact women who have come to the court for assistance over the last two years to request their participation in the study. In this way, a purposive sample of women might be developed.

Data collection

Effective methods for this piece of research would be semi-structured interviews with women who have experienced violence and focused discussion groups with service providers. Semi-structured interviews allow certain designated areas of inquiry to be explored with the interviewees. Focused discussion groups with service providers will allow information to be collected from all providers and for response strategies to be 'brain-stormed' in the group situation. This method will save time and money. Data from both chosen methods are most effectively gathered via electronic recording. Permission must be sought from participants to allow recording, and confidentiality of such highly sensitive material must be ensured. We have found it effective to use no identifying family names during interviews; this protects the confidentiality of informants when tapes are being transcribed by assistants.

Because qualitative interviews usually take more time than quantitative interviews, and elicit a great deal of rich data, researchers tend to do a smaller number of interviews. Students often ask, 'How many should I do?' The best response is that you should continue until no new data is emerging.

Data analysis

Once tapes are transcribed, you will find yourself with piles of printouts or data files—and no doubt a huge sense of uncertainty! However, you will have a sense of the key issues from your interviews. This is why qualitative researchers usually prefer to collect and analyse their own data. The research is an emerging process, which you should signpost by writing memos to alert you to significant features of the data. During the analysis phase, these memos form an important part of the coding process.

Your data should be coded around key issues and recurring themes. In this case, key issues might be the significant factors that have led to the violence, coping strategies, sources of help, issues of rurality that aid or constrain help, legal responses, effectiveness of protection orders, and suggested changes in response systems. The qualitative analyst looks for patterns of response around such themes to determine their findings.

Analysis of data from the focus groups should be a process shared and developed by the group. The group might have a series of meetings focusing first on what is happening now and the current responses. Further meetings might develop strategies for change to address the problem.

Reporting findings

The data gathered in a qualitative study are no less important than those gathered through quantitative research. Although this research has looked only at the town itself, it is also important for workers in other areas who may be facing similar issues and it is vital for policy development because it may have identified issues, that must be addressed at policy level. Your research should be widely disseminated through newspapers, journals, conferences or a book chapter.

A final word

In these examples, we have made a clear distinction between qualitative and quantitative methodologies for the purpose of illustrating and highlighting differences. Many researchers now incorporate both qualitative and quantitative aspects into a study in order to obtain a comprehensive understanding of issues. Thus, in this example, the committee might choose some quantitative analysis—analysing trends in violence—and some qualitative analysis—assessing the reality and impact of violence.

Summary

This chapter has identified the steps you should undertake to conduct a piece of research. Although these steps may vary by methodology, they generally include problem definition, literature review and research design stages of sampling, data collection, data analysis and reporting.

The stages in the research process have been illustrated by reference to research aimed at examining violence experienced by women in rural areas. What is important to note is the way qualitative research seeks to discover and explore issues in a different way to quantitative research. While quantitative research seeks to tabulate, quantify and discover cause-and-effect variables, qualitative research seeks to understand a situation from the inside by investigating the lived experience of research subjects. These are important concepts for beginning researchers to understand. Equally important is the fact that research projects may contain both quantitative and qualitative elements. In fact, we have often found that this may produce the most comprehensive results. Furthermore, despite any claims to methodological purity, experienced researchers will tell you that the type of research you choose to conduct is often determined more by pragmatic considerations such as time and resources than by any overriding methodological orientation.

Discussion questions

4.1   What factors might influence your research?
4.2   What are the steps in the research process?
4.3   How does the process of quantitative research differ from qualitative research?
4.4   How do methods of data collection differ in quantitative and qualitative research?
4.5   What means of data analysis would you use in qualitative research?
4.6   How might you analyse quantitative data?
4.7   What administrative arrangements should you make in order to conduct your research successfully?
4.8   What is the purpose of a literature review?
4.9   How and why should you report your research findings?

Exercises

4.1   In your work as a hospital social worker, you have become aware of an increasing number of patients presenting with AIDS-related illnesses. Consider how:
   (a)   a quantitative study could add to our knowledge of the problem
   (b)   a qualitative study might assist us to develop an understanding of the area.
   Outline the steps in your research process.
4.2   Part of your work in a local community centre is to construct a day-care program for the aged. You have become conscious of the difficulties experienced by carers. How might you:
   (a)   develop a quantitative study?
   (b)   develop a qualitative piece of research?
   Outline the steps in your research process.

Further reading

Morris, Teresa 2006, *Social Work Research Methods*, Sage, Thousand Oaks, CA. This book has several chapters detailing the planning and execution stages of a research project.
Smith, Roger 2009, *Doing Social Work Research*, Open University Press, Maidenhead. Chapters 8 and 9 address 'making it happen' and 'putting it all together'.
Yegidis, B.L., Weinbach, W.W. and Myers, L.L. 2012, *Research Methods for Social Workers*, 7th edn, Pearson, Englewood Cliffs, NJ.

PART II

Research methods for social work

5 *Sampling*

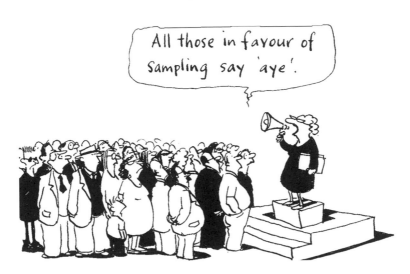

Sampling is about choosing who or what we wish to study in order to answer our research question. Sometimes these units of study are chosen randomly (more typically for quantitative research) and sometimes they are purposively selected (more typically for qualitative research). In any case, the way we choose the units of study will have a major impact on our results, so should be done thoughtfully and with a clear rationale.

Quantitative and qualitative research samples

It is important to note that quantitative researchers use probability sampling while qualitative researchers will more often opt for non-probability sampling. Quantitative researchers require a random or probability sample for the statistical processes they undertake (see Chapters 16 and 17). Qualitative researchers, on the other hand, use non-probability sampling because of the nature of their research, which is largely exploratory. Researcher bias is unavoidable, but the process allows a significant sample to be generated quickly.

Qualitative researchers often seek typical cases. Sometimes, however, they deliberately seek atypical, extreme or deviant cases as a means of shedding light on the typical or for their own intrinsic interest. Often sampling in qualitative research is controlled not by a need for statistical rigour but by the developing theoretical argument, so the sampling paradigm is sometimes referred to as *theoretical sampling*. In other words, the sample is chosen to help the researcher to understand the phenomenon under study and to illuminate the researcher's emerging theory. Because the type of research undertaken by quantitative and qualitative researchers is different, neither probability nor non-probability sampling is superior to the others—nor is one of them necessarily more effective.

Quantitative versus qualitative sampling

Quantitative

- Probability sampling
- Objectivity
- Representative
- Results generalisable
- Statistically rigorous
- Random sampling
- Claims no researcher bias

- All units equal or known chance of selection

Qualitative

- Non-probability sampling
- Subjectivity
- Non-representative
- Results not generalisable
- Not statistically rigorous
- Theoretical sampling
- Researcher is integral to sample selection
- No attempt to give units an equal chance of selection

What is a sample?

Once we have decided on our research question and other aspects of our research design, some thought must be given to the subjects, cases or events we wish to study. In order to be completely accurate, every person (or case or event) in the population under study would need to be surveyed. This is called a *saturation sample* or *census*. In practice, saturation sampling is rarely possible because of the nature of the study question, the size of the population, and time and resource constraints. Instead, we select a *sample* from the total population under study. In quantitative research, this sample is ideally chosen at random. As a result, researchers can claim that results are generalisable because inferences can be drawn from the research about the wider population (that is, the results from the sample are representative of results in the entire population).

For a sample to be representative, it must be chosen in such a way that subjects or cases have beliefs, attitudes or experiences that are similar to those of the population being investigated. Conventional social science wisdom suggests that a random sample drawn from the study population and selected according to sampling theory will reflect the characteristics of the entire population. In this way, the researcher is able to make informed statements about the group under study.

Let us look at an example to allow us to better understand the concept of sampling. Imagine yourself an employee of a government income-support organisation that provides payments for people who are unemployed, ill or unable to work due to disabilities. It also pays pensions to people of retirement age and income supplements to people caring for others full time, or for children with disabilities.

You are interested in examining the attitudes and experiences of clients coming to your agency for the first time. You are concerned that clients may find the experience humiliating and confronting. Your ultimate aim with such a study might be to make this experience easier for clients. To study such an issue affecting a very large group, you must draw a sample. First-time clients will represent at least several thousand people each week. Ideally you would study all first-time clients in every office of the income-support organisation across the country over a specific period of time. Pragmatically, you might choose a sample that is localised (first-time clients in your own office) and time-defined (for a one-week period). Such a sample may allow you to generalise beyond the subjects of the study but with a large degree of caution.

No doubt you have noted that drawing such a sample will have serious limitations. Can you generalise beyond the local area? Do your findings reflect the experiences of clients in branches in other locality areas? Will clients in small communities find the experience more difficult than those in larger, more impersonal offices? By confining your timeframe to one week, are you picking up on seasonal variations in the workforce? Are recent school leavers, for example, a part of your sample?

As you can see from this example, drawing a sample that accurately reflects the study population requires a great deal of thought. Because of pragmatic concerns such as time and resource constraints, you may have to make tradeoffs that reduce the generalisability of your findings. This is not to say that you should not undertake the proposed study. Your findings, and particularly any strategies you develop to improve client service, will be useful to workers in offices across the country.

Let us examine some of the most common types of sampling. First, you should note that sampling can be categorised as either *probability* or *non-probability* sampling.

Probability sampling

Probability sampling refers to sampling in which each unit of the population has an equal (as in the case of simple random sampling) or known chance of being selected for study. The units of the population under study are referred to as the *sampling frame*. The sample is chosen from the sampling frame in an unbiased and rigorous way, allowing a small sample to be used to assess or predict the studied behaviour in the larger population. Probability sampling is favoured by quantitative researchers as it allows a high degree of representativeness from which results can be generalised. The four main types of probability sampling are:

- simple random sampling
- systematic random sampling
- stratified random sampling
- cluster random sampling.

Probability sampling
- Each population unit has an equal, or known, chance of selection.
- There is a high degree of representativeness.
- Allows researchers to generalise results.
- Favoured by quantitative researchers.
- Four main types:
  - simple random sampling
  - systematic random sampling
  - stratified random sampling
  - cluster random sampling.

Simple random sampling

Simple random sampling is the most common form of probability sampling. There are several methods we might choose to select a simple random sample.

Let us use another example to illustrate the process of simple random sampling. Imagine you are working on a government policy research team and you are interested in assessing the effects of a new policy to move previously institutionalised people with psychiatric problems into group homes in the community. Your study is motivated by a number of violent incidents reported by police and causing community concern. Your sampling frame represents the entire population of people who have moved from institutions to group homes in the five years since the policy was adopted. Suppose you find that there are 10 000 people in your sampling frame and you choose to sample 1000 of them. We might first allot a number to each person on the list from 1 to 10 000. Numbers from 1 to 10 000 are then randomly drawn using a variety of methods that might include a computer sorting program or even numbers being placed in a container and selected (without replacement) until 1000 numbers have been drawn. Referring to your list, the numbers you have selected randomly are related to the people in the sampling frame. These 1000 can then be used as subjects for your study.

You are more likely to use a table of random numbers; these are readily available in many research methods textbooks or can be generated by a computer. Begin at a randomly selected point in the table and choose the first number on the table between 1 and 10 000. Work your way up (or down) the column, selecting numbers and relating them to your list of names. In this way, you can generate your sample of 1000.

Table of random numbers		
1986	3067	1309
2254	5321	0532
4763	9854	5643
1589	8623	2875
7415	9792	3261

A simple random sample may be chosen in a number of other ways, including by dates of birth or by initials. Any randomised technique is suitable.

Simple random sampling

- Sampling frame is identified.
- Desired sample number is identified.
- Numbers are assigned to subjects in sampling frame.
- Random numbers are selected in some way.
- Numbers are related to list of subjects.
- Sample is generated.

Systematic random sampling

Systematic random sampling varies from simple random sampling in that the chosen units are not independent of each other. For instance, you might decide to select every tenth person in order to generate your sample.

The size of the interval between chosen units is decided by dividing the total population, or sampling frame, by the desired sample size. Thus, using our previous example of previously institutionalised people (10 000) and our desired sample (1000), we decide the interval (x) in the following way:

$$x = \frac{\text{total sampling frame}}{\text{desired sampling}}$$

The first name on our list is chosen at random from those numbered from 1 to 10. Thereafter, we choose every tenth person. We will generate a sample list of 1000 using this method.

When using this method, we need to be careful that no unintended bias creeps into the sample. For example, by choosing every tenth name, we might be missing residents in smaller communities and in certain types of group housing. (If the initial list is randomly generated, this should not be an issue.) Once your sample is selected, carefully check that you have generated a sample that is not biased on certain variables that may be important to your study.

Systematic random sampling
- Sampling frame is identified.
- Desired sample number is identified.
- Numbers are assigned to each subject in the sampling frame.
- Sampling interval (x) is identified.
- First subject is chosen randomly.
- Every xth subject is chosen.
- Sample is generated.

Stratified random sampling

Stratified random sampling allows us to divide our sampling frame into various strata or groups before selecting our sample. This allows us to ensure that each group is represented proportionately or disproportionately to their numbers in the overall population. For example, we might decide that it is important to assess how the effects of group home living vary by gender. We divide our frame by gender and select a random sample of 500 from each group.

Alternatively, we might decide that age is a critical factor. We thus divide our sampling frame by age and select from each group. If we are to select a proportionate sample, then we choose a sample from the sub-group that reflects their numbers in the total sampling frame. If we choose to sample disproportionately, then we choose equal numbers from each group regardless of their relative proportions. Table 5.1 illustrates the way we might select a stratified random sample by age.

Table 5.1 Selection of a stratified random sample by age

	Number in sampling frame	1/10 proportionate sample	Disproportionate sample
Age 20–29	4 000	400	250 (1/16)
Age 30–39	2 500	250	250 (1/10)
Age 40–49	2 000	200	250 (1/8)
Age 50 +	1 500	150	250 (1/6)
	10 000	1000	1000

Whether you choose a proportionate or disproportionate sample depends on how valuable you feel the information from each group might be and what it is you wish to find out. For example, reported incidents of violence among deinstitutionalised people might be related disproportionately to the older age groups, in which case you might feel a disproportionate sample will be more valuable. To choose a disproportionate sample, the sampling frame is divided into age groups. The sampling fraction is used to decide the interval between chosen subjects. For example, in the 20–29 years age group, every sixteenth person is chosen; in the 30–39 years age group, every tenth, in the 40–49 years age group, every eighth; and in the 50+ age group, every sixth.

A proportionate sample, on the other hand, is selected by choosing every tenth person in each group.

Stratified random sampling

- Sample frame is identified.
- Desired sample is identified.
- Strata or groups are identified.
- Proportionate or disproportionate sample numbers are identified.
- Sampling interval (x) is identified for each strata or group.
- First name in each group is selected randomly.
- Every xth person is chosen from each group.
- Sample is generated.

Cluster random sampling

The final type of random sampling discussed here is cluster random sampling. Cluster random sampling is generally used when there is no sampling frame available—that is, we do not know who is in the group from which we are sampling as there is no readily available list of subjects. We also use this type of sampling when we are limited by resource constraints. Suppose, for example, that we wish to survey homeless street kids. We do not have access to a convenient list of names from which to draw our sample. What we can do is randomly select certain areas or *clusters* that are relevant to our research problem. For example, we might choose to survey kids in youth refuges in both city and country areas. While we cannot hope to survey all homeless youth in all areas, we can choose the areas, or *clusters*, that represent the sample under study. To reduce the possibility of sampling bias, it is a good idea to increase the number of clusters surveyed. In our homeless youth study, we might reduce bias by surveying in inner-city areas and in outer suburbs with high ethnic populations. We might also survey in regional cities and a selection of country areas, making sure we sample coastal as well as inland regions. Once our clusters or areas are identified, we then randomly choose our desired sample from the current population in the identified youth refuges.

Cluster random sampling allows us to systematically sample a population that is not readily identifiable. While it allows us to work within budgetary limits and other constraints, it does increase the possibility of sampling error. The only way to minimise this problem is to increase the number of clusters surveyed.

Cluster random sampling

- Sampling frame is unknown.
- Desired sample is identified.
- Clusters are identified.
- Random sample is drawn from clusters.
- Sample is generated.

Non-probability sampling

The second major category of sampling is non-probability sampling. Non-probability sampling generally is used in exploratory research and by qualitative researchers. It does not make any claims to be representative of the population under study, and therefore the generalisability of results is limited. This, however, is not the point of the research.

Non-probability sampling is very useful and justifiable when the researcher is seeking information in a new area and targets subjects or cases who typify the issue to be studied. Suppose, for example, you are working in a respite unit and wish to examine the pressures facing carers of AIDS patients. Because AIDS is a relatively new disease by global standards, little may be known about the unique issues facing carers. To explore this new area of investigation, you select a small sample (for example, ten) of carers known to you through your position in the respite unit. You will note that these ten cases will not be representative of all carers of AIDS patients because of the small sample number and because they are limited by locality. However, this sample will give insights into a previously unexplored area and will provide a qualitative researcher with a rich source of data.

The four most common types of non-probability sampling are:

- accidental (sometimes called convenience or availability) sampling
- quota sampling
- purposive sampling
- snowball sampling.

Non-probability sampling

- Each population unit does not have an equal chance of selection.
- There is no claim to be representative.
- Does not necessarily allow the researcher to generalise results.
- Favoured by qualitative researchers.
- Four main types:
  - accidental sampling
  - quota sampling
  - purposive sampling
  - snowball sampling.

Accidental sampling

As the name implies, accidental sampling is a sample you chance upon by accident. The sample is convenient or available to you for some reason. The most common form of accidental sampling is standing in a public place such as a supermarket or railway station for a certain period of time and interviewing people who walk by. For workers in the welfare industry, an accidental sample might be drawn from a worker's caseload or from clients coming to the agency. Suppose you are working in a women's refuge and wish to understand more about the difficulties women have seeking court protection orders. You might choose a sample from your case records or, alternatively, you might sample all new residents over a two-week period. In either case, your sample is not representative of the entire population of women seeking protection orders; however, it will give you valuable insights into the legal and court process and allow you to explore the problems facing women in this situation.

Accidental sampling

- Sample is drawn from available or convenient group.
- Sample reflects the problem being investigated.
- Number of subjects is determined by access and availability.
- Sample is generated.

Quota sampling

Quota sampling allows us to set quotas for sub-groups of our sample. Suppose, for instance, that we believe from our experience in the women's refuge that women with ethnic backgrounds find it more difficult to obtain protection orders because they are reluctant to approach the court system. We might then choose to study women from a non-English-speaking background as well as English-speaking women. We might also decide that it is important to survey women with children aged under five as well as those with no children or older children. We can draw up a matrix that will allow us to categorise women in the study.

Children under 5	Non-English-speaking background	English-speaking background
Yes	A	B
No	C	D

We must now decide how many women in each category will be surveyed. If we decide that all categories are important, we may seek equal numbers of subjects for each category. For example, should we seek a sample of 20, our matrix would look like this:

Children under 5	Non-English-speaking background	English-speaking background
Yes	5	5
No	5	5

Quota sampling allows us to target certain characteristics that are important to our research problem. Because it is a type of non-probability sampling technique, it does not claim to be representative of the population being studied. While it does allow us to make observations about particular sub-groups of the population, these results cannot be generalised with any degree of certainty.

Quota sampling
- Significant categories are determined.
- Quota is determined for each category.
- Quota is selected.
- Sample is selected for each category.
- Sample is generated.

Purposive sampling

This sampling technique allows us to select the sample for our study for a *purpose*. We may have prior knowledge that indicates a particular group is important to our study, or we select those subjects who we feel are 'typical' examples of the issue we wish to study. In our study of women seeking protection orders, we might decide that women from rural areas or out-lying metropolitan areas appear to have more serious problems and so we choose a sample from these clients in order to determine why the system appears to be letting them down. Alternatively, we might choose a sample of experienced women who work in refuges in these areas to allow us a different perspective to aid our understanding of the issues involved.

Purposive sampling
- Sample is chosen for a particular purpose.
- Sample gives insights into a particular issue related to the study area.
- Number is determined by the research topic and availability.
- Sample is generated.

Snowball sampling

Snowball sampling is used when we have no knowledge of the sampling frame and limited access to subjects who may meet the criteria for our research. Suppose we do not have access to women seeking protection orders as we do not have access to a refuge. However, we do know a woman who has taken out an order. We might approach her for an interview and ask her to nominate other women she might know in the same circumstances. We contact these women for interviews and they nominate further women. We continue collecting our sample in this way until we feel we have reached the stage where our sample is *saturated*. In other words, no new information is emerging from our research, so we determine our sample is complete.

Snowball sampling
- Contact a 'typical' case.
- Ask this person to recommend further cases.
- Continue until the sample is complete and saturated.

How big should my sample be?

One of the most frequently asked questions concerns sample size. Students and beginning researchers often beg for a magic sample size number. However, research is not as simple as that. Sample size depends on what it is we wish to know, how certain we want to be about our findings, the resources we have available, the research design and its purpose, the type of statistical analysis required and the degree of representativeness we consider desirable (Yegidis, Weinbach and Myers 2012). Naturally, to be entirely accurate we would need to survey the entire sampling frame. As this is rarely possible, you should note that, in general, the larger the sample is, the more accurate your findings will be, and the richer your data will be (Dudley 2011). Of course, you should also note that a small representative sample may be more accurate than a large unrepresentative one. It depends on the accuracy of the sampling technique. In general, you should note that, for small populations, you should choose proportionately more for your sample than for samples drawn from larger populations.

With quantitative research, sample size is related to the type of statistical analysis you may wish to undertake. A minimum size for adequate statistical analysis would be 30, although many texts suggest your sample should be at least 100 or 120. Dudley (2011) makes the important point that the larger the sample, the more likely it is to represent the population, but that we should aim for a sample with a margin of error of 5 per cent.

It is important that you understand the concept of *sampling error* in relation to sampling in quantitative research. We will explain this concept in detail in Chapter 17, once we have explained some basic statistical concepts. For now, it is important to know that sampling error is an estimate of the amount of error you could make if you used just one sample of a certain size from a population to estimate the results for the whole population. In Chapter 17 we show you that standard error or sampling error is inversely proportional to the size of your sample—hence you will have more confidence that your sample statistics will be closer to those of the population if you use a larger sample. The general principle is to take the largest representative sample you can.

Experienced statisticians have developed ways of estimating sample sizes that will give you a fairly accurate result based on the size of the population. One such table is reproduced here (Table 5.2) for your consideration. Note that the ideal sample size varies according to the confidence level required.

Confidence level (or confidence interval) refers to the level of confidence we have that the results accurately reflect the views of the population. A 95 per cent confidence level (or 5 per cent margin of error) means that our results could occur by chance only five times in 100 trials. You should aim to have a 95 per cent confidence level with a 5 per cent margin of error, meaning that the results will be out by 5 per cent only five times in 100 (Dudley 2011).We will discuss confidence intervals in more detail in Chapters 16 and 17.

Using Table 5.2, you can see that, should you wish to sample a population group of 100 with a 95 per cent confidence level and a 5 per cent margin of error, you would need to draw 79 of the members of that group into your research sample. If the population is 1 million, your sample size should be 384.

Social work students frequently do qualitative research where sample size is not such a big issue and relates more to convenience and availability. With qualitative research, you tend to continue to sample until no new information is emerging. Once you get to the point where you feel you've heard it all before, you know your sample size is complete.

Size of sample is also guided by the diversity of the population you are studying. If your target group is heterogeneous, you will need a larger sample size than if it were homogeneous. For example, if the target group is white, Anglo-Saxon and middle class you will achieve a high level of accuracy with a small sample. If the target group includes several ethnic groups and diverse income levels, you will need a much larger sample.

Table 5.2 Appropriate sizes of simple random samples for specific permissible errors expressed as absolute proportions when the confidence level is 95 per cent

	Sample size for permissible error				
Population size	0.05	0.04	0.03	0.02	0.01
100	79	86	91	96	99
200	132	150	168	185	196
300	168	200	234	267	291
400	196	240	291	343	384
500	217	273	340	414	475
600	234	300	384	480	565
700	248	323	423	542	652
800	260	343	457	600	738
900	269	360	488	655	823
1000	278	375	516	706	906
2000	322	462	696	1091	1655
3000	341	500	787	1334	2286
4000	350	522	842	1500	2824
5000	357	536	879	1622	3288
6000	361	546	906	1715	3693
7000	364	553	926	1788	4049
8000	367	556	942	1847	4364
9000	368	563	954	1895	4646
10 000	370	566	964	1936	4899
15 000	375	577	996	2070	5855
20 000	377	583	1013	2144	6488
25 000	378	586	1023	2191	6938
30 000	379	588	1030	2223	7275
40 000	381	591	1039	2265	7745
50 000	381	593	1045	2291	8056
75 000	382	595	1052	2327	8514
100 000	383	597	1056	2345	8762
500 000	384	600	1065	2390	9423
1 000 000	384	600	1066	2395	9513
2 000 000	384	600	1067	2398	9558

Note: This table was calculated for binomial distributions.

Source: Royse (2009).

Summary

When we conduct a piece of research, we are interested in a particular target group or population. It is rarely possible to survey the entire population so, using sampling techniques, we select a sample of this target group. This chapter has examined the types of sampling techniques we can use to generate an adequate sample. We have seen how a sample can be developed using either probability or non-probability techniques. Probability sampling is a more precise or non-biased method that allows a representative sample to be selected and results to be generalised. In order to use probability sampling, we should have access to the entire target group—this is called the sampling frame. Four types of probability sampling have been discussed in this chapter. They are simple random sampling, systematic random sampling, stratified random sampling and cluster random sampling.

Non-probability sampling, on the other hand, is less precise and involves researcher bias. It allows the researcher to carefully select the sample for a particular—usually theoretical—purpose. Non-probability sampling techniques are used for exploratory, qualitative and often feminist research. They include accidental sampling, purposive sampling, quota sampling and snowball sampling.

Decisions on sample size—which are particularly critical in quantitative sampling—are governed by the accuracy we desire and the degree of homogeneity of the group. In general, the larger the sample, the more confident we can feel about the generalisability of our findings. However, if the group is homogeneous we can feel confident about limiting sample size.

Non-probability sample sizes are not as critical as sample sizes are for probability sampling, as sample size is governed by the emerging data such that a researcher should continue sampling until no new data is emerging.

Discussion questions

5.1 Why can't I make it easy on myself and do a saturation sample?
5.2 What is the difference between probability and non-probability sampling?
5.3 Outline the four main types of probability sampling and provide an example of when each would be an appropriate choice.
5.4 Outline the four main types of non-probability sampling and provide an example of when each would be the most appropriate choice.
5.5 What issues affect the size of the sample you should take?

Exercises

5.1 Go to the library or your library website and find three social work research articles. List the article and the sampling technique used for each. Note whether you feel the sample is adequate for the research problem discussed.

5.2 Go to the library/library website, or a government department or their website. Locate a government report based on research that lists policy recommendations. Assess whether the report is based on an appropriate sample and whether the recommendations are well grounded in the research.

5.3 How would you develop a sample to study the employment status of graduates of your social work course?

5.4 How would you develop a sample to study the opinions of people about euthanasia?

Further reading

You will find that most research textbooks have a detailed section on sampling techniques. Select those that support your methodological position and review the discussion on sampling. There are many excellent discussions of sampling. We suggest the following:

Dudley, James 2011, *Research Methods for Social Work: Being Producers and Consumers of Research (updated edition)*, 2nd edn, Pearson, Boston, MA.
Royse, David 2009, *Research Methods in Social Work*, 5th edn, Thomson, Belmont, CA.

6 Systematic reviews

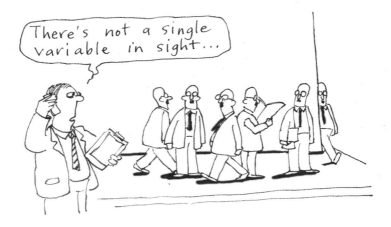

Systematic reviews are a relatively new form of social science research. Beginning in the late 1980s in the health sciences as a response to the explosion in readily available published research and the pressure for evidence-based policy and practice, systematic reviews are different from traditional or narrative literature reviews and have become a research methodology in their own right.

We have already discussed that reviewing the literature is an integral step in the research process (see Chapter 4)—all researchers need to be able to demonstrate that they know the scope of the research already in their field of study, the key debates in that literature and the major gaps that exist. Researchers use the literature review to argue for the value of the approach they have taken in a particular study, and to locate their research in the context of existing debates, definitions, gaps and approaches.

The problem is that with so much research now instantly available on the internet, with its search engines such as Google and library databases, it becomes almost impossible to discuss all the available literature in a given topic area. It also becomes very tempting for researchers to 'cherry pick' those research papers that support their chosen methodology, or make their approach look good. With the avalanche of published research online, how do you know that the literature review you are reading or writing is balanced, and at least offers a reasonable summary of the range of existing research findings and debates about this topic?

Systematic reviews offer a way for researchers to be more transparent about how they undertake literature reviews. Using the principles of systematic reviews, researchers create a path that others can follow, showing where and how they located the literature on which their research is based, and revealing the basis for their decisions about which research was included and which excluded.

Why do a systematic review?

For practitioners and consumers of research who face increasing pressure to demonstrate that their practice is evidence based, the problem becomes how to sift through all the evidence that is available about a particular aspect of practice. How do you know what all the evidence actually says about a practice or policy? How do you choose between competing or opposing findings? How do you keep up with all the evidence about your area of practice or policy? Seeking answers to these questions is just one of the reasons why people undertake systematic reviews.

Initially, systematic reviews were developed to overcome issues of bias in how literature reviews were presented (the 'cherry-picking' identified above). The aim of systematic reviews in the scientific tradition is to give a summary of *all* the research evidence using specific criteria in a transparent and rigorous way. This purpose is also about enhancing the reliability and validity of the findings of existing research. Traditionally, the purpose of systematic reviews was to answer the questions 'What works?' and 'What works in which circumstances?' (Hannes and Claes 2007)

Systematic reviews are used to assess the quality of existing research. They can identify existing gaps in the literature, help to avoid duplication and identify future research questions. They also have a 'translation function', synthesising large amounts of complex literature about specific questions. Systematic reviews are used to answer research questions, especially when there is conflicting evidence, uncertainty and debate. They can develop new knowledge when research methods are applied to the findings once all the available evidence has been accumulated (Hemingway and Brereton 2009; Victor 2008).

What are systematic reviews?

Systematic reviews are a type of secondary data analysis of existing research. They synthesise large amounts of existing literature using transparent methods that can be replicated. Although systematic reviews began in medicine and the health sciences, there is now a range of approaches that offer important research possibilities in the social sciences. Here are some examples of systematic review topics that are relevant to social work and/or published in social work journals. This small sample illustrates the range of research areas in which systematic reviews are used.

Examples of systematic reviews

- Exploring first-person accounts of the lived experience of heart failure and social work roles (Hopp, Thornton and Martin 2010)
- Recognising neglect in childhood and examining early response to neglect (Daniel, Taylor and Scott 2010)
- Kinship care for the safety, permanency, and well-being of children removed from the home for maltreatment (Winokur, Holtan and Valentine 2009)
- Domestic violence against women—prevalence studies (Alhabib, Nur and Jones 2010)
- Ethical considerations in the field of assistive technology in the care of community-dwelling older people with dementia (Zwijsen, Niemeijer and Hertogh 2011)
- Resilience amongst Latino immigrant families (Cardoso and Thompson 2010)

Types of systematic review

Victor (2008) identifies three main approaches to systematic reviews. She emphasises that, despite their differences, all these approaches share some common features:

- They try to be as comprehensive as possible.
- The quality of the papers to be included is assessed in some way.
- Findings/data synthesis is systematic.
- Processes are rigorous and transparent (can be replicated).
- They usually take considerable time and resources.

The three types of systematic review are:

*   traditional
*   extended (also called mixed methods)
*   integrated (also known as critical interpretive synthesis).

Traditional systematic reviews

The traditional systematic review was the first approach developed. It originated in medicine and the clinical sciences, and uses scientific methodology to answer questions about which medical treatment is most effective or to choose between conflicting claims (it is primarily outcome-focused). Traditional systematic reviews follow a rigorous set of steps with a hierarchy of evidence. In this type of review, the best or 'gold standard' of evidence is considered to be the randomised control trial (RCT), along with other systematic reviews that follow the scientific method. The 'data' presented in traditional systemic reviews are summaries of the articles selected for inclusion, which are tabulated and presented in order of their quality with traditional systematic reviews and RCTs at the top.

Examples include papers published in the Cochrane Library and Campbell Collaboration tradition. Typically, a traditional systematic review takes a great deal of time and resources: some estimates are that it takes two researchers around two years part time or nine months each full time to conduct a full traditional systematic review. To reduce the time and resources spent on systematic reviewing, a quicker type of traditional review, termed a rapid or brief review—which takes around two to six months to complete—is becoming popular in the health sciences (Hemingway and Brereton 2009). Abrami et al. (2010) provide clear guidelines for how to conduct quality brief reviews, concluding with the warning: 'Brief is not another word for careless. Brief reviews must use techniques that ensure replicability and objectivity within the constraints of time and money.' (2010, p. 384).

In the social sciences, which use very few randomised control trials, traditional systematic reviews and rapid or brief reviews are mostly used to assess impact of policy. Often the conclusions are as much about problems in the methodology of published studies and the paucity of existing research as they are about giving guidance as to 'what works'.

Example 6.1: Systematic review into kinship care

This traditional systematic review published in the Cochrane Library aimed to evaluate the effect of kinship care on the safety, permanency and well-being of children removed from the home due to maltreatment. Databases, relevant social work journals and reference lists of published literature reviews were searched and authors contacted to locate other research. Outcomes were analysed from randomised and quasi-experimental studies of children who had been removed from home and placed in kinship care, compared with children placed in non-kinship foster care.

Reviewers independently read titles and abstracts and selected appropriate studies from fifteen online databases, finding 4791 articles that matched the search terms. Of these, 263 met the initial criterion of being an empirical study on kinship care. Eligibility based on methodological quality was then assessed and only those studies that met the eligibility criteria were included. Finally, 62 quasi-experimental studies were included. Results from these studies were meta-analysed (using a computer data-analysis system called REVMAN).

Findings from these studies show that children in kinship care experience better behavioural development, mental health functioning and placement stability than do children in non-kinship foster care. While there was no difference in reunification rates for either type of care, children in non-kinship care were more likely to be adopted and more likely to use mental health services.

The authors conclude that kinship care is a viable out-of-home placement option, but urge caution due to the 'pronounced methodological and design weaknesses of the included studies and particularly the absence of conclusive evidence of the comparability of groups' (Winokur, Holtan and Valentine 2009, p. 50). Implications for practice and research are discussed in some detail.

Source: Winokur, Holtan and Valentine (2009).

Mixed methods or extended reviews

This approach adapts the traditional systematic review for social sciences to include a wide range of types of research in areas where randomised control trials are not used. It includes qualitative research more easily than the traditional approach, which tends to put qualitative findings at the bottom of the evidence hierarchy. However, the way in which qualitative studies are included/excluded is hotly debated—for example, see Norton's (2008) review of the major text in mixed methods design by Petticrew and Roberts (2005).

An extended or mixed methods approach includes research about processes and people's perceptions/experiences, whereas the traditional method is concerned with outcomes. It is more flexible than traditional reviews and includes a wide range of types of social research. Criticisms of this approach include that it can be less transparent and lose the clear focus of traditional approaches.

Example 6.2: Rigor in qualitative social work research

This extended review uses quantitative research methods to examine how qualitative social work researchers enhance the rigour of their work. The authors developed a template of nineteen strategies that qualitative researchers use to enhance rigour (or credibility), including strategies such as various kinds of triangulation, providing a rationale for sampling, member checking of results, specifying a theoretical framework and so on. They then took a random sample of 100 qualitative research articles from 27 social work journals, and mapped the strategies found in those articles against the template of nineteen strategies they had developed.

The results were analysed using the statistical package SPSS. As part of the review, the authors were careful to spell out both their methodology and their criteria for including or excluding articles. They also explained their own reliability processes (reviewing each other's work until they agreed on how to assess the article), and then having their results peer-reviewed by other researchers.

Some of the findings included that the most popular way of enhancing a qualitative social work study's rigour is to provide a rationale for the sample chosen (67 per cent of studies), with the next most popular strategy being analyst triangulation (having multiple perspectives or sets of 'eyes' interpret the results). Specification of research problems or limitations came next, followed by careful discussion of analysis procedures so that studies could be replicated. The fifth most popular strategy was having a theoretical or conceptual framework (51 per cent of studies). The authors noted that the average number of strategies used to enhance rigour in a qualitative social work study increased between the years 2003 and 2008 (from 1.4 strategies on average in 2003 to 2.4 strategies in 2007 and 2008). They were surprised that in the vast majority of articles (86 per cent), authors did not provide any information about themselves (a strategy termed reflexivity), despite the acknowledged subjectivity of qualitative research methods. They were also surprised that only 51 per cent of studies specified a theoretical or conceptual framework.

The authors conclude with recommendations for strengthening 'methodological awareness' in social work qualitative research.

Source: Barusch, Gringeri and George (2011).

Integrative approach

Also termed 'critical interpretive synthesis' by some of its champions, this type of systematic review is concerned with theory-building. It is different from the other approaches in that it views knowledge as being created in an integrative, rather than additive, way and uses qualitative methodology, building categories and themes from the research evidence to create theories. It rejects a staged approach to reviewing, seeing the various tasks of question formulation, searching, data selection, extraction, critique and synthesis as being 'iterative, dynamic and recursive rather than as fixed procedures to be accomplished in a pre-defined sequence' (Annandale et al. 2007). However, unlike other research in these qualitative traditions, this type of systematic review can include *all* types of research evidence: quantitative, qualitative and theoretical, not just qualitative papers.

This approach uses purposive samples of evidence, and can examine any question concerned with theory-building. The main drawback to this type of systematic review, according to Victor (2008), is that it does not have to be comprehensive and might be less transparent, making it harder for others to judge the validity of the findings.

Example 6.3: Gender and access to health care in the United Kingdom—a critical interpretive synthesis of the literature

This systematic review aims to develop a way of understanding gender issues in health care in the United Kingdom, following legislation making 'gender equality duty' mandatory. This policy came from a

United Nations directive to achieve gender equality, and to take account of women's and men's concerns and experiences in all policy areas.

Using the 'critical interpretive synthesis' approach outlined above, the authors synthesised a diverse range of research to develop an approach to gender and access to health care that they call 'critical gender awareness', based on an idea they developed and termed 'candidacy'.

By defining 'access' broadly, they included a wide range of types of research, including theoretical papers, in their review. Their sampling process—unlike the other approaches—followed a qualitative methodology, starting with purposive sampling and then using theoretical sampling to test, refine and 'saturate' the theoretical categories they were developing. Thus the sampling and theory-generation evolved in response to each other, in a cyclic process rather than as a linear, staged set of steps.

Papers were included or excluded in the review not just on the basis of whether they met criteria such as having clear aims and objectives, or whether the methodology was clearly specified and appropriate for the aims, but also according to whether a paper added an interesting idea or approach. This integrative approach focuses on being critical of assumptions—of how access was understood by the researchers—so that critical analysis forms part of the data analysis itself, and is not just the basis for the exclusion/inclusion of papers.

The aim of the review was to integrate or synthesise the evidence from research and theoretical papers into a 'coherent theoretical framework'. The authors used typical qualitative data analysis and software to do this. They emphasise that because they used these methods, which involved creative and interpretive processes, their methods are not as transparent and replicable as other systematic reviews. However, they did use various checks and balances—mostly discussing their categories and analysis with other members of their multi-disciplinary team (analyst triangulation) to ensure rigour.

Results of this review included rejecting the usual notion of 'service utilisation' as a way of measuring equality of access. The authors concluded that it is not possible to know whether high or low rates of utilising health services is a good or bad thing, or exactly what it means in terms of equality or inequality for men and women. Instead, they propose a construct they call 'candidacy', which is more dynamic and is about how men and women negotiate eligibility and access to services. Candidacy involves understanding help-seeking as a gendered activity, 'which is actively negotiated within the context of highly complex everyday lives' (Annandale et al. 2007, p. 473).

The authors conclude that so far research into gender and health care has been piecemeal, and that on the whole health services have been 'gender-blind' or unaware of or insensitive to the gendered assumptions that are built into the delivery of health care. Although they identify many challenges in attempting 'gender equality' for health services in the United Kingdom, they propose that an important first step is for service providers and policy-makers to develop 'critical gender awareness'. This is a critical and evolving process of understanding and negotiating between the care provider and the subject (not object) of that care. Annandale et al. (2007) emphasise that critical gender awareness is not a top-down strategy or set of clear rules that is put in place and followed to create gender equality; instead, they argue that developing a culture of critical gender awareness can help to address the problems of routinisation and over-simplification that can plague attempts to create gender equality.

Source: Annandale et al. (2007).

Types of systematic review

Traditional reviews

Use scientific method to answer questions about outcomes and effectiveness. Consider randomised control trials and other traditional systemative reviews to be the 'gold standard' at the top of an evidence hierarchy. Problematic for social work research, as so few randomised control trials are possible or necessary.

Mixed methods or extended reviews

Use a wide range of research evidence, including qualitative research. Address questions about process and people's experiences rather than outcomes. Drawbacks include that they can be less transparent than traditional approaches.

Integrative or 'critical interpretive synthesis' reviews

Focus on theory-building and use qualitative methodology. Can include all types of research evidence. Do not have to be comprehensive, and might be less transparent than the other two approaches.

Steps in undertaking a systematic review

The following steps involved in undertaking a systematic review draw on the work of Hemingway and Brereton (2009) and Victor (2008).

1   Define the question/s, scope and protocols for the review

The first step in any systematic review is to define the aims, questions and scope of the study. This includes deciding on which stakeholders (policy-makers, practitioners or service users) you might involve in the process. You also need to decide what types of evidence are best able to address the question you want to answer: qualitative, quantitative, theoretical or some mix of these. Part of this early planning is thinking about where you might find this evidence: which databases, individuals or organisations.

Once you have decided on the questions and type of evidence that will answer the question, it is important to write a protocol specifying the basis on which you will include or exclude studies. This is one of the features of systematic reviews that distinguishes them from narrative reviews. Having a detailed protocol ensures rigour, transparency and that the review is systematic. It allows a reader to assess whether bias exists in the kinds of evidence that are included and excluded, and to judge the appropriateness of the evidence that has been selected. Documented inclusion and exclusion criteria are an important part of the methodology section of all systematic review reports.

2   Search the literature

Systematic reviews document their search strategy for finding relevant articles to include. As you have read, no matter what type of systematic review is undertaken, it is important to be as comprehensive in your searching as possible. This means that not only databases are searched, but also 'grey literature' in your area (literature that is not formally published, such as government reports, technical papers, theses, conference papers), hand searches of relevant journals as well as reference lists of full-text papers. Direct contact with researchers, specialists or organisations in your chosen area may also be useful.

Once you have identified the possible evidence and screened it against your inclusion and exclusion criteria, you are ready for the next step.

3   Assess the quality of the included studies

When your list of studies to be included has been decided, each is obtained in full-text format and its quality is assessed. This step allows the researcher to make claims about the strength of the conclusions from the review.

The quality of the research can be assessed in various ways, depending on the type of the research. Assessing the quality of the evidence—particularly for qualitative research—has been the focus of hot debate by systematic reviewers.

In traditional systematic reviews, quality is assessed on the basis of methodology. As noted, there is a hierarchy of evidence, with RCTs and scientific systematic reviews at the top in the 'gold standard' position. Attempts to assess the quality of qualitative studies have varied—the example in the mixed methods research section illustrates one attempt using rigour as the measure of quality for qualitative social work research.

However you choose to assess the quality of the studies you include, this is an important step that must be explained fully and should include the quality of the processes of the systematic review itself (for example, the processes explained in the example of the integrative review). Most systematic reviews have their quality assessed by two reviewers, who cross-check their individual assessments.

4 Synthesise the results

Relevant data from the included studies is usually presented in table form, including sample size, data analysis and findings. The information is then synthesised to produce findings and conclusions, taking into account the quality assessment conducted in the previous step (the results of which may be included in the results table or a separate table).

The data from the included studies may be entered into various databases for data analysis by computer programs (known as meta-synthesis for qualitative data and meta-analysis for homogeneous quantitative data). More commonly, however—at least in social sciences research by students—tables of included studies are presented, with structured narratives linked to the tables synthesising the data, explaining how the conclusions are drawn.

Analysis of findings also depends on the research methodology used for the review. For example, the hierarchy of evidence strongly influences conclusions drawn about reviews of quantitative research (that is, the more RCT and/or systematic review evidence, the stronger the conclusion). On the other hand, thematic analysis of themes emerging from the included studies, linking findings to theoretical models, might be undertaken in integrative reviews, as shown in the example above.

5 Report the findings

Systematic reviews usually are undertaken to resolve an issue, or to make a choice about how to act. This means it is important that they are reported clearly, in plain English and with multiple audiences in mind. Victor (2008) notes that while it is important to include summaries of key findings that are accessible to a range of readers, it is also important to include the technical information later in the report that will enable other researchers to judge the quality of the review itself.

What to include in a report of a systematic review

- Abstract
- Introduction, aims, importance of the review
- Methodological protocol:
  - inclusion and exclusion criteria, search strategy including which databases and other sources of evidence were searched, which search terms were used
  - how quality of included articles was assessed, and what measures were taken to ensure quality of the review process itself
- Commentary on the nature of the evidence found and its quality
- Detailed findings (often in table form), conclusions and recommendations

---

Writing abstracts for systematic review reports

Traditional systematic reviews such as those published in the Cochrane Library follow a structure for writing abstracts that provides a useful template for all research abstracts. This structure includes:

- background
- objectives
- search strategy
- selection criteria
- data collection, analysis
- main results
- conclusion.

Steps in undertaking systematic reviews

1 **Define the questions**, scope and protocols for your review. Decide on research questions, what type of review you will undertake, and the 'rules' by which you will include or exclude studies.

2 **Search the literature.** Include a wide range of literature, not just database searches. Screen your findings against your inclusion and exclusion criteria.

3 **Assess the quality of the included studies.** Assess the quality of the articles and report how you did this.

4 **Synthesise the results.** The spectrum of data analysis for systematic reviews goes from simply recording summaries of the research included in order of the highest quality (according to the process used in step 3) and then drawing conclusions from that, through to computer programs using quantitative and qualitative methods to analyse the results.

5 **Report the findings.** Use the structure summarised in step 4 above.

Issues for systematic reviews and qualitative research

As a growing research area, systematic reviews offer plenty of opportunities for critical discussion. Even within the quantitative domain, questions are being asked as to how applicable findings from RCTs are in the 'real world', where medical practitioners and resources are scarce. As a senior professor of surgery and chair of various quality committees remarked recently: 'There is little evidence that the outcomes from so called "gold standard" RCT studies apply in contexts that are not as well resourced as the Mayo-type clinics from which they originated.' (Maddern 2011, n.p.)

In a related vein, Pearson and Coomber (2010) argue that traditional systematic review methods do not produce adequate guidance for policymakers in the area of substance abuse because there is too much emphasis on internal research validity, which produces a very narrow evidence base with too much focus on short-term interventions with individuals. These authors argue that systematic reviewers should be educated to pay greater attention to external validity and the wider determinants of health in order to produce a broader evidence base from which to make policy decisions. They also argue for the kind of qualitative methodology described in the example of integrative reviews, as a way of improving systematic reviews. In a related argument, Boaz and Pawson (2005) compare five systematic reviews of mentoring, each of which concludes with quite different policy recommendations. Indeed, recent articles propose a methodology of 'systematic reviews of systematic reviews' (see Smith et al. 2011) to overcome such problems.

Other issues arise when multi-disciplinary systematic reviews are undertaken. Curran et al. (2007) explore several of these issues, which range from practical problems relating to database compatibility and computer processing power to inconsistent definitions of social phenomena across disciplines, and different uses of key concepts and search terms.

One of the most hotly contested topics in systematic reviewing is in the field of mixed methods or extended reviews, and whether and how findings from qualitative and quantitative studies can be incorporated into a single review. Norton (2008), in reviewing the chief textbook for extended reviews by Petticrew and Roberts (2005), suggests that the type of knowledge used should inform the methodology of studies selected and that it is counter-productive to try to measure qualitative studies by quantitative benchmarks, as the qualitative studies always end up being assessed as inferior.

Instead of becoming trapped in assumptions about a hierarchy of knowledge that privileges scientific method, Norton (2008) proposes six basic principles which, if followed, will enable systematic reviews to retain their distinctive features—that is, transparency and focus—as against narrative reviews and which will also, he hopes, mean that systematic review is a useful research methodology for qualitative social work researchers. The six principles of systematic reviews he proposes make a good summary for all systematic reviewers (see box).

Six principles for undertaking systematic reviews

- Refined research question
- Transparent methodology
- Clearly defined inclusion criteria based on research question
- Clearly defined criteria setting out what is and is not acceptable (quality criteria) and what is 'fit for purpose'
- Clear procedure for analysis
- Specifying relevant databases, individuals and organisations to be searched/contacted for evidence

Source: Norton (2008, p. 385).

Hemingway and Brereton (2009) warn that good systematic reviews are complex exercises requiring high levels of skill. We recommend that beginning researchers join a team of experienced systematic reviewers for their first experiences of undertaking a systematic review. There are several online checklists for systematic reviews that offer useful guidelines.

Summary

Systematic reviews are a relatively new form of research that is designed to help social workers and human service workers to make sense of the vast array of existing research, to judge the quality of research evidence available, and in some cases to create new knowledge from existing research resources.

The hallmark of a systematic review, as opposed to the more common narrative review, is that it is comprehensive and explicit about the search strategy used so that others can replicate it or make judgements about its quality.

Originating within the medical and scientific fields (traditional systematic reviews), systematic reviews have been adapted for social sciences to include qualitative methodology (the extended and integrative types of systematic reviews). Traditional approaches to systematic reviews, which privilege other systematic reviews and randomised control trials, are undertaken in social work research areas. Choosing which approach to take depends on the type of research question the review addresses.

Six steps need to be followed to complete a systematic review:

1 Define the question/s, scope and search protocols.
2 Search the literature according to your protocol.
3 Assess the quality of the studies you have included.
4 Synthesise the results of the search.
5 Report the findings, including in your report:
    (a) structured abstract
    (b) introduction, aims, significance of review
    (c) methodological protocol, including inclusion and exclusion criteria, search strategy (keywords, databases and other sources searched), how quality of articles was assessed and how quality of review process was ensured
    (d) commentary on the nature of the studies included and their quality
    (e) detailed findings (often in table form), conclusions and recommendations.

Considerable debate and controversy surround systematic reviews, including which approach is most useful, and the value of their contribution to policy and practice. At a minimum, the advent of systematic reviews as a research method challenges all researchers to become more accountable and transparent in how they undertake literature reviews.

Discussion questions

6.1   How is a systematic review different from the 'usual' literature review conducted as part of a social research project?
6.2   What distinguishes a traditional systematic review from an extended or mixed methods review and an integrative review?
6.3   What are the steps involved in undertaking a systematic review?
6.4   What are the key elements to include in a systematic review report?
6.5   Outline the main subsections of an abstract for a systematic report.

Exercises

What type of systematic review would you undertake to explore the following questions? What databases, grey literature sources would you search and what key stakeholders would you consult?

6.1   What is the most effective form of early intervention for families whose children are at risk of abuse?
6.2   How should our organisation evaluate its disaster-relief efforts?
6.3   What in-home supports are most useful for people caring for loved ones at the end of life?
6.4   How can our organisation best support its workers?

Further reading

Overview of systematic reviews
Victor, L. 2008, 'Systematic reviewing', *Social Research Update*, vol. 54, pp. 1–4.

Traditional reviews
The Cochrane Library: http://onlinelibrary.wiley.com/o/cochrane/cochrane_search_fs.html?newSearch=true.

Extended reviews
Norton, M. 2008, 'Systematic reviews: Can qualitative social work research live up to the Zeitgeist?' *Qualitative Social Work*, vol. 7, no. 3, pp. 381–6.
Petticrew, M. and Roberts, H. 2005, *Systematic Reviews in the Social Sciences: A Practical Guide*, Blackwell, Oxford.

Integrative reviews

Annandale, E., Harvey, J., Cavers, D. and Dixon-Woods, M. 2007, 'Gender and access to health-care in the UK: A critical interpretive synthesis of the literature', *Evidence & Policy: A Journal of Research, Debate & Practice*, vol. 3, no. 4, pp. 463–86.

Dixon-Woods, M., Cavers, D., Agarwal, S., Annandale, E., Arthur, A., Harvey, J. and Sutton, A.J. 2006, 'Conducting a critical interpretive synthesis of the literature on access to healthcare by vulnerable groups', *BMC Medical Research Methodology*, vol. 6, p. 35.

7 Surveys and interviews

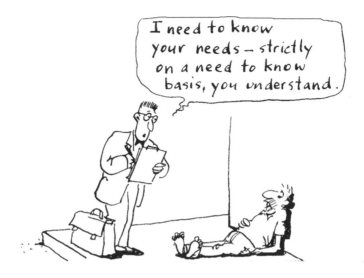

Having decided on your research questions, the basic design of your research (whether qualitative, quantitative or multi-method design) and who will be researched (your sample), the next step is to create your research instrument. In this chapter, we will consider the two most common forms of research instrument: surveys (or questionnaires) and interviews.

Surveys and interviews generally lie on a continuum, with surveys being at the more structured end and interviews at the less structured end. Usually, surveys are the research tools for quantitative methodology, with the design and questions being prepared well before the research subjects are contacted. Interviews, on the other hand, can be more flexible and are often the tools of qualitative research. Sometimes, however, surveys may be administered by an interviewer (structured interviews), and qualitative researchers can use surveys. We have already seen one example of how a mailed questionnaire was used in qualitative research in Chapter 3, in the evaluation of rural postnatal depression groups. Keeping these things in mind, the continuum of research tools from surveys to interviews is as shown in Figure 7.1.

Figure 7.1 Continuum of research tools

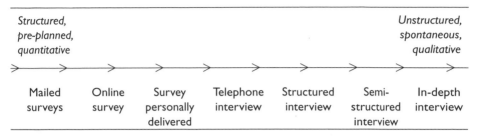

Structured, pre-planned, quantitative						Unstructured, spontaneous, qualitative
Mailed surveys	Online survey	Survey personally delivered	Telephone interview	Structured interview	Semi- structured interview	In-depth interview

Interviews can also be held with groups of people. Such interviews are often called focus groups and will be discussed at the end of this chapter.

Of course, there are many other research instruments as well as surveys and interviews, some of which are covered in later chapters.

Nevertheless, surveys and interviews are still the most commonly used tools in social research, and it is important to understand some basic principles for using them. In this chapter, we will first discuss surveys, including a look at issues common to both surveys and interviews. We will deal mainly with quantitative surveys in this section. We provide some tips on how to construct a questionnaire, then we discuss the sorts of questions you might include in your survey. The third section summarises the process of conducting a survey. Following this, we review different styles of interviews, including handy hints on interviewing, in-depth interviews and focus groups.

Surveys

In designing surveys for quantitative research, most of the hard work is done before you conduct the interviews or mail the questionnaires to the people you are researching. For the purposes of this chapter, we will assume that you have thought about your research topic and its general design, read about it and discussed it widely with key stakeholders and interested people, perhaps formed a steering committee or advisory group, and formulated your research questions (including transforming them from concepts into measurable variables). We will also assume that you have decided what the unit of study is to be, who the population is, and how you will design and find your sample.

Constructing your questionnaire
You need to address five aspects when constructing your questionnaire: the cover letter, the instructions, the structure of the questionnaire itself, layout and follow-up procedures.

Cover letter

The cover letter is essential and needs to be planned carefully if you want people to take your survey seriously and be willing to participate. The cover letter can make the difference between whether people will return their survey, or agree to a telephone or personal interview. Be prepared for many drafts to get the right tone and form for your cover letter.

Figure 7.2 Cover letter

Consumer Consultancies Inc.
PO Box 54
Country Gardens Inland City
Australia 8276
Telephone 09 33322111
Fax 09 33322211

20 February 2012

Dear Citizen,

I am part of a group of independent consultants who have been employed by the government income-support agency. We are conducting research on how people found their first visit to an office of this organisation.

Please fill in the enclosed questionnaire. Everyone who visited the agency for the first time this week has been given a copy. Your response will provide valuable information about the operation of the organisation. Answering the survey is entirely voluntary—you are not required to fill it in. However, if you do, you will help us improve the quality of service the agency provides.

You will see that although personal questions are asked, you do not identify yourself. The information you provide is completely confidential. Only your postcode, age and gender are requested so that comparisons can be made between regions, age groups and men and women. The agency will not know who answered the survey—it is sent to us, not the agency.

Please ring me on the above number if you have any questions about the survey.

Your time in filling in the questionnaire is greatly appreciated. It should not take longer than half an hour. When you have completed the questionnaire, please post it, in the Freepost envelope provided, by the end of the week. No stamp is needed.

Thank you for your time and cooperation.

Yours sincerely,

Miranda Bloggs

Principal Researcher

Figure 7.3 Consent protocol

This research project on the gendered impacts of climate variability in [your region] is being conducted by the Director of the Gender, Leadership and Social Sustainability (GLASS) research unit.

The purpose of the research is to assess how the impacts of climate variability might differ for women and men in your region. We are planning to interview key informants in three regions—one experiencing flooding, another water-logging and another drought conditions. They will be asked about their perceptions of impacts on women and men in their region. In-depth interviews will be held with key informants in local government, health and welfare services, civil society organisations and other representative organisations. These interviews will be taped, transcribed and analysed via computer. Questionnaires will be developed following these interviews for distribution to women and men in your community.

In order to ensure confidentiality, no person will be identified on the recording, and names will be changed where any reference is made to informants in the final report. Tapes will remain the property of the researcher and no other persons (other than the research assistant and the transcriber) will have access to the tapes.

Please note that should you have any complaints about the conduct of the research, you may contact the Executive Officer, Ethics in Human Research Committee on 099 654321.

Consent Form
Research Project: Gendered Impacts of Climate Variability
Principal Investigator:
Dr Miranda Bloggs
Gender, Leadership and Social Sustainability (GLASS) research unit
099 654321

I am willing to participate in this research project. I understand that I am free to withdraw my participation in the research at any time.

The purpose of the research has been explained to me and I have been given the opportunity to ask questions about the research.

I understand that any information or personal details gathered in the course of this research about me will remain confidential, and that neither my name nor any other identifying information will be used or published without my written permission.

I understand that if I have any complaints or concerns about this research I can contact the Executive Officer of the Ethics in Human Research Committee on 099 654321.

Signed:
Date:

Your cover letter should include a number of elements. Explain who you are, which agency you represent (and it is important to construct the letter on official letterhead to assure your legitimacy), what the survey is about and what it is aiming to achieve. It is also important to reassure people about their anonymity and confidentiality, and about their right not to participate. If you are using an identity number to follow up non-respondents, you need to explain its purpose, how it is used and how privacy will be protected. In mailed questionnaires, a reply-by date (usually two weeks) should be specified and a reply-paid or freepost envelope included. For interviews, the next stage of contact is explained. The cover letter must be as brief as possible, never more than a page. Your aim is to arouse people's curiosity and motivate them to become involved.

Sometimes the cover letter doubles as a consent form, especially in mailed surveys where consent is implied if people return the question-naires. At other times, it is necessary to include a separate consent form with your covering letter, and to make sure that respondents have read and signed it (that is, given their informed consent to participate in your study) before you proceed with any form of interview or questionnaire comple-tion. Figures 7.1 and 7.2 contain examples of a cover letter and consent protocol.

What to include in your cover letter
- Official letterhead of sponsoring organisation
- Introduction to yourself and your role in the study
- What the survey is for and why it is important
- How the person was chosen and why their response is important
- Measures to protect confidentiality or anonymity (explain identifying number if using one)
- Right to refuse
- General information about the research procedure (whether they will be contacted again, who will interview them, reply dates, etc.)
- Contact phone number for further questions

Instructions

There are three types of instructions that you need to give when sending a mailed survey, developing an online survey or conducting a structured inter-view. The first type involves general instructions about the whole survey. These are usually in the cover letter, with the most important instructions sometimes repeated in an introductory paragraph at the beginning of the survey itself. General instructions include who should complete the survey; how you want the questions answered and in what order; that there are no right and wrong answers; that all questions should be attempted; and how to return the questionnaire by what date.

The second type of instructions introduce different parts of the survey. These instructions also act as signposts and punctuate the 'flow' of the questionnaire (for example, 'In this section you are asked to answer some background questions so that we will know how different people think about this issue'). Remember to thank respondents at the end of the survey and to provide a contact number for further questions or information, if this is possible.

The third type of instructions are specific guidelines to answering different questions (for example, 'Please tick the box which corresponds most closely to your employment situation at present. Choose one option only from the following list . . .').

Simple, clear instructions are vital to the success of your survey, in relation to both the accuracy of people's answers and the response rate. If people are confused about what is expected of them and the general reasons for it, they may give up and not return the survey at all, perhaps only partially complete it, or answer a different question from the one you intended. Figure 7.3 provides an example of the first page of a survey, showing introductory and specific instructions.

Questionnaire structure

Good questionnaires are structured similarly to good conversations. Initially, it is important to establish rapport with the respondent by asking enjoyable, interesting questions that are not too difficult, challenging or personal. The researcher then 'takes the respondent by the hand' and guides them through a series of questions, which are grouped into topics or sections, providing brief rationales and clear instructions as discussed. Thus it is important that the sections or topics are meaningful, following a logical or sensible sequence, and that within each section questions follow a logical order.

Usually it is best to move from concrete to abstract, from easy to hard, from simple to complex, from impersonal to more personal or sensitive questions. This allows respondents who may not have thought about issues in detail to think through the topic as they go. Respondents are more likely to answer personal questions—including background information such as age, gender, employment or marital status, if these arise—further into

Figure 7.4 Example of questionnaire (page 1 only)

Questionnaire on quality of life

Introduction

This questionnaire deals with quality of life and access to education. You are asked questions about various areas of life, including your housing, health, education, work, transport and leisure.

Most questions just require you to tick or circle the answer that applies to you. Please write 'Don't know' if you do not know the answer to any question, and 'N/A' if it is not applicable. Leave blank any questions you do not wish to answer.

The information you provide is completely confidential. Only your postcode, age and gender are requested so that comparisons can be made between regions, age groups and men and women.

The questionnaire should take no more than half an hour of your time. Thank you for your assistance. The first section is about your housing and household.

Housing and household

1   Is your home in a:

☐ City ☐ Large town ☐ Small town ☐ Isolated dwelling
☐ Other

2   Your postcode is:_____(for regional comparisons)

3   Are you living in a:

☐ Caravan   ☐ Flat/apartment   ☐ Townhouse
☐ House   ☐ Farm   ☐ Hostel
☐ Institution   ☐ Retirement village   ☐ Boarding house
☐ College   ☐ Nursing home   ☐ Hospital
☐ Training facility ☐ Other (e.g. rehab centre)_____

4   Please tick whether you own, rent, pay board for your home, or whether it is free:

☐ Owned by self/spouse   ☐ Owned by self and others
☐ Privately rented   ☐ Public rent:
☐ Rented through organisation   Department of Housing
☐ Pay board to relatives   ☐ Pay board to others
☐ Free
☐ Other_____

5   How long have you lived here?

_____ years _____ months

the questionnaire, when they have become more comfortable with the process.

It is important not to waste respondents' time by asking them questions that are irrelevant to their situation. Written and online surveys and structured interviews avoid this by using filter and contingency questions, which direct respondents to other parts of the survey if a particular topic does not apply to them. These questions will be discussed in the next section.

Try to finish the interview or survey on a high note, leaving people feeling a little better than when they began the process. As most respondents volunteer their time to complete surveys or interviews, this is the least researchers can do. Asking people's advice about a particular topic and acknowledging their contribution are two ways to achieve this. Remember to thank them for participating. A reminder at the end of the last page to post the questionnaire is also a good idea.

Layout

In these days of computers and a discerning public, the layout and presentation of your questionnaire are increasingly important, especially for online and mailed surveys. It is now accepted that the presentation of your questionnaire, even down to the type of envelopes and colour of the paper, will affect your response rate. Paying attention to detail and presenting your survey as an important document that is worthy of the respondents' involvement (and also reflects the hard work you have put into it) has become a vital prerequisite for a successful survey. Online surveys need to be clear and well laid-out, and if there are links to other sections, these should be clearly signposted and must work!

For mail surveys, most researchers advise printing on one side of each page only, because people often miss the second page on the back of another. Having only one side of the page printed also allows room for extra notes to be made on the blank side. Take advantage of the different fonts now available to distinguish between instructions and questions. Make sure that filter questions and instructions about where to go in the questionnaire can be seen at a glance. Space the questions so that the page does not look crowded, leaving adequate room for answers to open-ended questions. Also, remember to leave a column on one side of the page for computer coding.

Layout is not so important for interview schedules, as these are usually for the interviewer's eyes only. However, it is important to leave plenty of room for comments and, where possible, guides to directly computer-code the respondents' answers on to the form. Spacing needs to be clear so that interviewers can find their place easily. On interview schedules, it is also possible to include extra suggestions about prompts and, in more qualitative, semi-structured interviews, probes to explore topics further.

Follow-up procedures

Whether interviewing or sending mailed questionnaires or emailing online links, you need to plan what to do in case of non-response. With emailed links to online surveys, it is relatively simple to keep track of non-responders and to send them a reminder. Many researchers label each of their mailed questionnaires with an identity number so that they can keep track of who has replied. Some researchers send a reminder postcard to all people in the sample a week after the survey was due, thanking those who replied and reminding those who have not. A week or so later, another copy of the questionnaire and a new cover letter are sent to non-respondents. Sometimes researchers also use follow-up reminder telephone calls. Of course, it is important to respect people's right not to participate in the study, and not to harass non-respondents who are actually refusals.

In the case of interviews, researchers often contact potential respondents by telephone soon after the initial letter or approach is made, to seek consent and arrange a time for the interview. Follow-up procedures for people who are not at home when the researcher calls, or who are not on the phone, also need to be planned.

Survey questions

Survey questions can be about *facts, knowledge, attitudes, beliefs, motivation, behaviour* and many other aspects of life. When formulating your questions, it is important to be clear which of these you wish to collect information about and word your questions accordingly.

Types of questions

Questions in surveys can be divided broadly into two categories: *open-ended* and *closed-ended*. In *closed-ended* questions, a range of answers is set out for the respondent: either a yes/no, or multiple choice, or a scale showing a range of responses. From the example of the government organisation providing income support in Chapter 5, some examples of closed-ended questions are provided.

Devising closed-ended questions is difficult and requires considerable work to make sure that a wide enough range of options is provided not to prejudice the results. Sometimes the options for closed-ended questions are created after extensive pre-testing and pilot testing (see next section), and are based on the results from earlier open-ended questions. One advantage of closed-ended questions is that respondents may be more inclined to circle a point on a scale, or to tick a box, than to take the time to write sentences or comments, especially about sensitive issues. A disadvantage is that closed-ended questions could reflect the reality of the researcher rather than the people being researched.

Examples of closed-ended questions, including scaled questions

1. Please tick the box that describes the social security payments you were receiving when you first visited the office of the Department of Social Security:

   Sole Parent Pension ☐
   Young Homeless Allowance ☐
   Aged Pension ☐
   Disability Support Payment ☐
   Special Benefit ☐
   Unemployment Benefit ☐
   Other ☐
   Not receiving payments at the time ☐

2. Please indicate how you felt about your first interview with departmental staff by circling a rating out of 5 for the following statements. On the scales, 1 = strongly disagree and 5 = strongly agree.

   From my first interview at the Department of Social Security I would say:

   a. staff listened carefully to what I had to say

   1_____ 2 _____ 3 _____ 4_____5
   strongly   neutral   strongly
   disagree   agree

   b. staff acted as though I was lying

   1_____ 2 _____ 3 _____ 4 _____5
   strongly   neutral   strongly
   disagree   agree

   c. staff treated me with respect

   1_____ 2 _____ 3 _____ 4 _____5
   strongly   neutral   strongly
   disagree   agree

---

d. staff attitudes need to improve

1_____ 2_____ 3_____ 4_____5

strongly   neutral   strongly

disagree   agree

e. staff provided me with the information I required

1_____ 2_____ 3_____ 4_____5

strongly   neutral   strongly

disagree   agree

f. staff understood my situation

1_____ 2_____ 3_____ 4_____5

strongly   neutral   strongly

disagree   agree

3. Were you told of your right to appeal decisions made by the department during your first interview?

   Yes   ☐

   No   ☐

When creating the options for closed-ended questions, three rules
must be followed. First, the options listed must cover all the possibilities
so that all respondents can choose an answer (thus sets of options are said
to be *exhaustive*). The second rule is that each category must not overlap
with any other (this is called having categories that are *mutually exclusive*).
Lastly, each set of categories should refer to only one dimension (this is
called *unidimensionality*). For example, a scale referring to the agency's
staff would *not* be: 'rude—aloof—courteous—punctual'. Note that when
using scales it is best to alternate between positive and negative statements
to avoid 'response bias' (respondents selecting answers in a set pattern).

Open-ended questions invite comments or opinions without anticipating
the results. They are used extensively in qualitative research, especially in
interviews. Open-ended questions in mailed surveys are best placed towards
the end of the survey, and should be used sparingly as they require more
time and effort on the part of the respondent than closed-ended questions.
Prompts can be added to clarify open-ended questions in mailed surveys. In
interviews, the interviewer can clarify, probe and prompt respondents about
open-ended questions. The advantages of open-ended questions include that
they make no assumptions about how the respondent will reply (allowing
for surprises that you may not have anticipated), and that they provide much
more scope for the respondent to express their thoughts and feelings.

Examples of open-ended questions
- What happened the first time you visited an agency office?
- Please describe how the staff behaved towards you during your first interview at the agency.
- How would you describe the attitude of agency staff towards you?

Two other types of question that are important in questionnaires are *filter questions* and *contingency questions*. These questions help respondents to avoid topics that do not apply to them and to move on to relevant parts of the questionnaire. In the income-support agency survey, a filter question might be: 'Do you have young children?' (followed by instructions such as: 'If yes, please answer the following questions, if no, please turn to Section 2 of this questionnaire.') The contingency questions following the filter question might be about taking children into an agency office—for example, 'Would you feel comfortable taking your children with you to an interview at the agency?' 'Could you suggest improvements we could make so that our office is more friendly to parents and children?'

Tips on wording questions
- Use plain, simple English; avoid jargon, acronyms and initials.
- Make questions as short as possible.
- Be clear and avoid ambiguity (check the cultural meaning of terms as well).
- Avoid double-barrelled questions (e.g. ask about mother and father separately, not parents).
- Beware of leading questions (e.g. 'Wouldn't you agree that all people on employment benefits are lazy?').
- Beware of the word 'not' (avoid negatives, especially in closed-ended questions—they can be very confusing).
- Beware of artificially creating an opinion. (Allow for the options of 'don't know' or 'no opinion'. Use filter questions to check whether people know about the topic you are researching. Decide whether wording should be direct or indirect ('Have you ever been unemployed?' versus 'Please list your employment history.')
- Decide whether wording should be personal or impersonal.

Source: Adapted from de Vaus (2002, pp. 97–9).

Steps in conducting your survey

There are several steps involved in designing a survey or questionnaire. Note that they overlap, and that many will be carried out concurrently. For example, as you design your sample you will also need to have in mind the method for your survey (mailed questionnaire, online survey, telephone interview or face-to-face interview) and your research topic. When you are constructing the survey and the questions you will ask, you will also be planning your data analysis.

Step 1: Define the research topic

See Chapters 2 and 3. Think about the problem, consult and read widely, formulate your research topic, decide on qualitative, quantitative or mixed design, formulate questions and hypotheses and operationally define variables (if quantitative).

Step 2: Choose the research instrument

Decide on the form your survey will take. Will you choose to mail out a questionnaire, send a link to the online questionnaire, personally deliver the questionnaire to individuals or a group, conduct a telephone survey or undertake structured interviews? Your decision will rest upon the aims of your project, the resources at your disposal, the sample of people you aim to research and the types of information you are seeking.

Generally if you are aiming to reach a large number of people and have well-thought-out research questions that have been operationalised into indicators, a mailed survey will be the most convenient and possibly most effective research instrument. On the other hand, for exploratory research on sensitive or complex issues, or for research with populations who have difficulty with written English, face-to-face interviews may be the most effective method. Telephone interviews can also be a useful strategy. Costing somewhere between interviews and mailed surveys, and allowing more flexibility than written surveys—though less than face-to-face interviews—they are also well worth considering. However, if doing telephone surveys, your questions must be kept simple unless you also mail people a copy of the questionnaire to look at during the interview. Another limitation of telephone interviews is that you will only be able to interview people who have a telephone. As you can see from this very brief discussion, there are advantages and disadvantages of each method. These are summarised in Table 7.1.

Table 7.1 Comparison of three survey research instruments

	Mail or online survey	Telephone survey	Face-to-face interview
Cost	Lowest cost	Middle cost	Highest cost
Response rate	Lowest response rate	Moderate response rate	Highest response rate
Coverage	Reaches greatest number of people yet only those with good literacy skills and motivation respond	Reaches respondents with poor literacy skills but only those who have telephones	Reaches smaller numbers but wide range of people whether illiterate, low income, without phone
Convenience	Respondent can complete in own time, at own pace	Can be completed quickly	Time-consuming for interviewer and respondent
	Quick results ready for computer entry	Direct computer entry of results possible	More time-consuming to code and enter data
Accuracy and type of information	Visual layout can help comprehension	Can clarify questions	Can clarify questions, probe and prompt
	Cannot clarify confusion, probe or prompt	Limited opportunity to probe and prompt	Can record non-verbal and other responses
	Cannot check whether right person answered the questions	Misses non-verbal responses	Can ensure the right respondent answers questions in the right order
	Cannot check whether questions were answered in the right order	Ensures questions answered in right order	Interviewer may misrecord response
	Partial response possible	Can't always ensure the right person answers the questions	Most likely that survey will be completed
	Needs to be short to ensure response rate	More chance that survey will be completed fully	Allows for longer, more open-ended responses
	Least chance of bias caused by interviewer attitudes, presence	Must use simple questions	Highest chance of interviewer bias
		Moderate chance of interviewer bias	
Anonymity	Highest level of anonymity/ confidentiality	Less assurance of anonymity	Less assurance of anonymity

Step 3: Identify population and sample

Review Chapter 5. In defining your population and the units of study, it is most important that you know who is included within the scope of your definitions—who is in and who is out. It can be easy to exclude people who should have been included, and thus weaken the impact of your results. As you design your sample and work out sampling procedures, you will also be thinking about the most effective research method.

Step 4: Construct draft questionnaire

Develop your questions, keeping in mind the objectives of your study, and the research questions and indicators you created as you operationalised your variables. As you work out the questions, you will also be thinking about how you will analyse the data you collect. *All* the variables you have come up with will need corresponding questions.

A good idea at this early stage is to draw up 'dummy tables' of the results you expect to get, to make sure that you are collecting the right information to explore the relationship between the variables that are most important for your study. Dummy tables are most helpful in explanatory research. They can assist you to think through whether your questions are at the right level of measurement, and have the right amount of detail, for the purposes of your study. Dummy tables are also useful in descriptive and exploratory research for checking that the questions you ask will provide the information you need to address your research questions.

Taking the income-support agency example from Chapter 5, suppose that you want to know whether clients have different experiences of the agency, depending on whether they live in the country or city. At this stage you are interested in whether the clients' experience was good, satisfactory or bad. In this case, it is implied that coming from the country or city will be the *independent* variable and clients' experiences the *dependent* variable. The first dummy table could look like this:

	Location	
	Rural	*City*
Experience at agency	%	%
Good		
Satisfactory		
Bad		
Total	100	100
	(n=)	(n=)

You will need to work out questions that measure whether respondents come from the country or city, and whether their experience of the agency is good, satisfactory or bad. The series of scales described in the section on question formulation can be transformed into a summary measure to suit this table.

Perhaps you suspect that the length of time people have been unemployed may also affect clients' treatment when they visit the agency's office. Length of time of unemployment would then be an 'interfering' or 'test' variable, because it may 'interfere' in the relationship you are investigating between living in the country or city and people's experience of the department. The dummy table for the interfering variable 'length of time unemployed' could look like this:

	Long-term unemployed		Short-term unemployed	
	Rural	City	Rural	City
Experience at agency	%	%	%	%
Good				
Satisfactory				
Bad				
Total	100	100	100	100
	(n=)	(n=)	(n=)	(n=)

As well as including questions about all the variables you have devised for your research topic (*independent, dependent* and *interfering* or *test* variables in the case of explanatory research), surveys include questions on *background* information such as gender, age, education, employment, marital status and ethnic background, again depending on the nature of the research. Such issues may affect the relationships you are investigating and also provide a baseline of information about the characteristics of your sample, which you can compare with the population you are studying. Generally you should include questions about these four types of variable in your draft questionnaire. At this draft stage, it is wise to have a few extra questions about each variable to try out during the next step of survey design.

Four aspects to include in questionnaire design

- Independent variables
- Dependent variables
- Interfering or test variables
- Background variables

Step 5: Pre-test questionnaire

Once you have your first draft of questions, including questions relating to each of the major variables and background variables, it is time to pre-test your questionnaire. Try out sections of it, or the whole thing, on friends, family, colleagues, experts and non-experts in the area of your research, to see whether the questions you have devised really elicit the information you want. Ask people whether the questions could be improved, and generally obtain as much feedback as possible.

This is one of the most important stages in the process. It can be very embarrassing to have the final version of the survey returned, only to find that the majority of respondents ticked the 'other' category for an important question. You would still be none the wiser as to what people thought about the issue! Thorough pre-testing will help you to pick up such difficulties early in the process.

Pre-testing also assists you to discard poorly worded or confusing questions, and questions that are repetitive or boring. During the pre-test, you may also discover that some of the language is offensive to the people you are researching. If so, change it immediately. It is important that only the most effective questions end up in the questionnaire, and that the survey itself is not too long while covering the essential aspects of the topic.

Step 6: Revise questionnaire

While you are pre-testing the questionnaire on a wide range of people, revise it and make changes, testing the new or revised questions as you go. At the same time as you are pre-testing the questionnaire, you will probably be working out how you will select your sample for the study. Once you are satisfied that the questions seem to work, and that you have drawn the sample you hope to interview or to whom you will send the questionnaire, it is time for the next step.

Step 7: Pilot the questionnaire

This is an important stage, particularly for written or online questionnaires. To pilot the questionnaire, you literally give the survey a 'test run', under the same conditions in which you intend to conduct the whole survey. Thus you use the sampling procedures you have worked out to try out the survey on a small group of respondents, just as though it were the 'real thing'. Have people test an online questionnaire for ease of understanding and to ensure all functions work.

During the pilot, you have the opportunity to fine-tune three main areas of the survey. First, you are checking the questionnaire design itself, including the wording of questions and scales, and the 'flow' of the questionnaire. Second, this is your chance to finalise field procedures, such as the number of call-backs you will make if the people you are interviewing are not at home when you call, or people do not respond to mailed or online surveys. The pilot may also allow you to gain an idea of how many refusals (to participate in your study) you can expect, and to form ground rules about how you will deal with this. Will you select a larger sample to begin with, to account for refusals? While all researchers would welcome a 100 per cent response rate, refusals indicate that respondents have genuinely been given a choice about being involved, and that those who do participate have given their informed consent. You also need to ensure that you only survey people once and don't double-count people in your sample. This can be a problem in large surveys or when you are constructing a sample from multiple lists of names, and is known as the issue of *coverage*.

Third, during the pilot you can test your definitions of population and sampling procedures to ensure that your sampling frame has allowed for all the people who should be included. You need to include enough cases in the pilot to cover the variability that exists in the total population. For example: Is the gender balance right? Is there provision for people from non-English-speaking backgrounds to be included? Is the right age range covered? This is called attending to the *scope* of the survey. Often researchers nominate a referee (it could be your advisory committee) to make decisions about problems of scope and coverage.

Another function of the pilot can be to test your tools for data analysis and make sure the questions provide answers with the right level of detail and measurement for analytical purposes. Thus you could use the data from the pilot to fill in the dummy tables and check whether the information gained will be sufficient for the statistics you wish to perform. You also trial your coding procedures at this time.

During the period of the pilot test, training for interviewers often takes place if there is to be more than one interviewer in your study. Feedback from interviewers during the pilot as to how the survey is received is invaluable. Many researchers devise evaluation sheets for their interviewers' comments during the pilot test (a survey within a survey!).

If the pilot test shows that there are only a few minor changes to be made (that is, if your pre-testing was thorough enough), then you can keep your pilot test results to include in your data analysis. If major changes are made to the questionnaire or sampling procedures, however, you may not be able to include pilot results in your final data analysis.

Steps 8–11: Data collection, coding and data entry, data analysis and interpretation, publication

These last four steps are covered in Chapters 14, 15, 16 and 17. Further references on surveys are provided at the end of this chapter.

Interviews

As we have seen, interviews are more flexible research instruments than questionnaires. They can be used for a wide range of research purposes: from very structured settings (literally as 'spoken questionnaires') through to unstructured in-depth interviews, and for both quantitative and qualitative research designs. In this section, we will examine some of the extra features of interviews that are different from surveys and provide some handy hints for conducting interviews. Note that many of the general principles identified for surveys, such as establishing rapport and being clear about your expectations, also apply to interviews and will not be repeated in detail here. The chapter concludes with a brief look at focus groups and other types of group interviews.

Before discussing the various types of research interviews you could use, we raise some of the issues with which social workers must engage when they are doing research interviews.

Your role as interviewer: Researcher or social worker?

Social workers undertaking research interviews face some interesting challenges—particularly if they are doing research as one of their work roles in an organisation in which they also do face-to-face or other client work. On one hand, they can use their communication skills to assist interviewees to feel comfortable, to be open and to explore their feelings about a research issue in depth. On the other hand, social workers must be very careful how they use their skills so that they do not 'lead the witness' in any way.

Social workers interviewing people with whom they have other relationships (for example, clients, relatives of clients, colleagues, supervisees or supervisors) must be aware of the power they hold and the political and ethical implications of their research, as well as its effects on the people they are interviewing. If you have something your interviewee wants, such as access to resources, or if they just want to please you because you are their counsellor and they like you, they are likely to tell you what they think you want to hear rather than their actual opinion about an issue. This applies particularly to social workers attempting internal evaluations of their own services. In such cases, other methods—such as anonymous questionnaires or using interviewers from outside your service who can guarantee some protection or privacy—are preferable to you doing your own interviews.

The ethical issues raised throughout this book are especially pertinent to social workers undertaking research interviews, particularly when they are in the dual roles of researcher and service provider. You must be sure that interviewees are not exposed to additional risks as a result of being part of the research. For example, how will you deal with a situation where an interviewee reveals something confidential during a research interview that impacts directly on whether they will continue to receive a service? In such cases, the issues of privacy, confidentiality, protection from harm and informed consent are of paramount importance. It is part of your duty of care as both a social worker and a researcher to have thought through such issues well in advance, and to have worked out strategies that will protect the interests of all the players. Many of these dilemmas can be solved in advance, particularly if representatives of the people you are interviewing are also involved in designing the research (for example, on the advisory committee). Another important way of preventing the dilemmas arising in the first place is to develop clear role delineations with your supervisors about the separate roles of practitioner and researcher.

A related dilemma faced by social work researchers when they are interviewing people is drawing the line between helping and research roles during the interview. Of course, this dilemma is not limited to social work researchers. Researchers doing qualitative research, for example, talk of the times when the people they are interviewing become emotional about a topic, or it becomes obvious that they need some assistance or information that the interviewer has. At this point, you the interviewer may decide to 'turn off the tape' and switch roles, becoming a social worker for a while and then returning to the research interview when it is appropriate. If such a situation arises, it is important to be clear with your interviewee what you are doing and what role you are undertaking at the time.

Researching sensitive issues

Most social work research involves sensitive issues. Usually these issues affect the people you interview, so the communication skills you have as a professional are particularly important. Just as we noted for surveys, it is best to locate discussion of sensitive issues around the middle of an interview. This gives you and the interviewee time to develop some trust and rapport to be able to discuss such topics, and also allows time for you to deal with any unexpected outcomes.

It would be disastrous to raise an emotionally laden topic towards the end of an interview, then finish abruptly leaving the interviewee distressed. Remember that as most research participation is voluntary, the least you can do is leave them feeling a little better at the end of the interview than they did at the beginning.

Diversity and interviewees in social work research

Because social work directs much of its effort towards improving conditions for people who are disadvantaged and disempowered, it is to be hoped that much of your research will include people from a wide range of backgrounds. An essential social work skill that is also a research skill is the ability to work with a diverse range of people, including people who come from different backgrounds from your own.

While we mention various aspects relating to differences between interviewers and interviewees throughout the rest of this chapter, we thought it would be useful to include a checklist of 'respectful communication' hints. This checklist was devised by Cindy Lesley, an Indigenous advocate for people with disabilities. Originally created as a tool for teaching students how to enter Indigenous communities and work with Indigenous people with disabilities, it is also useful as a checklist for respectful communication generally. It is relevant to situations in which the people you are interviewing are different from you, and may have different assumptions about the world and/or ways of talking about things. This includes differences such as culture, language, disability, sexual preference, age or gender. You will notice that it is as much about homework and preparing for the interview beforehand as it is about your behaviour during the interview itself.

Guidelines for interviewing people from backgrounds different from your own.

Note: As each situation is different, this is a list of questions and things to be aware of, rather than hard-and-fast rules!

When entering a new community

- Know the country/community you are visiting.
- How do the people of the community refer to themselves?
- Do you have permission to enter the community?

Dress sense

- What is respectful and appropriate dress for this community?
- As a general rule, don't wear glitz and glitter—usually basic wear causes less offence.
- Do not wear clothes that could be seen as sexually provocative.

Non-verbal communication skills

- Find out what is appropriate: should you use eye contact or not? How is other body language used (for example, head gestures)?
- What is respectful non-verbal communication?

Verbal communication

When people are from non-English-speaking backgrounds (including deaf people using sign language), or have learning disabilities, it is important to:
- use an interpreter whenever possible
- speak in plain English
- use minimal written material unless in the person's language
- use simple words without being patronising
- find out about and use respectful verbal communication.

Concepts and language about sensitive concepts

- Build trust and rapport before launching into delicate issues.
- What words do people use about concepts such as 'disability' or 'poverty'?
- How do they refer to these concepts within their community?
- Do you need to go around the issue rather than ask directly?

Gender

- What are the usual rules for speaking with people from your own and different genders?
- Do you need to take special measures in this community as a result of your gender?

Source: Lesley (2002).

Structured interviews

Structured interviews are usually questionnaires that are administered by an interviewer. In the strictest quantitative tradition, interviewers working with quantitative interview schedules try to use exactly the same wording, prompts and tone of voice for each interview, to ensure that every interview is conducted as similarly as possible. Nowadays, computer interviews provide the closest approximation to this ideal. In an interview situation with two human beings involved, it is virtually impossible to make each interview the same. This has its advantages, even in quantitative designs. The added flexibility of an interview allows misunderstandings to be clarified, and enables the researcher to ensure that the right person answers the questions in the right order. None of these advantages is available with mailed or online questionnaires.

The general rules for structured interviews follow the same principles as for questionnaires. Go over the section on surveys carefully if you are planning to use a structured interview as your research instrument. Depending on the design of the study, it is often possible to include more open-ended questions in structured interviews than in mailed or online questionnaires, as the interviewer can prompt the respondent, probe for more information and clarify what the questions mean. Structured interviews can also be longer than mailed surveys, as respondents will be more motivated to talk with interviewers than to complete lengthy pen-and-paper exercises, and there is less concentration involved if the interviewer is recording the answers.

Semi-structured interviews

As their name implies, semi-structured interviews fall somewhere between structured and in-depth interviews. Usually, semi-structured interviews follow a set outline of topics with some pre-tested questions and prompts in each section. These are the triggers for the main directions of the interview, and interviewers mostly are required to at least ask the questions on the schedule as they appear. However, having asked a particular question and recorded the answer/s, the interviewer is often allowed to explore additional information that the respondent has raised, to ask other questions, or to follow up issues that were not originally included in the interview schedule.

Thus the interviewer is allowed more initiative and has more ability to respond to the perceptions and priorities of the respondent. Semi-structured interviews vary enormously in the degree of structure and amount of initiative given to the interviewer. They can be ideal research instruments for exploratory and descriptive designs through which the researcher is finding out about a topic and/or has little prior knowledge of what the respondents think about it. Skilled interviewers are needed for semi-structured interviews because so much depends on the interviewer's ability to pick up, explore and accurately record additional information.

Typically, semi-structured interview schedules contain many open-ended questions, with lots of suggestions for prompts and probes. Probes can include reality checking responses, summarising statements or further probing about the issue being discussed, during which you ask further questions (for example, 'Can you tell me more about that?', 'What do you mean?', 'Can you give me an example?'). It is important to leave plenty of room on the page under appropriate headings for the extra information interviewers may collect. Sometimes semi-structured interviews are audio-recorded; however, due to the costs of transcription it is more usual for the interviewers to record the responses on the interview schedule.

Interviewers using a semi-structured approach need careful training about the aims of the research and the stance of the researcher, and to be skilled in interviewing techniques. The gender, age, class and ethnicity of interviewers can heavily influence how the respondent answers questions. This is more of an issue in face-to-face interviews than in mailed or online surveys or telephone interviews, in which the characteristics of the interviewer may not be as obvious. Sometimes feminist and other researchers deliberately match such interviewer characteristics with respondents, believing that respondents will be more open and honest with interviewers who are similar to themselves. This is an area of debate, as other feminist researchers believe that respondents are more likely to be honest with strangers or people who are different from them.

Depending on the ideology of the researcher, the ability of the interviewer to maintain 'objectivity' or 'neutrality' is considered to be more or less important, and more or less possible (see Chapter 1). Whatever the researcher's position on this, throughout the process of data collection regular checks with interviewers are needed to keep track of how the interview process is developing. After a few interviews it can be tempting for different interviewers to develop their own hypotheses about the topic, which they may indirectly 'suggest' to respondents. In some designs, this may be acceptable and even encouraged and shared with other interviewers; in others this is not so. In any case, the researcher should be aware of what is happening and be guiding the overall process. One way of achieving this is by holding regular group meetings with the interviewers, during which they discuss how the interviews are going.

In-depth interviews

In-depth interviews are the most flexible type of research instrument, and are used in qualitative research. Generally the researcher/s conduct in-depth interviews themselves rather than employing other interviewers. This is because the quality of data collected depends so much on the skill of the interviewer and their developing understanding of the issues being researched. Whereas semi-structured interviews include many open-ended questions, in-depth interviews are often seen as being more of a discussion, and ideally are guided by the respondent rather than the interviewer.

Some feminist researchers try to develop an 'equal' relationship with the people they are interviewing, rather than the traditional relationship of 'expert researcher' interviewing a subject or respondent. These researchers may include personal self-disclosure, provide information and answer questions as part of the discussion process. They may also conduct multiple interviews with respondents, using subsequent interviews to check the accuracy of their impressions and information, and to discuss the results and their meaning. Such researchers see themselves as being in partnership with the respondents (also called 'participants'), and may make conscious efforts to share control and ownership of the research process and results with them.

The structure of in-depth interviews depends on the nature of the topic, the context of the interview and the personality and skills of the researcher and the respondent. Although at one end of the spectrum of in-depth interviews it is theoretically possible to begin with absolutely no structure other than a general topic, most researchers arrive at in-depth interviews with a number of topics or areas that they wish to cover and a loose structure for how they anticipate the interview unfolding. This enables some comparison of what different respondents think about the same issues. It is also important, for ethical reasons, to be able to foreshadow the general content of the interview and the way it will be conducted, in order for the respondent to give their informed consent to the research.

During an in-depth interview and in follow-up interviews, new issues that may emerge can be fully explored. The aim of an in-depth interview is to see the world from the eyes of the respondent as much as possible, to explore with them their thoughts and feelings and to thoroughly understand their point of view. Whatever structure is planned before the interview is less important than capturing the 'reality' of the person being interviewed, including their own language and use of words.

A critical skill in in-depth interviewing is the ability to establish a relationship with the respondent in which they feel free to openly express their inner thoughts and feelings. The social work skill of demonstrating *empathy*, in which the person being interviewed feels heard, accepted and understood, is vital to in-depth interviewing. Empathy is a complex skill that involves the researcher's own characteristics (age, gender, socio-economic status, etc.) as well as learned communication skills. As early second wave feminist researcher Reinharz (1992, p. 26) once commented: 'every aspect of the researcher's identity can impede or enhance empathy'. Another feminist researcher, Nancy Naples (2003, pp. 61–5) explores this notion of empathy in greater depth. She notes that a feminist researcher 'broadens the ground upon which individuals will share deeply felt experiences'. She argues that the ethic of caring implicit in feminist research breaks down barriers and power differentials between researcher and researched. She articulates the notion that this ethic is what sets feminist researchers (and, I would argue, social work researchers as well) aside from others and enables them to address inequalities—'how we draw on our capacity for empathy and dialogue is directly related to this political project'. This argument is further developed by Smith (2009, p. 74), who notes that 'empathy and unconditional acceptance have been at the heart of [social work's] key principles' and therefore lead us more naturally to this form of data gathering. This thinking about method leads back to our original thoughts on emancipatory research discussed in Chapter 1, and the notion that social workers tend to conduct research that aims to enhance and empower. Thus, as with feminist researchers, social work researchers tend to favour empathetic listening and unconditional acceptance, and this leads us more naturally to interviews.

Communication skills involved in empathy include attending to the respondent's verbal and non-verbal messages, displaying attentive, respectful listening, and accurately reflecting back the content and feeling of what has been said, including the 'message beneath the message'. Accurate empathic listening is a powerful way to help respondents clarify what they think and feel, to explore it in more detail and to become more specific. Empathy can be built up over several interviews.

Generally, due to their flexibility and the huge amount of information that is collected (typically an interview will last from one to three hours), in-depth interviews are audiotaped by the interviewer. This allows the interviewer to focus on the respondent and the interview process, rather than having to attempt to record data at the same time. Questions have been raised about the effects of the microphone on the respondent and the data collected. In reply, qualitative researchers maintain that they have effective techniques for overcoming reticence on the part of the respondent, and that once the interview is underway most people forget about the microphone.

Clearly, given the nature of in-depth interviews, the researcher must have exceptionally good interviewing skills, a highly developed theoretical understanding of research methodology and considerable experience in this method before they attempt it without close supervision. Researchers using in-depth interviews can experience high levels of stress, which can adversely affect the quality of the data they collect. For example, some researchers find themselves avoiding painful issues with respondents, cutting them off with comments such as 'I know what you mean' because they cannot cope with the distress or painful nature of the material being discussed. Interviewers must be aware of their own sensitivities and responses, and how these are affecting the interview process, if they wish to use in-depth interview techniques.

This section on interviews concludes with a list of 'handy hints' for interviewers. These hints apply to all forms of interviews, although obviously some will be more important in structured, and others in unstructured, formats.

Handy hints for interviewers

Arranging the interview

Send introductory letter covering the same issues as for a survey cover letter. Then follow up with a phone call. Sometimes you need to obtain prior written consent before further contact; sometimes a phone call is made to explain the purpose of the research, obtain consent and organise the interview. Make sure that both interviewer and respondent are clear about the place, time, purpose and approximate length of the interview, and that these are at the respondent's convenience. Try to organise a time and place that will be private and have minimum interruptions.

Beginning the interview

Dress in a culturally appropriate manner to show respect and avoid offence. Introduce yourself. Begin with a clear (re)statement of purpose, timeframe, general outline of process and content of interview, as well as confidentiality precautions. Make sure appropriate consents have been signed, including the way in which the data will be recorded (notes, tape-recording, video, etc.). Establish rapport, perhaps begin with some small talk. The same principles apply as for surveys: easy,

---

interesting questions assist in developing motivation and trust at the beginning of an interview.

During the interview

Be sensitive to the respondent's state of mind. You have an ethical duty of care not to upset or cause distress to respondents. Have open-ended questions, prompts and probes prepared. Place difficult or potentially sensitive questions in the middle of the interview so that there is time to deal with any repercussions before the end of the interview time.

Closing the interview

Finish on a high note. Clarify permission for follow-up procedures, further interviews, call-backs, and so on. Tell the respondent how they can contact the researcher for more information, or for anything further they wish to say. Arrange for other follow-up such as results to be sent. Don't make promises you can't keep. Thank the respondent.

Focus groups

Interviews can also be conducted with groups of people. Focus groups are groups that parallel the range of interviews, from semi-structured to in-depth interviews. Structured interviews are also often administered in groups, but these are not focus groups because the role of the interviewer is to administer the questions on the questionnaire, and the role of the respondents is to answer the questions as presented.

In focus groups, the researcher is usually prepared with some structure, a list of topics and trigger questions, but also aims to use the group discussion to explore the topic further. People in the focus group are often specially chosen because of their interest, involvement or knowledge in relation to the research issue. The group process during the discussion allows people to develop their ideas with each other, and to 'brainstorm' different options or opinions. With skilled facilitation, focus groups can come up with ideas and solutions that none of the individual members had thought about beforehand. Focus groups can be an economical means of gathering data. On the one hand, they can produce creative ideas; on the other, 'group think' can operate so that individual members feel afraid to voice their true opinions and diversity is lost. Much depends on the skill of the group facilitator.

Summary

In this chapter, we have considered a range of research tools, beginning with more structured quantitative surveys and moving through a range of research formats, finishing with in-depth interviews. The advantages and disadvantages of each method have been discussed, along with key techniques and handy hints. Of course, it is possible to mix these methods. Combining methods, if approached thoughtfully, can lead to much better results. For example, focus groups can be used following individual in-depth interviews to report back results and discuss their meaning. Your choice of research tool will largely depend on the topic, the design of your study and the type of sample you are using.

Discussion questions

7.1   What are the three types of instructions that are used in surveys?

7.2   What are the two broadest categories of questions in survey research? Give examples of each.

7.3   What is wrong with the following questions?

(a)   Please tick the box that corresponds most closely to your marital status:

Single   ☐
Married   ☐
Living alone   ☐
Cohabiting with a partner   ☐
Other   ☐

(b)   Please indicate your opinion of the government's actions to cut interest rates on the following scale:

1_____   2 _____   3
bad   very bad   terrible

(c)   Wouldn't you agree that the savage beating of innocent children should be punished by more than a 'holiday at the taxpayers' expense' (i.e. prison)?

Yes   ☐
No   ☐

(d)   When you last visited a police station, was the duty officer polite and did he or she deal with your request to your satisfaction?

7.4   List four advantages/disadvantages comparing mailed or online questionnaires, telephone interviews and structured interviews as methods of conducting surveys.

7.5 What is the difference between a pre-test and a pilot test?

7.6 When would you use structured compared with in-depth interviews?

7.7 How would you record information from an in-depth interview?

7.8 What are some of the differences between semi-structured and in-depth interviews?

7.9 Give some examples of non-directive probes that could be used in interviews.

7.10 List some of the ways in which you could establish rapport with an interviewee.

7.11 What is empathy? In which types of interview is it most frequently used? What is its purpose?

Exercises

7.1 Devise a questionnaire to examine the influence of media on the body image of teenagers. Assuming that this is an explanatory study, write questions around the following variables:
- dependent variable
- independent variable
- interfering or test variables
- background variables.

Include examples of open, closed and scaled questions, and at least one example each of a filter and contingent question.

7.2 List some strategies for pre-testing this questionnaire.

7.3 Draw some dummy tables to show the relationships you are investigating.

7.4 Write a cover letter of no more than one page, including the aspects listed in this chapter.

7.5 How will you pilot this survey?

7.6 What ethical issues are raised in this study?

Further reading

Babbie, E. 2010, *The Practice of Social Research*, 12th edn, Wadsworth, Belmont, CA. See Chapter 9 on survey research, and Chapter 10 on qualitative field research.

Babbie, E. 2011, *The Basics of Social Research*, Wadsworth, Belmont, CA. See Chapter 9 for a detailed discussion of survey research, interviews and online surveys and Chapter 10 on qualitative field research.

de Vaus, D.A. 2002, *Surveys in Social Research*, 5th edn, Allen & Unwin, Sydney. Chapters 7 and 8 provide an excellent guide to designing and administering questionnaires that remains current.

Engel, R. and Schutt, R. 2010, 'Survey research', in R.M. Grinnell and Y.A. Unrau (eds), *Social Work Research and Evaluation*, 9th edn, Oxford University Press, New York.

Gochros, H. 2010, 'Qualitative interviewing' in R.M. Grinnell and Y.A. Unrau (eds), *Social Work Research and Evaluation*, 9th edn, Oxford University Press, New York.

Hardwick, Louise and Worsley, Aidan 2011, *Doing Social Work Research*, Sage, London. Chapter 5 provides an interesting discussion of social work interviews and questionnaires.

Naples, Nancy 2003, *Feminism and Method*, Routledge, New York. This book provides a very interesting understanding of feminist research. Chapter 4 relates the insider/outsider debate with an informed discussion on empathy. Chapter 9 discusses empowerment.

8 Assessing community needs and strengths

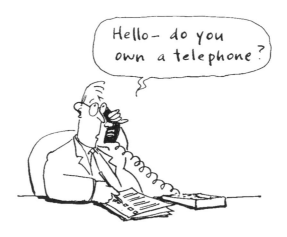

In this and the following five chapters, we introduce you to research methods that will be useful for you as a social work practitioner. We begin with identifying and analysing community needs and strengths, one of the most common types of research undertaken by social workers (Marlow 2011). While needs and strengths assessment is one of the most useful tools in the planning process, it is often done poorly or avoided due to the many pressures that organisations face (Dudley 2010; Moore 2009). These pressures include funding deadlines and the mistaken belief that anecdotal evidence provides the answers so there is no need for a more formal assessment process (Dudley 2010; Moore 2009).

Part of your role as a community social worker will most likely include identifying the needs and strengths of your community or target group, and analysing these with a view to determining priorities for action. While needs and strengths assessments can be seen as legitimate research activities in their own right, they can also be viewed as a first stage in the process of evaluation. Evaluation is discussed more fully in the next chapter; however, you should be aware that needs and strengths assessment can lead to the development of new programs or the overhaul of existing programs and services that may be evaluated further using the strategies discussed in Chapter 9.

Traditionally, needs analyses or assessments have been an essential part of the community social worker's research toolkit. Needs assessments form the basis for knowing what needs groups or communities have, where the inequalities and service gaps lie, the extent to which people are having their needs met and what our priorities should be. Nearly all funding applications require some form of needs assessment. If you can't demonstrate that your idea is needed, it won't be funded.

Because it is so value-laden and non-objective, needs assessment is a complex and potentially dangerous task. On one hand, it can 'reduce the community to a repository of problems and confirms hopelessness and desperation' (Homan 2008, p. 111). On the other hand, needs assessment can empower communities and services to make strategic changes to improve health and well-being, and to tackle issues that previously may have been seen as insurmountable. To make sure that your needs assessment makes a positive contribution, it is important that you are aware of your own fundamental values and the perspectives that guide your work. It is just as important that you can identify the values behind the assessment itself. Before you begin any assessment, you need to be clear about *who* the assessment is actually for and *why* it is being done. Addressing these values issues up front is a critical part of needs and strengths assessments (Marlow 2011; Wadsworth 2011b).

Two developments have become increasingly important strategies to limit the more destructive unintentional consequences of traditional approaches to needs analysis. These are, first, to involve the people whose needs are being assessed as partners or directors of the process; and, second, to assess the strengths and resources of the community being investigated at the same time as you assess the needs.

Ife (2010) warns that conventional approaches to needs definition and assessment are inherently disempowering because they privilege the experts' ideas about how to define and justify needs. Traditional approaches to needs assessments, he maintains, rely on 'top down' quasi-scientific methods when actually only the most basic of human survival needs, such as the needs for food and shelter, can be objectively shown to be 'needs'. All other needs, such as the need to belong, to be respected and to be included, are constructions that vary depending on their cultural, social and political contexts. This means that it is very important to establish who is constructing or defining needs.

Ife (2010) points out that statements about community needs or human needs tend to imply an 'ought'—that is, they tend to be normative. When we say that a high school is needed, we are implying that it should be provided. Further, there is usually an unstated question about why it is needed. Once we ask why, we bring in the idea of rights. For example, the right to adequate education is implied in the statement that the community needs a high school. Thus, ideas about rights and needs are intertwined, and as both are constructions, again it becomes very important who is defining these ideas.

With a vision of 'human rights from below', Ife (2010) argues that in order for needs assessments to be empowering, the people whose needs are being involved must be the ones directing the process. He lists some fundamental questions that must be answered when designing needs assessments (2010, p. 134):

- Who is defining the needs or rights (and who is excluded from the act of definition)?
- On what information do they base this definition?
- What processes do they use?
- In what context(s) does the definition take place?

If you are able to answer these questions so that the people whose needs are being assessed are in charge of the processes and goals of the needs assessment, or are at least key decision-makers, then you will be well on your way to ensuring that the needs assessment is empowering. Viewing the community and its groups as senior partners in the process, rather than as passive recipients of your expertise, is crucial. This makes the composition of the steering committee or reference group that we introduced in Chapter 2 a critical element of all needs and strengths assessments.

The second strategy for minimising potential damage arising from needs assessments is to include investigation of the strengths or resources that exist in a community, but may not have been identified as resources up to this point, as part of the assessment. For example, if a community has experienced closure of industry such as a steelworks, so that a large proportion of its male workforce is unemployed, this group of men can be seen either as a drain on the economy (welfare dependent) or as a potential resource of skilled volunteers who suddenly have time available for community-based activities. Strengths-based approaches are familiar to many social workers, though relatively new in the needs assessment area (Engel and Schutt 2009).

Community development workers Kretzmann and McKnight (1993) were the first writers to propose a model of mapping community assets. They developed this as an antidote to what they identified as the negative, deficit orientation of traditional needs assessments, which ignores the 'gifts, skills and capacities of the community's residents', especially of 'those who find themselves marginalized by communities ... who have been labeled mentally handicapped or disabled, or those who are marginalized because they are too old, or too young, or too poor' (Kretzmann and McKnight 1993, p. 6). These writers argue that strong communities are those that identify and mobilise the capacities of marginalised people so that they are partners in the community-building process, not just clients or recipients. Several writers in needs assessment (e.g. Homan 2008) now advocate inclusion of strengths as part of the process.

What is needs and strengths assessment?

There are many types of needs and strengths assessment, and many things that they can do. Homan (2008, p. 111) describes a needs and strengths assessment as being 'to help the community effectively declare what it needs, so these needs will be considered important enough to be met, and discover and build its resources, so the community can act to strengthen itself'. Homan suggests that the kinds of questions a needs assessment addresses are: 'What's not here that should be here' or 'What's not happening that should be happening?' (2008, p. 113).

Needs and strengths assessments must build 'a comprehensive picture of conditions' (Moore 2009). They should be conducted regularly and broadly based so that the information collected can be used to determine community and service priorities, to apply for funding from various sources, and as a basis for evaluating services or interventions. There are two parts to the process of assessment. *Needs and strengths identification* is a process of identifying health and social service requirements in a geographic and social arena, and the resources already present about which the community may not be aware, whereas *needs and strengths analysis* is a process of synthesising the information you collect and then prioritising the identified needs and actions that are to follow. This includes deciding how the community's identified resources and strengths can be used to help address the needs or resolve issues. Thus there is a two-stage process where we (in partnership with the community or group) identify needs and strengths and then make value judgements about which actions will be prioritised, or which needs will be addressed first.

What is needs and strengths identification and analysis?

Needs and strengths identification is a two-stage process involving:

- collecting information about the needs and resources of a community in order to improve community well-being and address disadvantage
- analysing the information and determining priorities for action.

What do we mean by needs and strengths?

To adequately identify and assess need, we must understand what it is we mean by need, and be aware that this will differ depending on who is defining need. The classic typology developed by Bradshaw (1977) is important in any discussion and definition of needs because it establishes that there is more than one kind of need. Bradshaw describes four types of need: *normative need*, which is the standard or expected need defined by professionals or others in authority; *felt need*, which is the 'wish list' of the target group and which equates with want; *expressed need*, which is the need of the target population expressed overtly in some form (for example, waiting lists for services); and *comparative need*, which is the need of the community or group determined through comparison with other communities or similar groups or national or state norms.

As you can see from this typology, need can be defined differently by professionals/experts (normative and comparative) and by the community (felt and expressed). In the years since Bradshaw developed his classic typology, writers have developed different compressed versions (e.g. see McArdle 1998; Brueggemann 2006). However you define needs, it is important that you take into account the various kinds of need and that you don't rely on just one type. Expert opinion may be misleading because it is not based on lived experience and is limited by the perspective of the expert. However, it may provide a broader view of need. Community opinion, on the other hand, will be grounded in experience but may also be unrealistic. In any needs analysis project, you should incorporate the different levels of need. Your ultimate aim is to work towards a *convergent needs analysis*, which is a comprehensive assessment of different types of need, based on the perspectives of as comprehensive a range of the stakeholders in a community as possible.

Just as there are many approaches to defining needs, there are different ways of defining strengths. Kretzmann and McKnight's (1993) process of mapping community assets focuses on three key levels: gifts of individuals, citizens' associations and local institutions (described in Sullivan and Rapp, 2009). Typically, strengths assessments focus on auditing community capital. Healy (2006) lists five types of capital: *human capital*, the skills and capacities of individual community members; *social capital*, the networks and local organisations in which people collaborate to achieve common goals; *financial or economic capital*, the money and credit sources available to the community; *physical capital*, the buildings, roads and housing that might be useful; and *environmental capital*, natural resources such as rivers, mountains, clean air or open spaces that might attract tourists or be useful for the community. To this list Homan (2008) adds *human development capital*, the ability to recognise and develop talents and skills; *political capital*, including decision-making and policy structure; *information and communication capital*, local information and communication strategies and resources; *cultural capital*, the arts and music, identity and emotion expressed in rituals and traditions; and *spiritual capital*, including how the need for meaning and connectedness is expressed, how religious groups cooperate, and how spirituality is valued and expressed in the community.

Why do we conduct a needs and strengths assessment?

Needs and strengths assessments are undertaken for a number of reasons:

- to empower the community to seek action by providing a 'snapshot' of the community's needs
- to determine whether services exist in the community and who uses them
- to find out whether a new intervention is needed
- to allow us to advocate for change and provide information about gaps in service
- to determine what barriers to service use exist
- to find out whether existing informal resources are adequate
- to justify an action we wish to take
- to identify and mobilise community resources (adapted from Homan 2008; Dudley 2010; Marlow 2011).

A comprehensive needs and strengths assessment allows us to work for change, secure in the knowledge that we are working with the community's priorities and towards its sustainability. If the motivation for conducting the analysis has been to support or promote a political cause, or the agenda of some organisation, rather than the priorities and expressed needs of the community members themselves, then you should re-examine your motivation. It can also be very tempting to 'prove' a need just because the funding for some service is available. Be wary of such dubious reasons for conducting a needs analysis—tempting though they can be.

Before you begin

Because there is no set formula or guide to conducting a needs and strengths analysis, you must start with basic issues in order to establish what it is you wish to know and the most feasible way to gather that information. We have already established that before you start you must clarify the values and purposes driving the assessment. Several other issues also need to be addressed before you begin.

Your design necessarily is constrained by the resources available to you (including your time), so your methods of gathering information must fit the available funds and other resources. Determine what resources are available to you before you design your analysis. With community involvement in your project, you may be able to count on extra resourcing and help. Your first task should be to draw together a steering committee or reference group (as discussed in Chapter 2) which represents the community first and foremost, as well as service providers and funding bodies. Strengths-based approaches in particular emphasise gathering people together who don't usually talk to each other, such as representatives of funding bodies and local people who are usually the recipients of services.

The critical point is that the strongest voices on this group should come from the community with whom the assessment is being conducted. It is important that the community 'owns' the data produced in the needs and strengths analysis process. This committee should decide early what it wants to know and why, and what will become of the data.

Before you design your needs and strengths analysis, you need to know exactly what the community is that you are assessing. Clear definitions are essential. Normative data about population characteristics such as from Census records and other sources like local government websites will be helpful. You will need to assess available services—the criteria for clients to be accepted, service capacities and whether the services are locally relevant. Social plans done by local government authorities are excellent places to begin your data collection. Seek advice from others about the important issues and identify existing community strengths. This inventory of resources allows you to analyse the services currently available to the target population, who is providing them, which services are under-utilised and where gaps exist.

When you conduct a needs and strengths analysis, it is important that you assess the problem in question carefully before trying to determine solutions. A lack of services for the aged or the disabled does not necessarily imply a need for more residential nursing homes. Similarly, a lack of services for carers of HIV/AIDS sufferers may not necessarily call for more respite services. What you should do is determine what services would *best* afford the frail aged, the disabled and carers an improved quality of life, and what hidden resources already exist in the community, waiting to be discovered and brought into play to address the issue, as well as what resources can be brought in from outside the community.

Ethical considerations must be acknowledged before you begin your analysis. These might include the need to ensure confidentiality for participants and the need to gain permission from agencies to examine client records if these are to be used for gathering information. In most agencies or departments, you will be required to submit your needs analysis proposal to the research ethics committee for approval. Your research plan should be comprehensive, taking account of resource and time restrictions. Consequently, it will include a detailed timeline that allows the steering committee and the community to understand the time commitment expected and the approximate time when findings will be released. It will also include an outline of methods and a list of responsibilities of staff and project personnel. The final step before you begin gathering data is to conduct a detailed literature review to ascertain what information is already available, where other studies have been undertaken and how these results might influence your study.

Before you begin

- Determine what resources (time, staff and funding) are available.
- Define the community whose needs you are documenting.
- Establish a steering committee that is representative of most groups in the community.
- Identify the range of needs you will explore.
- Be conscious of ethical concerns.
- Submit a proposal to the ethics committee.
- Draw up a research plan (including a timeline).
- Conduct a literature review.

Case study 8.1: Asset-focused health needs assessment in rural India

Lady Willmingdon Hospital (LWH), is a surgical mission hospital and Indian not-for-profit organisation that has operated for more than 70 years in Kullu district, Himachal Pradesh, India. It was invited to construct and open a rural clinic 100 kilometres away in a small village called Jibhi, on land donated by the community. In 2006, project co-leaders JM and KM were appointed to start a community health program, the Jibhi Community Health Action Initiative (Jibhi CHAI).

They formed a steering group (membership not stated), developed a mission statement, and agreed on values, methods, objectives and an implementation plan. KM and JM, who lived locally, were committed to having the community actively involved in defining problems and strengths, and in designing genuinely community-based responses. The project combined elements of rapid participatory appraisal, which emphasises community participation and assessment of assets, with health needs assessment methodology, which assesses formally defined deficits. The principles from these approaches that guided the project were clearly set out in a table.

The community requested active participation in the assessment. Key ethical concepts included informed consent, sharing of findings with participants and active participation by the community. While this was not a formal research project, and so did not need written ethics permission, verbal consent was obtained from representatives of community groups for participation, use of the findings generated and publication.

The community was clearly defined as being Jibhi.

Source: Mathias, Mathias and Hill (2011).

Case study 8.2: Urban Indian voices—community-based participatory research health and needs assessment

The Indian Health Care Resource Center of Tulsa (IHCRC) in Oklahoma, USA is a non-profit, comprehensive health-care facility offering culturally sensitive health services, including mental health, to the American Indian population in Tulsa. In 2005, it received funding to undertake a needs assessment as part of a project designed to expand and develop comprehensive and culturally appropriate mental health services for the American Indian community. Staff from IHCRC joined with the University of Oklahoma–Tulsa for this project.

The first step was to create a community advisory board to provide input on the research purpose, design, methodology, instrument development and results. The community advisory board included tribal elders and leaders, youth, parents, IHCRC staff and board members and other members of the local community, such as police, teachers, social workers and religious leaders. The advisory board met monthly and was open to the public. Meetings were advertised in a variety of local media. Between fifteen and 35 people attended the meetings.

Ethics approval for the project was gained through the University of Oklahoma.

Source: Johnson et al. (2010).

Conducting a needs and strengths analysis

When devising a plan to conduct a needs and strengths analysis, you would do well to revisit Bradshaw's (1977) typology of needs discussed earlier in this chapter. In any assessment of need, we should attempt to examine normative, felt, expressed and comparative levels of need. This is a form of triangulation that brings together different kinds of information and increases the rigour of our research. Similarly, it is important to collect comprehensive data on the various forms of capital to identify the community's strengths. If we neglect any significant area, our results will not provide a comprehensive analysis. This section will examine methods of gathering information under three different groupings: *social indicators analysis, surveys* and *community group approaches*.

Social indicator analysis

In order to understand the nature of your community, social indicators are used to provide an overall picture of the population, its characteristics, the size of the community in relation to the general population, the size of the potential at-risk categories and, consequently, the potential service users. Social indicators, which are available at the local, state and national levels, can also be used to investigate historical trends and population changes. The most accessible form of social indicator is the national Census records, which can be broken down to regional level to reveal demographic details such as age composition, ethnicity, gender, occupation, income levels, education, marital status and religion. Other types of accessible records include police crime and local court statistics, Bureau of Statistics information on special groups, Health Department indicators, local government social plans and other government statistics. Government departments at the local, state and national levels have records and reports containing vast amounts of quantitative information that may assist you to develop an understanding of the nature of your target group. Social indicators are a useful first step in analysing your community, and in identifying characteristics of the target population. This data can be used to determine risk factors within your group that may provide a preliminary indication of the potential use of services at the local level. For example, if your service deals with young people aged under 18 who are unemployed, social indicator analysis of Census material will give you the size of this target population in your community. Members of this group are all potential users of your service.

Social indicator analysis can also be used to compare regions or communities with others to determine area variations and target group variations. This information is useful when comparing different levels of services and support available. While social indicators provide valuable background research information, you should note that such information should be carefully scrutinised for reliability and validity. Census material that is collected every five years may quickly become dated—particularly if your community has a high transient population. Also be aware that people may not be entirely accurate with the information they provide. On examination of Census data from an isolated rural area of Australia, Margaret Alston noted that 6 per cent of the population had claimed that they travelled to work each day by tram. As the nearest tram was 500 kilometres away, we realised that much of the data should be treated with caution! Be cognisant of the purposes for which the data you are examining was collected. This may influence what is reported and, more importantly, what is not. Be cautious if you are relying on this information to tell you whether there are enough clients for a potential new service. You should also note that social indicator analysis helps you outline the problems in a community but does nothing to assist with the development of solutions.

Case studies 8.1 and 8.2

Both the mental health needs assessment conducted in Tulsa, Oklahoma, with an urban American Indian community and the rural needs assessment undertaken in Northern India used detailed social indicator analysis to introduce their research, establish the context and parameters of the communities and outline the key issues and problems faced by these communities. These studies also used social indicator information to compare the communities being studied with other groups in the wider society.

In their analysis of findings, both studies compared the data from their own needs and strengths assessments with information from social indicators. For example, where possible the Jibhi CHAI project compared official social indicator statistics from various Indian government sources and websites, and sources such as World Vision surveys with information gathered from local services including the government primary health centre, *panchayat* secretaries, Banjar hospital and local health services, as well as with the data they obtained from informant interviews and group meetings.

Sources: Johnson et al. (2010); Mathias, Mathias and Hill (2011).

Social indicator analysis

Sources

Census, government departments (national, state and local), police and court records.

Outlines

- Population characteristics
- Target group size
- Characteristics of target group
- Comparisons between regions and communities
- Historical trends
- Size of potential service users

Surveys

Surveys are used to determine felt and expressed levels of need. These techniques are useful for estimating which of a range of possible solutions or services may be the most appropriate. They do this by providing information on people's opinions, priorities and ideas around strengths. Surveys can include an analysis of the demand for services, an examination of the resourcing of existing services and a study of the experiences of people who use the services. It is important to get the community involved in the steering committee to identify what kinds of questions should be asked and which areas explored.

Community surveys

Community surveys will elicit information about *felt* needs and about ongoing social problems as well as community perceptions of strengths. These surveys may be either random community surveys or surveys targeted specifically at an identified target group, and are designed to determine the level of need and ideas about resources. Community surveys may be conducted as mail surveys, personally administered surveys or via interview. In each case, you will need to carefully select a representative sample of the target group. Re-read Chapter 5 on sampling and Chapter 7 on surveys and interviews before you conduct a community survey.

Analysis of service resources

While community surveys identify felt need, surveys of services explore expressed need. It is important to examine the range of existing services to ascertain what services exist; existing service use; services that are popular; the level of inter-agency cooperation; where there is any overlapping of services; and gaps in service delivery. This information is best gathered from service providers, management committee members and agency records that may reveal historical trends in service use. Such data may be collected by interview or survey with agency personnel. If it is detailed and comprehensive enough, and used in conjunction with other assessments of need, this information can form a basis for assessing the effectiveness of current services.

Barriers

Surveys elicit information about the demand for, and extent of, services and the level of felt need in the community. When compared with data from social indicator analysis, this information may reveal discrepancies between the potential and actual service users. Consider Table 8.1, which outlines the service users of our fictitious family services program and compares these data with population statistics.

Table 8.1 Client users of family services program

	Clients	Census population (%)
Clients using the service during a twelve-month period	783	
Female clients	564 (72%)	51
Clients from non-English-speaking backgrounds	32 (4%)	28
Indigenous clients	25 (3%)	19
Low-income clients	595 (76%)	28
Aged clients	89 (11%)	15

You will note from the table that the client base of the service is skewed towards women from low-income families. By comparison with the population statistics, the service is not good at reaching Indigenous clients, clients from non-English-speaking backgrounds and aged people. As a result of this information, you may wish to examine the barriers preventing others from using the service. It may be that those on higher incomes do not realise they are eligible for assistance; there may be language barriers; or transport may be a problem, given the location of the service. The service may be too expensive and have long delays, making it less desirable. Additional problems may be the times and availability of the service, a lack of awareness that the service exists and even a lack of acceptability of the service because of its philosophy or service delivery style. This type of information is important for assessing who uses the service and in alerting you to potential barriers to service use.

Of course, you should also directly seek information from the community about the barriers as its members perceive and experience them. In any case, your needs analysis should isolate factors that are barriers to service accessibility.

Case study 8.2: Urban American Indian voices—community-based participatory research health and needs assessment

Five community-developed research questions guided this needs assessment:

- What do community members perceive as the greatest social/health problems facing American Indians in Tulsa?

- What wellness and social programs are desired?
- How connected and safe do American Indians feel in the community?
- What strengths does the Tulsa American Indian community possess?
- How do adults and youth differ in their perceptions of problems and needs?

The community advisory board, IHCRC staff and university staff worked together to develop a telephone script and two surveys— one for adults and one for youth (which was shorter). They reviewed existing surveys and needs assessments, and constructed original questions as proposed by community members. The surveys went through a number of revisions until all partners agreed on the content.

The surveys included information on physical and behavioural health, wellness, demographics, community services and supports. The surveys contained both Likert scales and open-ended questions, resulting in quantitative and qualitative data.

Participants were recruited in various ways: through letters of invitation, advertisements in the media, and in-person requests at various meetings and events. Surveys were conducted by interview, either by telephone or in person. As there is a lower than average rate of telephone and internet usage amongst American Indians, more interviews were conducted in person than originally planned.

Source: Johnson et al. (2010).

Surveys
- Community surveys identify felt needs and assets.
- Agency surveys explore expressed needs, demand for services and analysis of service resources.

Methods

Interviews or surveys with community residents, leaders and representatives of key groups in the community with agency personnel, management committee members, workers.

Aspects determined

- Felt needs
- Assets and resources

- Services available
- Service use
- Inter-agency cooperation
- Overlap of services
- Gaps in service delivery
- Agency profiles
- Barriers to service use

Community group approaches

Community group approaches are essential when identifying community strengths. They are also useful when a rapid appraisal of community need is necessary and/or resources are limited. Used in conjunction with the approaches already outlined, community group approaches can give a clearer idea of a community's priority of needs and strengths because they elicit qualitative information as opposed to the quantitative data gathered through previously discussed methods.

Community forums

Community forums are open meetings of community members called to discuss a particular issue or to map community assets. As a tool for needs and strengths analysis, a community forum provides an opportunity to gather information and to construct an inventory of community strengths. All community members are invited and meetings should be widely publicised to ensure a cross-section of the community is represented.

An assets audit consists of four steps (Healy 2006, p. 251):

- engaging the community
- constructing an inventory of community strengths
- gathering data and listening for strengths
- recognising strengths to create action.

Community forums to assess strengths can also be held as small focus groups, or any other type of group such as cultural groups. During the meetings, a strengths-focused researcher is searching for possible resources that can be turned into an inventory of available community capital. This can include different types of capital, such as:

- individuals, their skills and capacities (human capital)
- associations

- institutions
- physical characteristics (natural and human made)
- businesses (Central Coast Community Congress Working Party, 2003).

Whatever the size of the group, remember your group-work skills, and use these to help people feel confident to speak up, to prevent the silencing of less powerful members, to encourage respectful diversity of opinion and disagreement without personal attack, and to deal with conflict constructively. Group-work skills are just as important in working with research groups or meetings as they are for any other group of people.

Nominal groups

The nominal group approach was developed by Delbecq (Seigel, Attkisson and Carson 1987). It allows the generation and evaluation of ideas from group members while avoiding problems that may result from normal group processes. In this approach, a group of key informants (people with expertise and unique knowledge about a particular situation), clients and service providers is brought together to discuss problems and pose solutions. Nominal groups follow a highly structured format, which includes breaking initially into small groups of up to ten members. Each person is given a list of questions to which they must write responses during a silent period of ten to fifteen minutes. These questions might include ideas about service needs and community problems. Group leaders then record answers on a flip chart, with each participant giving one response in round-robin fashion until all ideas have been listed. Discussion is discouraged at this stage to ensure everyone's opinions are recorded.

A discussion period follows during which ideas are clarified, new ideas are added and others are combined. Participants are then asked to privately select five or more ideas of the highest priority. These are handed in and results tabulated on a display chart. In a needs analysis, the prioritised, identified needs provide a useful basis for program planning.

The nominal group method has proved a popular and useful technique for ranking needs among key stakeholders. Each member is assured that their ideas have been acknowledged and recorded.

Delphi panels

Delphi panels are a systematic, time- and cost-effective way of reaching consensus among a panel of selected key informants or experts. The group is chosen to reflect expert or key informant knowledge of a particular issue. In the case of needs analysis, the group would consist of experts, service personnel, clients and community representatives. A questionnaire is developed by the project team to gauge opinions on key issues such as service needs and use of services. The questionnaire is distributed to the Delphi panel for response. Returned questionnaires are tallied and redistributed with collated responses noted, and this process is continued until consensus is achieved and responses are no longer altered.

Delphi panels have the advantage of being quick and easy, of ensuring anonymity and of allowing consensus to develop through reasoned responses. They are a useful way of determining and ranking community need among key stakeholder groups.

Focus groups

As discussed in the previous chapter, focus groups are small, homogeneous groups that are representative of the target population and of key informants brought together to discuss pertinent issues. In needs analysis, focus groups are conducted to discuss community needs and priorities. Various focus group discussions, with ten to fifteen members, may be held with community members, with service providers, with target group members, with carers and with any other relevant group of stakeholders. The number of groups held depends on the issues and the degree of consensus achieved. Issues are recorded and collated, and the degree of convergence between groups is noted.

Case study 8.1: Asset-focused health needs assessment in rural India

The Jibhi CHAI project team's work lasted four months. The team consisted of five members, all of whom spoke Hindi and three of whom were community members. They conducted key informant interviews with 26 community members who represented a cross-section of decision-makers in health, health workers, business people, administrative bodies and community leaders. Jibhi CHAI team members also visited and observed health practices in a variety of health settings, and ran a number of community meetings. Findings were developed as the project completed its different phases, and these were fed back to team members and the Ghyagi women's and high school teachers' groups.

Team members attended local leadership groups and several women's groups, and organised community meetings in eight villages. These meetings were usually held in the village square and were facilitated by the local Jibhi CHAI team member. An introduction outlined the meeting's purpose, a broad definition of health, background information about the project, roles of the assessment team and hoped-for input from the community. The floor was then opened for discussion. At the end of each meeting, the results were summarised and reflected back to the people at the meeting, to clarify understanding and to further verify information.

Source: Mathias, Mathias and Hill (2011).

Community group approaches

- Community forums
- Nominal groups
- Delphi panels
- Focus groups

Convergent analysis

Each of the methods of gathering data about community needs and strengths discussed in this chapter is an important technique by itself. However, they all focus on a particular aspect of need or resource, and hence have some inherent bias. For example, demand for service analysis will determine the expressed community need while a focus group with service providers may determine normative need. To improve the comprehensiveness of your needs and strengths analysis, and to achieve a convergent analysis, you should consider using multiple methods or triangulation. Triangulation involves the use of more than one method to increase the validity of results and to synthesise results from different sources. Of course, although the use of multiple methods is inhibited by time and cost constraints, you should endeavour to ensure that your methods have determined the normative, felt, expressed and comparative needs of your community, as well as the strengths (including previously unnoticed resources) that the community possesses. Locating untapped potential is an inspiring experience for communities, as is working out that some of the answers to entrenched problems may lie within the community. Convergent analysis ensures that you have gathered information from a variety of sources and from various levels of government, community and services personnel. As Homan (2008, p. 11) points out: 'A needs assessment can help give you an issue focus; a resource or asset assessment gives you the energy.'

Case study 8.1: Asset-focused health needs assessment in rural India

Data analysis and results: Setting priorities

Information from the meetings and informant interviews was grouped into themes and tallied. Ranked themes were re-presented to a women's meeting and a high school teachers' meeting for verification. Both groups supported the lists and rankings as representing their felt needs. The team also sought to triangulate the data by cross-checking it with different informants, and verifying information from different sources.

Once the eight key problems that had been identified were ranked, they were matched against organisational capacity, and also community assets and resources, that had been identified. The resulting matrix became the basis for developing a two-year pilot program in community nutrition.

With the information from social indicators and organisations, the researchers drew a comprehensive picture of the community, its environment, and normative, comparative and expressed health needs. They were surprised to find a strong alignment in the eight ranked felt needs discussed by key informants and at the community group meetings. Once a convergent needs and strengths analysis was complete, priorities were set.

Comprehensive primary care was the highest felt need. Not wanting to replicate government services, the Jibhi CHAI project used the community assets it had found (educated, young, unmarried village women and good mobile phone coverage) to train young women as community health-care workers with mobile phone back-up to the doctors at the centre. Among other initiatives, they also trained women as nutrition promoters, and formed a village street theatre team to promote health messages.

The authors concluded that unexpectedly, by using a wider definition and involving the community as partners, the community became empowered to use its own assets to address health issues. For example, it became aware that children were under-nourished and that young women could be great health assets.

Limitations and conclusions

Three limitations were identified in this study:
- The community was not included in the design and analysis of the assessment, as was preferred, and a wider cross-section of community members could have been included.

- The more powerless sub-communities, such as the Dalits, were not included.
- The poor quality of health data and information was limiting.

The authors concluded that the flexibility was suited to this situation of limited resources and a small team, and that notwithstanding the limitations, this methodology was 'an empowering development tool that puts health within the community's reach, using their own assets'.

Source: Matthias, Matthias and Hill (2011).

Summary

This chapter has examined the processes of needs and strengths identification and analysis by focusing on the typology of need developed by Bradshaw (1977) and strengths or community assets mapping initially developed by Kretzmann and McKnight (1993) to determine the type of information required to ensure that a comprehensive needs and strengths assessment is conducted.

Critical things to remember when undertaking a community assessment are, first, to clarify the values behind the research and to be able to answer the following questions: Who is the assessment for? What is its purpose? Who is defining the needs and strengths? Ensuring that the community is an active and respected partner in the assessment process, and that strengths as well as needs are included, will help ensure that your assessment is a useful and constructive activity.

Three types of analysis—social indicator, surveys and community groups approaches, each incorporating a number of methods—have been discussed. It is important in any community assessment to work towards a convergent analysis of the community's needs and strengths.

Discussion questions

8.1 What is a needs and strengths assessment?
8.2 Why would you conduct a needs and strengths analysis?
8.3 What issues need to be addressed before you begin your community assessment?

8.4   What are the four levels of need identified by Bradshaw (1977)?

8.5   What are the three approaches to needs analysis discussed in this chapter?

8.6   What are the key features of a community strengths audit?

8.7   What is a social indicator analysis and what information does it provide?

8.8   What are the different types of surveys discussed, and what are the types of needs and strengths about which they elicit information?

8.9   What are community group approaches? Describe a situation where this would be an appropriate method to assess needs and strengths.

8.10   What is convergent analysis and why is it important?

8.11   What ethical considerations are important in a community assessment?

Exercises

8.1   Examine the needs and assets analysis conducted in rural India and discussed in this chapter. How might the methods, data collection and recommendations have been different if they had involved a steering committee representing key community members?

8.2   Download from your library online journal collection the needs assessment from Tulsa, Oklahoma that was Case study 8.2 in this chapter (Johnson et al. 2010). How were the strengths that were identified used in this analysis? How could they have been used? What were the main conclusions from this study? How does the methodology used in this US study compare with the methodology used in the study of Northern India?

8.3   Go to the library and find another journal article that describes a needs and strengths analysis. Examine the methods used, the process undertaken and the final recommendations. Has the researcher used appropriate methods, and are the recommendations well grounded in the data? Were community assets considered? What might have been done to improve the study?

Further reading

Homan, M.S. 2008, *Promoting Community Change: Making It Happen in the Real World*, 4th edn, Thomson Brooks/Cole, Sydney. Chapter 5, 'Knowing your community', explains how to undertake a combined strengths and needs assessment.

Marlow, C. 2011, *Research Methods for Generalist Social Work*, 5th edn, Brooks/Cole, Sydney. Chapter 5, 'Designing needs assessments', covers needs assessments extensively, but does not include strengths assessments.

Tutty, L.M. and Rothery, M. 2010, 'Needs assessments' in B. Thyer (ed.), *The Handbook of Social Work Research Methods*, Sage, Thousand Oaks, CA. This chapter extensively covers needs assessments but does not include strengths assessments.

The internet has a wealth of downloadable 'How to' guides for conducting community needs and strengths assessments. For example:

- Australian Institute of Community Practice and Government (AICPG) Help Sheets: *Conducting a Community Needs Assessment*, <www.ourcommunity.com.au/management/view_help_sheet.do?articleid=10>.
- Australian Institute of Community Practice and Government (AICPG) Help Sheet: *Auditing Your Community Assets*, www.ourcommunity.com.au/management/view_help_sheet.do?articleid=9.
- Moore, P. 2009, *Community Needs Assessment Toolkit*, Missouri Association for Community Action, http://scholar.googleusercontent.com/scholar?q=cache:jnBKDEsvLoIJ:scholar.google.com/+community+needs+assessment+toolkit&hl=en&as_sdt=0,5.

PART III

Evaluation

9 How do I evaluate my program?

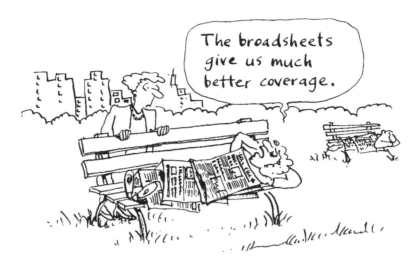

Evaluation and accountability have always been important concepts for social workers. Handled well, program evaluation gives us the means to develop techniques for ensuring our practice is enhanced and effective, and allows us to incorporate accountability and transparency into what we do. Program evaluation can help us to think retrospectively about how things have gone, as well as to plan ahead for how we want things to be.

Evaluation increasingly is becoming a requirement for ongoing funding of programs and services (Carson, Chung and Day 2009; Sullivan 2011). Not only are evaluations required from existing services, but a proposal for a new service is unlikely to be funded unless you have included an evaluation strategy (O'Leary 2010). Evaluation is a highly political activity (Dudley 2010), which can be seen as a tool of the funding bodies and policy-makers who follow an 'economic rationalist' or neo-liberal' agenda. This agenda emphasises so-called economic efficiency over other goals such as social justice, access and equity: 'It's said that all research is political, but none more so than evaluative research.' (O'Leary 2010, p. 141)

This chapter is designed to assist you to become familiar with ways and means of assessing your programs in order to determine whether they are effectively targeted, whether they are being conducted successfully, whether they are achieving quality outcomes and, finally, whether they provide an adequate cost–benefit ratio. The chapter will equip you with skills to enable you to produce the program evaluations required by your agency, department, funding body, community or client base, as well as to enable you to critically assess evaluations conducted by external evaluators.

Why do we do program evaluations?

Program evaluations are conducted for a variety of reasons, particularly the need to be accountable for our service and our practice. This need is driven both by the requirements of program and service funders for responsible spending and streamlined service, and by an increasingly powerful consumer movement that demands adequate services and accountable providers. While some of the motivation for our acquisition of evaluation skills has come from outside the profession, much has come from social work's desire to deliver high-quality responsive services in the most appropriate way.

We conduct program evaluations to improve the efficiency of our service and to cut out any overlapping programs. This need for efficiency of service provision can only have positive benefits for practitioners, who become more aware of the programs on offer, and for clients, who are assured of a more professional service.

Program evaluation also assists us to plan more effectively, and allows us to develop programs on the basis of a well-documented need for services. It is a valuable tool for improving existing programs in response to careful assessment of the delivery of and responses to our service.

Evaluation should be embedded in your daily practice, and not left to an annual review of your programs. Ideally, evaluation should include both qualitative and quantitative methodologies, and involve the perspectives of all the people involved—especially the service users or clients, who normally have the least power in decision-making about service directions. Dullea and Mullender (1999, p. 96) exhort us to empower our clients through our evaluation practices: 'There is no excuse for not seeing people as the experts in their own lives.'

Why we do program evaluations
- Accountability
- Efficiency

- Planning
- Development of appropriate programs
- Improvement of existing programs
- To maintain or increase funding

What is program evaluation?

Program evaluation is defined by Yegidis and Weinbach (2009, p. 286) as 'the application of both quantitative and qualitative research methods to evaluate the merit, worth or value of a program'. Both Wadsworth (2011b) and O'Leary (2010) emphasise the notion of value in their definitions. For example, Wadsworth (2011b, p. 14) writes: 'To "do an evaluation" is actually to do a piece of research or inquiry, but with the focus or emphasis on finding out what *value* people place on things.' Program evaluation is applied research that is designed not to uncover theoretical relationships, but rather to focus on and improve human service delivery. Dudley (2010) distinguishes between *program evaluation*—which is research into social programs to determine whether they are needed, working well and/or are effective—and *practice evaluation*—which is research into a practitioner's interventions. We explore practice evaluation in Chapter 11.

Before you begin

Before you being an evaluation, there are some fundamental questions you need to address.

Why evaluate?

The first question to answer is *why* an evaluation is being done. Clarifying the fundamental purpose is an essential task before you begin any evaluation (Wadsworth 2011b). What do you want to happen as a result of this evaluation? What key issues are you addressing?

Part of clarifying the fundamental purpose is to identify *who* the evaluation is for—which group of people it will benefit. Wadsworth (2011b) terms this group the 'critical reference group'. These are the people whose needs the program is intended to address, who make the final judgement about whether the program 'got it right' and whose voices are fundamental to any evaluation. Clarifying who constitutes the critical reference group is an important part of determining the purpose of an evaluation.

Who is involved?

Once you have determined the purpose of the evaluation and who it is for, it is important to ascertain who is involved and what is at stake for each party. If you are conducting an evaluation, be sure to include all stakeholders from the beginning. Wadsworth (2011b, p. 24) lists four conceptual groups of stakeholders that have to be taken into account in any evaluation:

- those who the evaluation is for (the critical reference group)
- the evaluator/s
- the evaluated
- others who the evaluation is also for (including service providers, funders, staff and others who act for the critical reference group or who provide the program).

These groups can all overlap, but it is important to think about each of them when you are conceptualising your evaluation. Whose interests will the evaluation serve, and whose perspectives will be taken into account? Is this evaluation from the funding body's perspective only? From that of the clients who use the agency? From the viewpoint of the critical reference group more generally? From that of the agency and its staff? Some combination of these? Answering these questions is the first step in coming to terms with the politics that inevitably surround evaluations.

As mentioned in earlier chapters, a steering committee with members drawn from the funding body, the staff, management and the critical reference group is one strategy to keep stakeholders informed about and involved in the evaluation. There is potential for conflict between the evaluators and the staff because staff may see their positions as being under threat and their work as being scrutinised. If this is the case, they may be inclined to withhold information or be circumspect about the information that is given. Similarly, clients of a service may fear the loss of the service if they voice complaints, and so are reluctant to criticise it. A steering committee can act as a communication channel about the evaluation between you and other parts of the organisation and service user groups, and help to dispel doubts and fears about the process. It will also ensure that all people affected by the evaluation have a voice in it. Plan the steps in the evaluation process in advance (see chapter 4) so that you have agreement about what is happening and clarity about the aims of the evaluation. Other basic questions that need to be addressed are discussed below in the section on planning the evaluation.

Be sensitive to the ethical and political implications

Even this early discussion should alert you to how politically sensitive, how value laden, an evaluation can be. Before you begin any evaluation you need to be comfortable that the purposes and processes are ethical and worthwhile. Once you have decided to go ahead, it is important to identify the ethical and political issues that might arise during the evaluation, and to develop strategies to keep the evaluation on track.

From the outset, if you are the evaluator it is important to state clearly your role in relation to the funding body, clarify the data you require and how this is to be disseminated, and set up an ongoing consultation process with staff. Negotiate with the staff for access to their files and any other data you require, and be clear about who owns the final report. At all stages of the evaluation process, give brief reports to staff and discuss your interim findings. If changes are called for, decide how this might proceed in consultation with staff.

Internal or external evaluations?

Whether an evaluation is conducted by an internal or external evaluator is a matter for the agency, but the following points should be noted. Evaluations conducted internally within the agency or service have the benefits of saving time, reducing costs, allowing change to be implemented effectively and allowing staff to 'own' the data. As well, an internal evaluator knows intimately the organisational culture that affects the program's success or failure. The disadvantages of internal evaluation include the fact that the evaluation may not be objective, it may brush over problems and it may be considered less valid by outside agencies such as the funding body (Logan and Royse 2010). While external evaluators may be considered less biased, they are likely to be viewed as 'outsiders' by agency staff. This can cause problems if the staff are unwilling to cooperate. External evaluations may also contain bias. Consider, for example, a case where the evaluator is seeking to maintain good relations with the funder of the research in order to secure further contracts.

Before you begin

Before you begin an evaluation, it is important to establish the following:
- What is the purpose? Who is it for?
- Who are the key stakeholders?
- What are the ethical and political implications?
- Is this an internal or external evaluation?

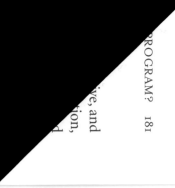

ng an evaluation

ion, there are four stages that you must go through: e information, analysing the data and reporting your are part of a continuous evaluation cycle. When eval- am processes, findings can be used to make changes ins again.

Planning

During the planning stage, work to develop stakeholder cooperation and set up your steering committee. The two key questions about purposes and who the evaluation is for will guide other questions in the planning phase. These include: What type of evaluation are you doing? What level of information is required? How will you gather your data? What data do you require and who is able to give them to you? How will you analyse the data and how will they be reported? To whom will the report be distributed and what are the interests of the key stakeholders in this report? What resources are available to you for the evaluation and how much will it cost?

Finally, and most importantly, you must work through the ethical issues involved in the evaluation, discussed above. Practical ethical issues include: Is there an ethics committee to which you must report? How will you ensure client confidentiality? Are you able to examine client records? Your planning stage allows you to negotiate these issues and to overcome any constraints that may affect your service evaluation.

Data collection

During the data-collection phase, decide the ideal ways to gather the data. Appropriate methods include interviewing or surveying key workers, clients and/or target groups, examining records, and observing work practices and intervention strategies. They might also include negotiating access to the records of other similar organisations.

A combination of qualitative and quantitative methods may prove to be the most effective way of gathering the data. Whatever you choose to do, bear in mind what the objectives of your evaluation are, and determine the best ways to gather the data that will meet these objectives.

Analysing the data

Various methods to analyse your data are discussed in Chapters 14, 15, 16 and 17. Your task is to organise and display your data in an easily interpreted presentation that will be useful for the people for whom the evaluation was done. Your findings and recommendations should be constructed around the fundamental purposes and goals of the evaluation.

Reporting your findings

An integral aspect of your evaluation is the way you produce your findings, as well as how quickly this can be achieved and to whom the information is disseminated. Remember that any research report is politically sensitive, and you must ensure that the information is easily accessed by key stakeholders. Your report should provide practical and useful feedback about the program strengths and weaknesses, as well as providing information about next steps (Logan and Royse 2010).

Stages in an evaluation

- Planning
- Data collection
- Data analysis
- Reporting the findings

Types of evaluation

Program evaluation techniques can be used to assess a program, a service, an agency or even over-arching policies. There are many types of program evaluation (e.g. see Wadsworth 2011b, pp. 130–206). In this introduction to research, we discuss five types. You have already learned about needs assessment in the previous chapter; as we noted, this may be the first stage of a program evaluation, leading to the development of a new program. Further types of program evaluation to be covered in this chapter are evaluability assessment, process analysis, outcome analysis and cost–benefit analysis.

These 'types' of evaluation are not discrete frameworks, although in the past they were considered to be quite distinct. For example, outcome evaluation was strictly concerned with whether a program 'worked', and only looked at outcomes. How the program got to these outcomes was a 'black box' that was the domain of a different type of evaluation: process evaluation (Engel and Schutt 2010b, pp. 274–5). These days, evaluations may include aspects of all five types, with the different types being incorporated into different phases of the evaluation cycle.

Types of program evaluation
- Needs analysis
- Evaluability assessment
- Process evaluation
- Outcome evaluation
- Cost–benefit analysis

Evaluability assessment

Evaluability assessments are carried out to determine whether, in fact, a program has been developed in such a way that it can be evaluated (Owen 1993). It requires 'an intense analysis of the program' by evaluators and all the stakeholders in the program. This usually involves reviewing program documents, conducting site visits and interviewing program clients, staff and managers (Hall 2008, p. 132).

Sometimes services develop in an ad hoc way with a poor conceptualisation of the objectives of the service and an equally poor framework for assessing outcomes. Such services are noted by a lack of clarity of objectives, by a failure to define key concepts clearly and by a lack of standardisation of treatment. For example, Carson, Chung and Day (2009) raise many questions about whether it is possible to evaluate domestic violence programs in Australia with a systematic, macro-level approach, given the complexities and differences in the way community-based domestic violence services operate. This is in spite of similar funding and evaluation requirements from the joint Commonwealth, states and territories Partnerships Against Domestic Violence Program, under which all the programs are funded. In particular, they highlight the difficulties inherent in evaluating outcomes, when the contexts within which each program operates can be so diverse. If programs are responsive to their environments, they are likely to be quite different, so outcomes are difficult to compare and contrast. Even aspects of the programs that were supposed to have been standardised, such as assessment procedures of perpetrators, and practices associated with adherence to the Duluth model, were not consistent or failed to provide enough data to enable evaluation.

Management structures that are not delineated clearly can also lead to ad hoc service delivery. Agencies must clearly outline their management process to ensure the funding body and workers are clear about who has responsibility for delivering the proposed service. Roles need to be defined so that accountability is assured.

Case study 9.1: Evaluability assessment of the Rape Prevention and Education Program

In the United States, the Center for Disease Control and Prevention (CDC) took over from another department to provide national leadership on sexual violence prevention by supporting Rape Prevention and Education (RPE) programs in all states and territories of the United States. PRE programs aim to raise awareness about and prevent sexual violence through educational programs, information, hotline operations and programs with target populations, such as youth and people with disabilities. The CDC wanted to establish a baseline understanding of the current activities and goals of the program, revisiting and updating program performance measures and identifying opportunities to provide training and assistance.

Three goals for the evaluability assessment were set:

- documenting goals and objectives of the RPE grant program
- assessing use of funds within states/territories
- assessing aids, barriers and needs in relation to implementing RPE grant.

Methodology included a web-based survey sent to all state Departments of Health and other state agencies to gain the perspectives of all states and territories, then site visits to a sample of fourteen states, at which in-depth face-to-face interviews were conducted with staff from these organisations. Focus groups were held in five of these sites with RPE providers.

Findings were reported against the goals of the study.

Goals

Across all sources, it was concluded that the perceived goal of all RPE programs was to reduce and prevent rape and sexual assault, primarily through funding educational and awareness-raising activities. However, there were high levels of variation in understanding what the goal meant, and how it should be implemented. Program strengths were identified, including the availability of specific funding for prevention of sexual violence, the high level of accessibility of CDC and other critical stakeholders and the ability to increase program capacity through partnerships.

Use of funds

Funds were used primarily for educational programs and informational material. The study detailed what groups were serviced by RPE programs and what activities were undertaken. One finding was that evaluation was not done very well across the sector.

Aids, barriers, needs

The strongest barrier to the RPE programs was community sensitivity around sexual violence. Other barriers included the political environment in the states, and access to and quality of data. The strongest aid was collaboration with other community-based agencies. A list of training needs was also identified.

An important finding was that many respondents suggested that CDC should no longer collect statistics incidence of rape and attempted rape, as definitions varied so widely, and as the statistics were so unreliable due to the high level of non-disclosure. Instead, they suggested collecting data on prevention programs and their effectiveness, as well as on the curricula of the prevention programs.

Recommendations included changing the reporting requirements for RPE staff so there were not so many duplications in reporting requirements, and making information about the wider context within which the services operate available for planning and evaluation purposes. More training and technical resources were also recommended, to build capacity for evaluation amongst other things. It was recommended that core practice components of the program be identified, to enable better evaluation. A strategic planning process was introduced, and there was more funding to develop modules on sexual violence and intimate partner violence, and for 'empowerment evaluation'.

Source: Basile et al. (2005).

How do we conduct an evaluability assessment?

In conducting an evaluability assessment, it is important to observe the day-to-day functioning of the agency program or service in order to determine what the agency objectives appear to be, and what the desired client outcomes are. You should also note the structure of the agency and the responsibilities of various agency personnel. This early observation is an important first step in your evaluation of the program. Further, you should be clear about the program's boundaries. For example, in Case study 9.1, the evaluators were careful to distinguish departments of health from the specially designated RPE staff and RPE's own discrete program objectives. The boundaries of your assessment should not stray beyond the service itself.

Your next step involves analysing the policy and procedural documents, mission statements, management structure agreements and any other relevant program documents to allow you to assess whether what is being undertaken within the agency is what originally was intended. Sometimes confusion results from the different perceptions of management and staff about the intended program outcomes, as was revealed in Case study 9.1. Involving program staff in the evaluation process allows you to develop a model of the link between program objectives and the program as it is implemented.

The next stage of the evaluability assessment is interviewing key stakeholders about their perceptions of the program's objectives. You should endeavour to interview not only staff, but also members of the funding organisation and clients (see Case study 9.1, for example). These interviews allow you to assess whether the key stakeholders view the program in the same way. Conflicting expectations may mean that the program objectives are not clearly defined or that the program has not achieved its initial objectives.

Your assessment must include an examination of the ability of the agency to meet its objectives. For example, does it have sufficient resources to succeed? Finally, you should write up your evaluation report and include detailed recommendations about how the link between program objectives and implementation might be strengthened.

Stages of evaluability assessment

- Observe
- Clarify the boundaries of your evaluation
- Analyse agency documents
- Involve program staff
- Interview key stakeholders
- Assess agency resources
- Make recommendations in a report

Process evaluation

Process evaluation is undertaken at the level of practice, and is used to investigate how the program is operating (Engel and Schutt 2010b). A process evaluation offers a 'snapshot' of a program at any given time, and is concerned with identifying program strengths and weaknesses (Logan and Royse 2010). We use process evaluation to assess overall program quality, to look at what is going on inside the organisation. The focus is on the process of the program and how it can be improved, rather than its outcomes. According to Owen (1993, p. 129), a process analysis is conducted:

- to examine program implementation in order to improve or review outcomes
- when developing and refining new programs
- when practitioners are concerned about the quality of the program being provided at agency level.

Program evaluations can be used to provide a context within which to interpret different program outcomes—for example, why one domestic violence program has different outcomes from another. They can provide comprehensive pictures about programs and offer lessons so that other programs won't make the same mistakes.

Key questions

To conduct a process evaluation, we must be aware of key questions that relate to the effectiveness of the service or program being analysed. In particular, we must note the target group for whom the program was intended and ask who is using the service and why. Who is being excluded and why? Who is failing to return and why? These questions will allow us to assess how effectively the program is targeted.

We need also to consider the service delivery itself by noting who is delivering the service, how effective they are and what the program actually involves. Is it being conducted in a specified manner and is it effective? How are the staff selected and trained? In particular, we should look at the costs and resourcing of the program.

How do we conduct a process analysis?

One of the optimal techniques involved in process analysis is observation. Observation allows the evaluator to examine the program or service in practice by noting the clients using the service, the suitability of the program's location, the way the service is delivered and its effectiveness in meeting its objectives. Where observation is not possible because of issues of confidentiality or impracticality, agency records may be examined to assess client response. Further information can be obtained from the workers providing the service, through interviews and by asking them to keep detailed, expanded records in the form of data forms or logbooks for a specified period of time. Information on the success of the service in effectively reaching its target group can also be obtained by some form of community survey. This will allow an analysis of barriers to service use. Client satisfaction surveys will help determine the effectiveness of the services being provided. A combination of some or all of the above methods will provide comprehensive data about the program, which must be analysed to determine whether what is happening in practice is consistent with program guidelines. The final process analysis report should relate to the key questions listed above, and make recommendations to improve the actual implementation of the service.

Stages of process analysis

- Observation
- Analysing agency records
- Interviewing workers
- Analysing data sheets or logbooks
- Community survey
- Client satisfaction surveys
- Assessing agency resources
- Making recommendations in a report

Case study 9.2: Domestic violence perpetrator program evaluation

Domestic violence is an entrenched, widespread and gendered social evil. In 2007, the Australian Rotary Health Research Foundation joined forces with a local Rotary Club and a non-government provider, Life-Works, as well as research team from Monash University to evaluate the effectiveness of two programs: the Men's Behaviour Change Program, and Couple Counselling (Brown and Hampson 2009). The evaluation was to include process and outcome elements, comparing the process and outcomes of both programs. They wanted to explore the clients' views of the program and whether they were satisfied, the staff's views and also the views of the partners of men in the Behaviour Change Program. In addition, they wanted to assess the outcomes of the program and whether it was successful in overcoming the men's violence. Brown and Hampson (2009) identified a gap in the existing literature in relation to process evaluations of such programs, and evaluations including the experiences of the participants of perpetrator programs.

In the first part of the evaluation, Brown and Hampson (2009) set out to study and compare the two processes of each program, including program goals, policies and procedures, program components, theoretical underpinnings, actual operations, locations, staffing and client groups, including the partners of the perpetrators and survivors of violence as well as the perpetrators.

They examined the extensive documentation about the programs from LifeWorks as well as Rotary, and information from staff, clients and partners. They visited the four sites where the programs were conducted, and made contact with staff, clients and partners. They held meetings with staff as a whole and in groups at each site over the months of the project.

The research team attended group meetings of the Men's Behaviour Change Program at the four sites to explain the research, seek participants and obtain information. Participants were interviewed individually, and the groups also provided valuable information through discussions. Team members contacted the perpetrators' partners separately by telephone, informing the men that they were doing so. In total, they interviewed 25 men and ten partners.

Only three couples were interviewed from the Couple Counselling program. Reasons for so few referrals included that in counselling the violence did not emerge until later in the process and then, when it did, the man would be referred to the Men's Behaviour Change Groups.

The report documented extensively on how the two programs operated. The evaluation found that this was a well-documented program with a strong theoretical base similar to that of the Duluth model. Client satisfaction was very high, with the main issue being men's fears about their behaviour once the program ended. Several program changes were recommended, including establishing follow-up services once the group program ended, incorporating individual-focused components in the group program and attending more to the children in the program. The evaluation also recommended more funding for such services and closer links with the criminal justice system. Changes were introduced to program operations, including clients being offered a wider and more flexible array of services including both Couple Counselling and Men's Behaviour Change Group instead of the previous approach of either one or the other.

Source: Brown and Hampson (2009).

Outcome evaluation

An outcome evaluation is conducted to determine whether stated objectives have been met, often looking at variables such as behaviour change (Logan and Royse 2010). Key questions include: How successful is the program? Are clients satisfied? What barriers have prevented optimal outcomes? Is the service targeted effectively? Are the intervention strategies effective?

An outcome analysis is important for assessing whether a program is worth continuing. It measures the success or otherwise of the program and, if results are positive, it will add justification for submissions for further or increased funding of services, and for continuation of the program. However, Logan and Royse (2010) note that one of the critical issues in evaluation is related to finding out for whom the program works best and under what conditions. To answer this sort of question, many program evaluations combine process and outcome approaches. Other critical issues for outcome evaluation noted by these authors are the timing of measuring the outcomes—as effects may be short term or long term—and the way measurement is carried out. For example, in measuring outcomes of domestic violence, is complete cessation of violence or reduction in violence a measure of success? If reduction of violence is accepted, what level is judged as 'success', and who makes this judgement?

How to do an outcome analysis

In order to conduct an outcome analysis, you must be very clear about the original goals and objectives of the program. Working from these, you must determine the most appropriate way to measure the outcomes, bearing in mind that this is not always as easy as it sounds. Data may be difficult to assess because of the nature of the program, the sensitivity of the issue or because of a lack of standardised records. Case study 9.2 illustrates this point.

Further sources of data for an outcome analysis may come from the workers, from formal systems (such as the court records), from the clients themselves, or from others such as partners. If possible, it is important to ask the clients what they value about the service and how it could be improved. It is generally acknowledged that client satisfaction surveys invariably reveal very high levels of satisfaction. The reasons are varied and include the fact that clients very often have little choice of service, have no knowledge of other services with which to compare the services being evaluated, and may be worried about criticising a service they desperately need. It may also be that those who remain with a service are the satisfied ones while the dissatisfied drop out. Given this information, you should treat client satisfaction surveys with some caution.

In analysing your data, you should note what the service has achieved, what support has been provided and how successful the service has been in meeting its objectives. Has it produced positive changes for the target population, and if so, how great are these changes? You should also note any gaps in service, any groups that are under-represented, any areas where services are lacking, agencies that might benefit from cooperation and whether the service is adequate to cater for the demand. Look beyond the obvious statistics and records and ask who might be missing out and why. Further, you should examine the management structure of the service to determine whether information is flowing freely through the system. An inadequately managed structure will have a detrimental effect on service.

How to conduct an outcome analysis

- Be familiar with the objectives.
- Analyse service records and statistics.
- Interview workers.
- Survey clients if appropriate.
- Examine the management structure and flow of information.
- Determine success in meeting objectives.
- Determine gaps in service provision.
- Analyse whether inter-agency cooperation should be developed.
- Report findings in terms of success in meeting objectives and areas for improvement.

Case study 9.2: Domestic violence perpetrator program evaluation

Brown and Hampson (2009) discuss how measuring outcomes in this situation is sensitive and difficult. The obvious outcome is the stopping or reduction of the domestic violence. However, assessing the perpetrator's behaviour is complex. Perpetrators are not likely to give reliable information as their consistent denial of their own behaviour is acknowledged to be a major part of the problem. Additionally, partners are thought to underestimate and even deny the extent of the violence, so relying on information from partners is also likely to be unreliable. Court records could be used, but only certain types of violence reach the courts, and in any case the perpetrators involved in the LifeWorks programs had not been through the courts as this and other domestic violence programs sit outside the criminal justice system.

Another difficulty in measuring outcomes is deciding how to assess the changes in the perpetrators' behaviour. Domestic violence covers a wide range of controlling behaviours. If an evaluator measures a range of indicators of domestic violence before and after the intervention, how are they to judge whether one indicator decreases (for example, hitting the partner) but another increases (such as denigration)? Brown and Hampson (2009) note that even though it is difficult to interpret, reviewing such behaviours is important.

Another issue is the timing of measuring outcomes. Brown and Hampson (2009) note that evidence is emerging that the longer researchers leave it after completion of a program to measure behaviour change, the more reliable the information is likely to be. Early studies in the United States of the impacts of domestic violence reduction programs were discounted because the information was collected too soon. Later research has also shown that improvements can continue to occur for at least four years after the program, suggesting that outcome evaluators should follow up the participants for many years to properly assess outcomes. As part of their review of existing research, Brown and Hampson (2009) also noticed that drop-out rates plagued outcome evaluations.

Notwithstanding these and other difficulties, Brown and Hampson (2009) found that the LifeWorks program was successful in stopping violence for 69 per cent of the clientele and reducing it for a further 22 per cent. Only 7 per cent of men reported no improvement at all. The research challenged many beliefs about perpetrator programs. It found that the programs provided services to both survivors of violence and perpetrators, rather than only to perpetrators, thus bringing relief to women and children when the violence stopped. The study also showed that the violence addressed in these programs is serious and life-threatening—not inconsequential, as has been claimed. Further, all forms of violence were reduced; the men did not replace one form of violence with another.

Source: Brown and Hampson (2009).

Cost–benefit analysis

The final type of program evaluation to be discussed here is cost–benefit analysis, an analysis of the overall benefits of the program relative to the costs of the service. Coming from the market economy, cost–benefit analysis is controversial in the human services (Wadsworth 2011b), with debates about what counts as 'costs' and 'benefits' and how to measure these. How does one determine an indication of benefit if one is dealing with the long-term unemployed, for example? It is very difficult to nominate an indicator of service provision that can be measured in monetary terms. How does one give value not only to the immediate service benefit but also to the indirect outcomes of an intervention for the family or group and for society? Wadsworth (2011b, p. 146) notes that in practice human service managers are rewarded for spending less money rather than being rewarded for increasing service, thus 'ensuring the most service for the least outlay can mean it is better to have an *appearance* of a service (even if it is dangerously thinly spread, and there is no real follow-through)'.

Logan and Royse (2010) highlight a number of challenges in relation to cost–benefit analysis, including that standard cost estimations of a program do not always reflect the true costs. For example, programs might work cooperatively, operating in conjunction with each other, and these costs will not be included in cost–benefit analyses. A comprehensive cost analysis would include things like opportunity costs—such as time and efforts of people referring clients to the program—and other costs for which the program does not actually pay, but which are needed. Similar challenges arise when benefits are analysed, as noted above.

In selecting indicators of cost–benefit you should be careful to evaluate the effectiveness of the service in terms of both cost and quality. For instance, you might improve the throughput of a skills training program for long-term unemployed people by reducing the program's duration from six weeks to four. You are thus able to demonstrate that more people are taking the program for the same cost. However, is the program as effective and is it producing the desired level of training for the clients? Always analyse your cost–benefit data with a careful eye to quality.

How to conduct a cost–benefit analysis

- Use observation to assess effective cost of service delivery.
- Compare agency costs and client statistics with those of other, similar agencies.
- If records are inadequate conduct a time budget survey.
- Use the same indicators for each agency.
- Calculate cost per hour, per client and per case.

Case study 9.2: Domestic violence perpetrator program evaluation

Cost–benefit analysis was not included in the domestic violence perpetrator program. If it had been, it might look at budgetary allocation to the services, and examine staffing profile and costs, types and numbers of services, numbers of clients, and numbers and types of incidents of services. It might compare this cost with estimated costs if there had been no interventions—for example costs in terms of medical and housing expenses, lost income, imprisonment, split families, and the inter-generational costs of child victims becoming perpetrators. Comparisons could be made with the cost-effectiveness of similar services.

Source: Brown and Hampson (2009).

Summary

This chapter has outlined the various types of program evaluation that might be conducted by social workers. With economic accountability now a determining factor of human service delivery, it is important that you are able to both conduct your own program reviews and assess the credibility of external reviews conducted for you.

Questions about purpose, who the evaluation is for and who is to be involved must be decided as part of planning your evaluation. A four-stage process of planning, data collection, data analysis and reporting was outlined. Altogether, five types of program evaluation have been discussed, which form part of a continuum of appraisal. Needs analysis was discussed in detail in the previous chapter. This chapter has examined evaluability assessment, process evaluation, outcome evaluation and cost–benefit analysis.

An overall program evaluation may contain all of these stages. You should be aware of each of these aspects of service delivery, because the success or failure of a program may be influenced by any of these.

You should also understand how politically sensitive an evaluation is to key stakeholders, and ensure that all are kept informed of the process and outcomes. Being able to understand and conduct evaluations of human service programs is a critical tool for astute social work practitioners in a climate of increasing accountability.

Discussion questions

9.1   What is a program evaluation and why is it necessary?
9.2   Outline the five types of program evaluation and detail when they would be used.
9.3   Why would you conduct an evaluability assessment?
9.4   What is process evaluation?
9.5   How would you conduct an outcome evaluation?
9.6   What measures would you use to determine a cost–benefit analysis?
9.7   What are the benefits of using an external assessor versus an internal assessor?

Exercises

9.1   Visit a human service agency and ask whether they have program evaluation reports you might read. Identify the type of evaluation conducted, and consider the appropriateness of the methods used and whether the recommendations are well grounded in the data.
9.2   Interview a worker in a human service agency about the types of programs and services provided by the agency. Ask about the quality improvement strategies built into the programs, and whether the programs are evaluated regularly. Inquire about the types of evaluation that have been conducted, who was involved, what recommendations were made and whether these were acted upon.

Further reading

Dudley, J. 2011, *Research Methods for Social Work*, 2nd edn, Allyn and Bacon, Boston, MA. See Chapter 16, 'Program and practice evaluation'.

Engel, R.J. and Schutt, R.K. 2010, *Fundamentals of Social Work Research*, Sage, Thousand Oaks, CA. See Chapter 10, 'Evaluation research'.

Logan, T.K. and Royse, D. 2010, 'Program evaluation studies', in B. Thyer (ed.), *The Handbook of Social Work Research Methods*, 2nd edn, Sage, Thousand Oaks, CA, pp. 221–40.

Marlow, C. 2011, *Research Methods for Generalist Social Work*, 5th edn, Brooks/Cole Cengage Learning, Sydney. See Chapter 6, 'Designing program evaluations'.

Wadsworth, Yoland, 2011, *Everyday Evaluation on the Run*, 3rd edn, Allen & Unwin, Sydney.

IO *Action research*

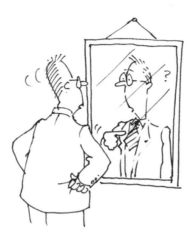

According to the definition of social work research we use in this book, and to a lesser extent our definition of social research (see Chapter 1), all the research in this book is about action research. Because social work research implies action, it is by its nature action research. Action research involves learning by doing, reflection and action in a continuous cycle to improve practice. The people involved in the research are usually the ones who will be vitally involved in what happens as a result of the research, and in carrying out the recommendations. Action research has strong emancipatory and participatory elements, with a focus on social justice, human rights and addressing issues of power.

Coming from the critical and emancipatory traditions, action research involves many traditions, disciplines, theories and approaches. There are different accounts of how it emerged, how it is defined and the focus of its efforts. Action research occurs across a diverse range of contexts and methods: for example from community development projects in countries in the global South to organisations in the global North where workers and the people they work with get together to examine how to improve services, and to international disaster recovery efforts (discussed in the following chapter). This diversity has led Reason and Bradbury (2006, p. xxi) to argue that action research is more of an orientation towards inquiry than a methodology in itself.

The purpose of this chapter is to highlight some of the key elements of action research. With ever-present pressures to adopt positivist approaches to evidence-based practice, it is important to reaffirm the values of social work research that is also action research.

Why do we do action research?

Throughout this book, we have identified many reasons for undertaking action research. One important reason is that the values underpinning action research resonate with social work's value base (AASW 2010). Principles of social justice, working for human rights and well-being, and working collaboratively to acknowledge and address power imbalances are all compatible with social work's general approach. While there can be many reasons for undertaking action research, notions about democracy, anti-oppressive and emancipatory approaches usually underpin projects in this tradition.

Why do action research?

- To work together with people to change ourselves, and the structures around us
- To empower people to become partners in the research process
- To address inequalities and pursue social justice
- To solve social problems
- To encourage the democratic process

What is action research?

The action research cycle

Yoland Wadsworth, a respected Australian action researcher and author, emphasises the cyclical nature of action research, as well as how action and research are two sides of the same coin:

> Action research or action learning . . . is action that is intentionally researched and modified, leading to learning what to try in the next stage of action, which

is then again intentionally examined for further change and learnings, and so on as part of the research itself. Life itself is a kind of action research project when you think about it this way! (Wadsworth 2011b, p. 132)

Wadsworth argues that traditional research is only half of the full inquiry cycle. She argues that by not closing the cycle between action and research, linear research falls prey to two dangers that can lead to defensive reactions from the people being researched. First, if the hypotheses driving the research are not grounded in the 'value-driven and experience-based' theories or hunches of the people involved, services are likely to conduct irrelevant research that is not worth the time and effort involved. Second, if research conclusions are merely presented in a report, that they do not take seriously the matter of putting the research's conclusions to a practical test, and thus can't get beyond defensive reactions when things are not going well. If the recommendation were put into practice and this becomes part of the inquiry cycle, then by getting back to reflecting on the positive values and desired states being sought, the defensive response could be addressed. An adaptation of Wadsworth's depiction of the action research cycle is shown in Figure 10.1.

Figure 10.1 The action research cycle

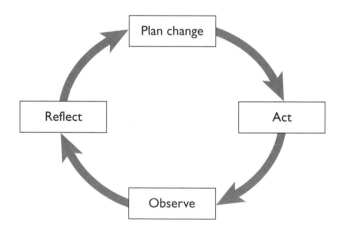

Source: Adapted from Wadsworth (2011a, p. 60).

Critical reflection and participation

Social workers value reflection—particularly critical reflective practice (Fook 2002, p. 41), which is also at the heart of action research. Action research is a 'bottom-up' strategy, based in a commitment to research as an empowering activity for everyone involved. As noted, it comes from the critical and emancipatory traditions we discussed at the beginning of this book (Morris 2006). Action researchers are oriented towards researching *with* people rather than doing research *to* them. Thus partnerships, collaborations and participation by all the people involved in the process—especially those being researched—is a high priority. Some schools of action research term this participatory action research to emphasise the collaborative, democratic and empowerment aspects of action research. Denzin and Lincoln's (2005) use of the term 'participatory action research' is discussed in Chapter 11.

Action researchers with a critical perspective will be sensitive to the structures and processes of power and oppression operating in a given context, and are committed to research that will improve the lives of people who are marginalised and excluded. A critical perspective will also influence the focus of the research. For example, a school social worker researching how to improve social inclusion of students with disabilities, if working from a non-critical and non action-research perspective, is likely to focus her research on how to improve the social skills of the students with disabilities. The social worker might administer questionnaires, conduct interviews and focus groups, assess the students' social skills, analyse the data and report her findings to the principal or other body.

A school social worker researching this issue from a critical action research perspective instead might want to examine the structures that support the social exclusion: the attitudes of teachers and 'able-bodied' students, and elements of the physical environment that set students with disabilities apart. Before the social worker 'did' anything, however, a great deal of consultation would take place, with as many members of the school community as possible. While ideally all stakeholders are included in participatory action research, time and resource limitations usually mean that this is unrealistic (Blum, Heinonen and White 2010).

Most likely a steering committee with representatives of all the key stakeholder groups would participate in the decisions about the research. Various consultation and communication strategies would be employed so that the school community 'owns' the process. Once the recommendations have emerged, the school would embark on another cycle of implementing the changes, observing their impact, reflecting on what this means, planning more changes—and so the cycle would continue.

Greenwood and Levin (2007) use a definition of action research that involves the three elements of action, research and participation. Their definition of action research captures the participatory and empowerment elements that are important in social work action research (Greenwood and Levin 2007, p. 3):

> Action research is social research carried out by a team that encompasses a professional action researcher and the members of an organization, community or network ('stakeholders') who are seeking to improve the participants' situation. AR [action research] promotes broad participation in the research process and supports action leading to a more just, sustainable, or satisfying situation for the stakeholders.

Which research methods do action researchers use?

Throughout this book, we argue that action researchers can choose from the wide variety of research methods available across the qualitative and quantitative spectrum. There is no one method of going about doing action research. This makes the other chapters of this book all potentially relevant if you want to undertake effective action research. Which methods you choose will depend on the nature of the issue being tackled, the context of the situation you are in and the purpose of the action research.

We do not agree with the view sometimes found in the literature that action research is part of the qualitative tradition. As long as it involves the key elements of a focus on action/change, using the action-reflection cycle and participant involvement as co-researchers or colleagues, action research can be as diverse as the people who practise it. Indeed, one of its strengths is its capacity for creativity and transformation. Good action research is as rigorous as any other method, and leaves a clear trail showing how it was carried out so that others may learn from its successes and failures.

In conclusion, we have identified a number of elements that together make up action research. These are shown in the box.

Action research involves
- the intention to change or improve a situation
- Active collaboration with participants as co-researchers
- a continuous cycle of planning, action, critical reflection and observation
- whichever research methodologies are most appropriate

How do we do action research?

In practice, action research can begin at any point in the action–observation–reflection–planning cycle identified above. Wherever you begin, the elements of working together with the people affected by the outcomes of the research and/or those involved in the practices you are investigating, reflecting with them about the process each step of the way, and having some kind of action or change at the heart of the research, are what sets action research apart from other methods.

Instead of an identified method, there are several principles or suggestions from other action researchers that you could incorporate into your practice; these are listed in the box.

Some principles of action research

- Involve the people in the research process as co-researchers in all decisions—about content and method—in the reflection phases.
- Get started quickly.
- Start small—do it yourself and gain momentum.
- Be explicit about collecting data.
- Seek out contradictions.
- Be explicit about power relations.
- Engage with the politics.
- Ensure the validity of the research by moving between reflection and action several times in your inquiry cycles.

Heron and Reason (2006, pp. 145–6) identify four phases of the action research cycle for cooperative inquiry groups (see below). They discuss how co-researchers develop their original ideas or test new ones during the next inquiry cycle. In order to enhance the validity of the findings, they recommend repeat cycling through these four phases. Cycles may be long or short—Heron and Reason report that six to ten cycles may take place over a short workshop, or over a year or more, depending on the nature of the inquiry.

In Case study 10.1, we present an example organised into each of Heron and Reason's (2006) phases, showing how the cycles of learning, action, observation and reflection worked out in one instance that led to changes in practice. This case study is from an action research project in social work field education. It demonstrates the way practice evolves as the inquiry cycles progresses. While it is not possible to show the repeating cycles in detail, we hope the general flavour is conveyed. At the time of writing, the networks developed as a result of this project were just being established.

Phase 1: Co-researchers meet and agree on the focus of the inquiry and the methods they will use to collect data

Case study 10.1: Online Student Supervision Project

The Combined Universities Field Education Group (CUFEG) is a network of Australian social work and welfare academics in New South Wales and the Australian Capital Territory who have been meeting together for many years to share ideas and improve field education (also known as practicum or professional field experience). They wanted to address issues such as improving access to training, resources and support for the social workers who supervise students on placement (termed field educators) in order to increase the pool of trained field educators, particularly in rural and remote areas where there is a shortage of health and welfare practitioners.

The project team agreed to develop an online student supervision program that would be accessible and that would meet the requirements for field educator preparation no matter which university hosted the placement. They wanted to develop shared standards in postgraduate education for student supervision, which would incorporate industry and professional requirements. Part of the project would involve seeking a strategy so that the resources developed could be shared cooperatively. As well as university educators, practitioner representatives from industry and the professional body were involved. It was agreed early on that existing resources would be examined in order to find 'common ground' from which to structure the program.

Source: Bowles et al. (2011).

Phase 2: Co-researchers become co-subjects—they engage in the actions to which they have agreed, and observe and record the process and outcome of their own and each other's experiences

Case study 10.1: Online Student Supervision Project

At their first meeting in 2008, the CUFEG project team and a major industry representative shared their supervision approaches and resources. The project team realised that, because they came from only two states, anything they did would not include the perspectives of educators, employers and practitioners from the other states.

The members of the project team decided that instead of developing a detailed program themselves, they would seek the views of as many universities as possible to find out whether a national online program would be useful, and if so what would be included. In the meantime, they met monthly to examine the data from their own resources to find common principles, conducted a literature review and investigated strategies to enable whatever was developed to be shared across the sector. Notes were taken and resource files compiled.

A national workshop about the project was held immediately following the national social work conference at the end of 2008. Twenty people participated, including practitioners, representatives of employers and the professional body (AASW), and field education academics from thirteen of the 26 schools of social work. People shared their approaches to supervision training and developed guiding principles for the project.

Source: Bowles et al. (2011).

Phase 3: Co-subjects become fully immersed in and engaged with their action and experience

Case study 10.1: Online Student Supervision Project

During 2009, the project team worked with the materials provided by their organisations and participants at the national workshop to develop the online program. They abandoned various legal agreements they had trialled in order to be able to share the new resources, opting to use the Creative Commons licence under which their sponsoring body, the Australian Teaching and Learning Council (ALTC), operated.

The online program was piloted with fourteen experienced social work practitioners from around Australia, along with one of the project team members who participated as well. The project team presented a progress report at another national meeting, with feedback on the pilot and the principles that were being developed. This meeting strongly endorsed the goal of developing national standards with social work peak bodies, along with the idea of a shared online program. As the pilot project was reviewed at successive discussions of the project team and modified in the light of the feedback, new theoretical insights—including definitions of supervision in field education—emerged.

During this phase, it became clear that some rural and remote social workers would not be able to access online materials because many areas of Australia still had no access to the internet. A written resource was produced, and a limited number of copies published for peer review by universities, employer groups and the AASW.

Source: Bowles et al. (2011).

Phase 4: Co-researchers reconvene to share their practical and experiential data and to consider their original ideas in the light of them

Case study 10.1: Online Student Supervision Project

Another national workshop was held in 2010, towards the end of the funding period for the project. This time, representatives from 23 of the 26 schools of social work participated, along with representatives from the peak bodies including the professional body, practitioners and employers.

During the day-long workshop, small groups reviewed the printed resource in detail, leading to a complete overhaul of its structure. New content on culturally competent and safe practice was recommended and other resources were offered. There was unanimous support for the new version of the book to be printed and distributed in addition to it being available for download from the internet, with agreement that people would use it in their own workshops with field educators and students.

Two peak bodies agreed to take over aspects of the project so that it could continue as a national conversation, developing standards and good practice in field education. The AASW agreed to establish a National Field Education Sub-Committee to advise on field education matters as well as take over the management of the online program. The Australian Association of Social Work and Welfare Educators (AASWWE) agreed to establish a broadly based inclusive national field education network to continue conversations about field education across the sector, which would involve all the groups involved.

Source: Bowles et al. (2011).

We conclude our review of action research with a case study from Australia that highlights the emancipatory and participatory nature of action research.

Case study 10.2: Listening to the stories of Australian Indigenous social workers—a report of a collaborative research partnership

Over an eighteen-month period during 2000–01, a collaborative research project was undertaken to explore the nature of Australian Indigenous social work practice. The research initially was conducted by a non-Indigenous social work practitioner and, following the pilot interview, evolved into co-research involving this Indigenous practitioner from the pilot and, later, the other participants. The aims of the research were to identify how Indigenous social work practitioners reconcile their Indigenous identity with their social work roles; balance their cultural knowledge and practices alongside a social work discourse that reflects the dominant culture; and construct their personal and professional boundaries.

An initial number of Indigenous social workers were invited to participate in the research. They were asked to identify others who might be interested in being interviewed. Each participant was sent a transcript of their interview and encouraged to change any aspect of the data. Once the interviews were completed, the researchers then undertook a joint thematic analysis of the data. Participants were informed of the involvement of the co-researcher. They were invited to collaborate in the research process. The researchers met with members of the community and participants to discuss the research and to gain feedback at regular intervals.

The six Indigenous social workers who participated in this study came from Queensland, New South Wales, the Northern Territory, the Australian Capital Territory and Western Australia. They were qualified social workers with two to six years' practice experience ranging from child protection, family support, income support, child and adolescent mental health and juvenile justice to social policy, research and teaching. The participants worked in both Indigenous-specific and mainstream positions, exposing them to practice with Indigenous and non-Indigenous clients and communities. They were aged in their thirties and forties. Two men and four women were interviewed.

Participants expressed their excitement that the research was being conducted in a collaborative and culturally appropriate way. It was an opportunity for them to be truthful about 'the lifting of the secret'. Additionally, the research was deemed timely and necessary to challenge the value system and theories that inform Australian social work practice.

The results of the research reveal some of the tensions of being an Indigenous social work student. Some areas covered were: being taught Indigenous subjects by non-Indigenous lecturers; and the isolation of being one of the few students from a culturally diverse background—and often the only Indigenous person.

Different features of Indigenous social work practice were also explored. These included investigating the effect of personal experiences in Indigenous communities and the impact this has on being an Indigenous social worker. Notions of obligation, kinship ties and identity contribute to the complexity experienced by Indigenous social workers in their professional lives. These factors conflict with the dominant social work discourse regarding personal and professional boundaries.

There have been a number of outcomes from the research process. These include an opportunity for researchers to learn from each other in terms of cultural knowledge and research theory; the participants being given the opportunity to explore their cultural, personal and professional identities and their fit with social work; the ability to increase Indigenous networks; and the opportunity to challenge the social work profession to incorporate Indigenous values within theory, practice and self.

Source: Bennett and Zubrzycki (2001).

Summary

Action research is characterised by its commitment to action and by the incorporation of stakeholders as co-researchers and co-subjects in the research process. The action research process is often viewed as a cycle of planning, observation, reflection and action, moving into a new planning phase. We recommend several cycles through these phases to increase the validity of the study. Action research does not end with a report listing recommendations; it consciously goes on to ensure the implementation of the actions and a renewed study and evaluation of the results as part of the 'inquiry cycle'.

Action research is especially important for social workers because of its theoretical grounding in critical and emancipatory approaches, and its resonance with social work values and approaches. Action researchers are concerned to address inequities, and they seek to change the social system as well as critically reflecting on their own practice as part of the research process.

The methods used in action research may be any from the conventional toolkit of social science research. The researchers must, however, consciously remove themselves from the role of expert and become an involved facilitator, colleague or co-researcher and co-subject, empowering others to work with them for change.

Discussion questions

10.1   What is action research? What are the elements of the action research cycle?
10.2   How does action research differ from other forms of research?
10.3   What stages do action researchers cycle through during the process of action research?
10.4   What are the most appropriate methods for action research?
10.5   Why is action research important for social workers?
10.6   Which of the case studies in the previous two chapters on program evaluation and needs and strengths assessment would you class as action research? Why or why not?

Exercises

10.1   Define a problem in your organisation or institution that impacts adversely on the way you work. It might be an issue about eligibility for service, or a staff or student policy. Outline how you might conduct a piece of action research that could lead to changes in the policy.

10.2   Imagine you are a worker in a nursing home. You are concerned about the over-medicalisation of patients. How might you conduct action research to effect change?

Further reading

Blum, E., Heinonen, T. and White, J. 2010, 'Participatory action research studies', in B. Thyer (ed.), *The Handbook of Social Work Research Methods*, Sage, Thousand Oaks, CA.

Greenwood, D. and Levin, M. 2007, *Introduction to Action Research Social Research for Social Change*, 2nd edn, Sage, Thousand Oaks, CA.

McNiff, J. and Whithead, J. 2006, *All You Need to Know About Action Research*, Sage, London.

McTaggart, R. (ed.) 1997, *Participatory Action Research: International Contexts and Consequences*, State University of New York Press, New York.

Reason, P. and Bradbury, H. 2006, *Handbook of Action Research Participative Inquiry and Practice*, Sage, London.

Wadsworth, Y. 2011, *Do It Yourself Social Research: The Bestselling Practical Guide to Doing Social Research Projects*, 3rd edn, Allen & Unwin, Sydney.

I I *Best practice evaluation*

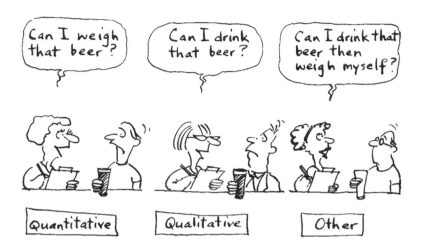

While in previous chapters we have discussed methodologies and methods suitable for social workers undertaking research and evaluation projects, in this chapter we turn to a discussion of ways in which we can use this knowledge and these skills to evaluate our own practice. Effectively, we are considering ways to turn the research spotlight on ourselves and how we operate in the workplace. Social workers traditionally are poor at drawing on research and evaluation to assess their own practice, preferring—as Gray and Schubert (2010) note—to draw on their humanistic values, diverse theories and client-centred approaches. Going further, Gray and Schubert argue that many social workers see their work as an art rather than a science, with all the nuances of difference that that portrays. Drawing on research to inform and assess our practice, or practice evaluation, is not so much about creating new knowledge as it is about assessing whether we have made a desirable difference. Proving this demands that we undertake a systematic evaluation rather than rely on an instinctual understanding of our skills. The questions we must ask are: Are the processes we use and the outcomes we achieve effective, efficient and competent? Is our practice based on a well-grounded evaluative process?

Did it work?

Are we achieving best-practice standards? In plain English, are we doing a good job?

To date, our discussion has located research activities as projects undertaken as part of the social work professional role. A more fundamental issue now emerging for many professionals is how well they are performing in this social work role. Evidence-based practice is now firmly established in social work, and the impetus to develop an 'evidence-based culture' is an expectation of many social work organisations. In the United States, the Social Work Policy Institute holds a number of references and tools on its website on evidence-based practice. Centres such as the Centre for Evidence-Based Social Services (CEBSS)—funded in the United Kingdom for several years to establish an evidence base for social services practice—and international organisations such as the Cochrane Collaboration have encouraged practitioners to use the results of research in their practice, to become informed consumers of research and to undertake research as part of good professional practice. In Australia, the Australian Association of Social Workers (AASW) has established an interest group in evidence-based practice and provides updates of events.

Just what constitutes evidence-based practice is a matter for debate—particularly the place of qualitative research and whether, as some claim, randomised control trials (RCTs) are the 'ultimate' in evaluating social work practice effectiveness. This debate mirrors somewhat Gray and Schubert's (2010) notion of art vs science and the evidence-based understanding we bring to our work.

This chapter will not only provide you with a range of ideas for evaluating your own practice, but also offers several entry points into the debate about best practice and evidence-based practice. This debate is one of the hot topics for social work in the twenty-first century, largely because we are expected to be accountable for our actions and our ethical principles demand that we do no harm. Proving this becomes a significant factor in our work.

In the previous chapter, we saw how one type of action research is devoted to workers evaluating their own practice. This chapter turns us inward, suggesting additional ways to reflect on the practices and methods we might use to evaluate our work. Such a task requires us to do more than outline a series of methods. It also calls on us to reflect on the social work profession, on its place in a postmodern world, on our values and our role in a rapidly changing political and ideological landscape, and on best practice standards and the most effective strategies to achieve those standards. These are big issues, and it is well beyond the scope of this chapter to explore them fully; nevertheless, it is important that we address them briefly if we are to reflect on our practice and competently self-evaluate.

Social work practice in the twenty-first century

Like most professions in the postmodern era, social work has lost its sense of certainty and its faith in rationality. The acceptability of a body of knowledge and the role of the professional as expert have both been called into question. Payne (2008) notes that adopting a post-modernist stance will enable social workers to critique, analyse and adopt various theories that assist with their work. In a subsequent work, Payne and Askeland (2008) also note that social workers must deal with greater complexity in increasingly managerialist organisations, and thus must have the capacity to justify their work from a secure knowledge base rather than from any assumed notion of professional expertise and status.

Those who operate outside the norms of expected human behaviour become marginalised, and are the targets of social work intervention. Social workers are thus part of the power relations operating in society to enforce certain mores and values, and their interventions may result in some groups being labelled, targeted and disempowered. Social workers have significant power to construct situations as social problems needing radical interventions, which may make them complicit in inequitable relations. They may, in fact, be maintaining structural inequalities or shaping new inequalities based on a sense of moral virtue not underpinned by a solid evidence base. If this is the case, then we need to reflect seriously on the basis from which we draw our practice interventions before we can evaluate how competently we practise.

Before we can do this, we should first address such questions as: What are the problems with which we are dealing? Under whose reality are we operating? What are the optimal outcomes we are working towards? Who is the client? Do we see the client as the expert in her/his own situation? Where are we focusing our actions? Are we aware of the power relations operating in the situation? Are we marginalising people by labelling them only because they are operating outside a currently acceptable norm? Do our language and terminology disempower clients? Do we pathologise difference and explain deviance by a concentration on individual pathology?

These are big questions that require us to be critically aware of the frameworks that bind our practice before we can evaluate how well we practise. We do not intend to engage the reader in a philosophical and ethical debate, but we would urge social workers to engage in a constant process of self-reflection. Building on the discussion in Chapter 1, we urge you to consider the following issues.

Theoretical and ideological position

The practice of social workers is necessarily embedded in a theoretical and ideological framework. Each practitioner holds a theoretical position with which they are most comfortable, and through which they interpret the social world around them—it may be feminist, social constructivist, postmodern, neo-Marxist or any one of a number of others. Our ideological position also shapes what we determine to be an ideal social world. This may be conservative, radical, neoliberal or any one of a range of positions through which we gauge the way we operate in the world and what we view as an ideal world. The way in which we interpret and view the world frames as much as anything the way we approach practice, the methods we use and the outcomes we are seeking.

In evaluating our practice, we must be able to articulate, as well as defend, the theoretical and ideological framework/s guiding our practice so that we can self-consciously reflect on our effectiveness. At the same time, we need to be aware of the methods we use to achieve our desired outcomes. Most workers have a preferred practice method or methods—be it narrative, systemic or psychoanalytic. Our reflection on practice must allow us to interrogate the methods and styles that we use, and to be genuinely evaluative of our approach. This self-conscious understanding of our position and practice methods is the first step in undertaking practice evaluation.

Performance criteria

When assessing practice performance, carefully defined performance criteria are essential to best practice. Determining such criteria is not as easy as it may sound, as we must first determine the criteria by which we are judging ourselves, our services and our practices. For example, when assessing our practice we may be more concerned about optimal client outcomes, client satisfaction and/or a reduction in recidivism. If we are concentrating on the services we provide, we may be more concerned to demonstrate that our service is effective for clients, that our response times are minimal or that we have used our resources effectively and so are providing a cost-efficient service. You should note that the desired outcomes, and hence performance criteria, will differ depending on the practice situation you are evaluating and the theoretical/ideological position within which you are based.

Equally perplexing is the dilemma of accountability in practice. We should, of course, be accountable for our actions—but accountable to whom? Is our main responsibility to our agency hierarchy, our clients, our colleagues, policy-makers or other professionals? You will note that each of these groups will require different measures of practice effectiveness—the agency hierarchy wants to know that the service is being delivered professionally and cost-effectively; the clients that their situations are improved; our colleagues that we are acting according to our professional codes; and policy-makers that we are reinforcing existing policy guidelines.

Another dilemma we face when assessing practice is whether to collect evidence that is quantitative, and therefore measurable, providing objective evidence against established criteria. On the other hand, qualitative evidence may be more subjective but provide a rich source of evidence of effective practice. Perhaps the most effective response is to gather a wide variety of data that will give a comprehensive picture and meet the needs of a variety of audiences.

You can see from this discussion that it is important to carefully define what the criteria against which we wish to measure ourselves may be, who are the key stakeholders and how we might most effectively measure performance. In relation to practice effectiveness, these measurements should be conceptualised through a process of self-reflection on practice in a political and ideological context.

Issues influencing practice evaluation

- Theoretical position
- Ideological position
- Preferred methods
- Desired outcomes
- Stakeholder groups
- Accountability measures for different stakeholders
- Type of qualitative and quantitative evidence needed to test outcome and accountability measures

---

The reflective practitioner

Fook (1996, 2000), Fook and Gardner (2007) and Thompson (2009) urge us to be self-reflective when attending to practice parameters. Fook (1996, 2000) argues that the reflective approach rejects the scientific, positivist and rational approaches in favour of more emancipatory and participatory approaches. A self-reflective practitioner will acknowledge the power differentials inherent in practice, will note the contextual issues and will view the client not as some marginalised 'other' but as the expert in their own situation and as a collaborator in determining optimal outcomes. A self-reflective practitioner will question their own role in maintaining marginality, their claim to professional expertise and their collusion in framing what is normal behaviour. A self-reflective practitioner will analyse the implications of policy for creating unequal power relations and challenge constructions of language that disempower. Thompson (2009) further urges us to be self-reflective practitioners while at the same time reaffirming our professionalism and resisting managerialism in order to address the challenges of social work practice.

A short example may assist in our understanding of the reflective process. The discourse and language surrounding mothers has changed in recent times in response to a conservative leaning in Western society. The label used to describe women who raise children on their own, 'single mothers', creates a situation of inequality. There is no similar popular terminology for mothers in a marital relationship, such as 'married mothers'. Through language and discourse, single motherhood is problematised. Welfare-to-work policy relating to mothers raising children alone, introduced under a conservative government in 2006, was directed towards increasing the incentives for women to participate socially and economically in society. Again, there was and is no such urgency for 'married mothers', and no expectation that a workplace commitment—although desirable—is expected. Discourse and language, and the resultant power relations, create a view that certain groups acting outside societal norms are a social problem to be dealt with through social policy. Social workers are used as part of the apparatus of power relations that is assigned to address these 'problems'. We must be able to critically reflect on language and discourse, and the resulting policy, if we are to be an able reflective practitioner.

A self-reflective practitioner is one who is good at self-evaluation and will constantly monitor their practice, will think critically about their own biases, will use their failures to improve their practice, will use evaluation techniques to determine whether to change their interventions, will use the knowledge gained through evaluation to assist the development of the profession and will include clients in any self-evaluation design.

Social workers need to respond to client situations in a self-consciously self-reflective way, questioning the way discourse shapes and directs policy, and empowering some and disempowering others. In working to become reflective practitioners, we should question the very nature of our practice, how we define social problems, what power relations are operating and the language and discourse of social work. Only then can we determine the desirable outcomes. Ideally, this is done in consultation with the experts— the clients themselves.

This lengthy introduction has been essential to an understanding of best-practice evaluation. We cannot evaluate our performance if we do not question our knowledge, values, status, power and discourse, and what our proposed outcomes might be.

A reflective practitioner

- Is aware of the assumptions and biases underlying different evaluation methodologies
- Views the client as expert
- Acknowledges power differentials
- Self-consciously questions their own role
- Notes conceptual issues
- Considers context
- Analyses the implications of policy
- Challenges the construction of language and discourse

Guidelines for conducting evaluation research

There are a number of methods available for assessing practice, some of which are more effective than others. These range across the spectrum of methods from the experimental design to qualitative models of assessment. We have taken the position that we should present a variety of methods, allowing the reader to come to their own conclusion about the effectiveness of each. We would argue that some methods are inadequate when used in isolation, and some have questionable validity. However, if used in combination and in accordance with the guidelines outlined below, there is some value in all of them.

First we would urge that any method adopted be client-centred. Ensure that clients agree on outcomes and on what is being measured, are engaged in design, agree on the goals and see the research as worthwhile. Ensure that performance criteria are developed in response to client-established targets. We would also urge that any method be used in a self-reflective way. Be aware of contextual issues and power relations and, finally, use a combination of methods. If these guidelines are followed, then methods can be adapted, used in combination and tailored to meet the needs of the context and practice issue.

Guidelines for conducting evaluation research

- Ensure that methods are client-centred.
- Engage clients in the design of the research where appropriate.
- Ensure that performance criteria are developed around client-defined outcomes.
- Be a reflective practitioner.
- Use a combination of methods.

Best practice evaluation methods

During the latter part of the twentieth century, the use of experimental methods gained popularity in response to the dominance of the scientific, rational model of empirical design. Many social work research texts outline practice evaluation techniques that are grounded in a scientific, rational approach. In particular, the use of experimental methods using strict scientific design came to be seen as the optimal design model. This approach relies on certain conditions and objective measurement to determine whether practice is effective. Objective measures are often favoured by managers, and this adds to the pressure to produce transparent outcome measures. Basing practice decisions on measurable outcomes has led practitioners to seek quantitative indicators of success, and could even influence the types of outcomes or goals that are acceptable. As a result, there has been growing criticism of the scientific, rational approach as an adequate way of assessing practice performance. As our previous discussion suggests, the scientific rational method has a number of drawbacks that do not necessarily capture the effectiveness of social work practice. Relying on quantitative measures risks obscuring the objectives of practice in favour of scientific method, and may interfere with optimal service delivery. While quantitative methods may in some cases be easier, faster and cheaper, workers who lack the necessary research skills may not undertake their research accurately or collect the data systematically.

In this section, we will outline some common quantitative methods. Given our criticism of the scientific approach as a useful way of evaluating practice, we would urge caution. However, if used in conjunction with our guidelines for conducting such reviews, they have some value—particularly if used in combination with other methods.

Quantitative methods

Experimental design

Before describing the various quantitative methods of practice-based evaluation, we introduce the principles of experimental design. In social work, experimental design is not often appropriate or possible. However, the quantitative methods that we can use are derived from this design, so it is important to understand it and the various compromises that have to be made when we use other quantitative methods.

Experimental design involving control groups has been used in the social sciences (beginning with psychology and education) since 1901, when Thorndike conducted some large-scale experiments to demonstrate that teaching Latin and shopwork had similar effects on increasing intelligence. Among other things, he used these results to argue that universities should not exclude potential students on the grounds that they had studied shopwork rather than Latin (Kerlinger 1973). Controlled experimentation without control groups goes back much further, however, with reports of Pascal using it as early as 1648 (Kerlinger 1973).

Experimental design aims to establish causality—that is, to establish that changes in the independent variable X cause changes in the dependent variable Y. The main elements of experimental design are:

- random assignment of subjects to control or experimental groups
- manipulation of the independent variable
- observation of the results on the dependent variable.

The simplest experimental design can be depicted thus:

$$RO_1 XO_2$$
$$RO_1 O_2$$

In this diagram, R indicates that subjects (usually clients) are *randomly* assigned to two groups—the experimental group (top line) and the control group (bottom line). A measurement of the independent variable is taken in both groups (O underscore 1) then the independent variable (X). The independent variable X is manipulated in the experimental group (that is, the experimental group undergoes some intervention) but not in the control group. A second measurement of the dependent variable is taken after this (O underscore 2). With large enough groups, random allocation to both groups means that there are equal chances that other factors (interfering variables) will affect both groups (theoretically, all possible independent variables are controlled). Therefore, any change in the experimental group compared with the control group (measured on the dependent variable Y) can be attributed to changes in the independent variable X.

For example, say we randomly select two groups of 20 six-month-old babies. We administer a controlled crying program to one group for one week at night and do nothing with the other group. At the end of the week, we measure how long the babies in both groups are sleeping at night. If the babies in the group with the program are sleeping through the night and babies in the other group are not, we could attribute this difference to the controlled crying program. We could say that the controlled crying program caused babies to sleep through the night.

Mostly, however, we cannot randomly assign subjects from a defined population to experimental and control groups. Usually we have non-random assignment of subjects, in that our clients are selected on the basis of eligibility and the need for a service, rather than random allocation. This means that technically we cannot generalise the results of our experiments beyond the sample of clients whose outcomes we are evaluating.

One way of improving generalisability, if we cannot randomly assign subjects to experimental and control groups, is to replicate studies at different times and/or at different places or with different subjects. If the relationship holds up in different conditions, we can be fairly certain that the variables are correlated. This means that the variables appear to be related but this does not mean that one variable causes the other. For example, we might note that children who watch more television achieve poorer grades. This does not mean that excessive television watching causes poor grades. Correlation may imply causation but doesn't prove it.

Another 'compromise' human services workers may have to make is that it may not be ethical to use control groups—that is, to have a group of people who do not receive a service. (In some situations, people may volunteer to do this, but normally social workers are dealing with people who have approached their organisation because they want a service. In any case, if people volunteer to be controls, randomisation is again lost.) In these situations, social workers may use the clients themselves as a type of control—observing changes in the clients before and after intervention.

The following examples of quantitative evaluation designs illustrate how compromises on the classic experimental design are made. Note that it is because these compromises are made that we cannot make claims generalising our findings outside our cases, without strong theoretical or other arguments for doing so. Some writers refer to these designs as quasi-experimental designs.

The single–system design

Adopted for social work evaluation, the single-system or single-subject design gained extraordinary popularity in the United States and became part of the curriculum in schools of social work. The single-system design focuses on a single, observable target behaviour such as binge eating, bullying or school avoidance behaviour. It takes as the objective measurement of success of the intervention a reduction in the observable problem behaviour. Repeated measurements of the pattern of problem behaviour (the dependent variable) over time are graphed to indicate success or otherwise of the treatment intervention (the independent variable). Before treatment is commenced, several measures of the problem behaviour are taken to establish the *baseline* measure.

To illustrate this method, consider the example of Susan, a ten-year-old girl suffering school phobia. When Susan presents for treatment, she has a pattern of school absence averaging three days per week. Her mother notes that on these days Susan suffers nausea and crying in the morning that are sufficient for her mother to keep her home from school. Before the social worker begins her treatment, she asks Susan's mother to keep a diary for two weeks noting the ongoing pattern of behaviour. This data provides the baseline data against which treatment outcomes will be measured. The diary suggests that on three mornings in the first week and four in the second, Susan is unable to go to school. Once treatment commences, the social worker tracks changes in Susan's school-phobic reactions and graphs the number of times the child attends school. The graph in Figure 11.1 illustrates the pattern of behaviour. Note that weeks one and two are the baseline period.

Figure 11.1   Susan's treatment phase

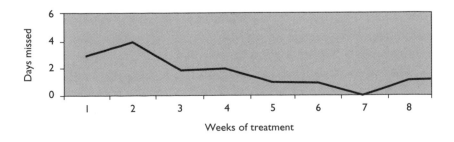

Weeks of treatment

The graph illustrates that the treatment period represents a marked improvement on the baseline data. This would suggest that the treatment given by the worker has been successful. However, caution would suggest that the target behaviour should be one chosen by the client, that it should be one causing most concern for the client and that it be relatively easy to measure.

You should note that this type of design is called an 'AB design'. That is, the A period represents the baseline and the B the treatment period. There are variations on this design, including the 'ABA design', where A is the baseline, B the treatment period and the second A represents a baseline reading taken some time after treatment. Using the example of Susan and her absence from school, an ABA design would be represented by a baseline period A, followed by a treatment period B as illustrated in Figure 11.1, followed by a further measurement period some time after treatment has ceased, to determine whether there had been a period of sustained improvement in Susan's school phobia.

The 'ABAB design' is another variation of the single-system design; it includes a baseline period represented by A, a treatment period B, another baseline period A some time after treatment ends and B, a new period of treatment. 'ABC design' represents a period of baseline assessment (A), with B being the treatment period and C a period of a different type of treatment. 'ABCD design' represents a baseline period A and three types of treatment.

Single-system designs are useful ways of assessing whether one or another type of treatment is effective with a particular client, whether the client's problem behaviour returns over time and whether the intervention used by the worker is effective. They have been popular because of the simple design, and because they do not require detailed knowledge of statistics.

There are, however, serious limitations to single-system designs. First, the choice of behaviour focused on and the best way to measure changes represent quite serious problems. What is being measured and is it an adequate representation of the problem? Who is measuring the behaviour? If it is the client or a member of their family, are we able to assess the accuracy of the information? Are they reporting socially desirable outcomes rather than what is really happening because that is what they feel is expected?

In addition, the different phases should be of equal length to allow adequate comparison. This may be difficult to achieve in practice, and may also result in periods of non-treatment that may present some risk to the client. It may be that treatment should start immediately, thus eliminating the period of baseline comparison and rendering the quasi-experimental design inappropriate.

Additionally, the results may be ambiguous. There may also be limited or no controlling for intervening variables. Taking Susan's case, there may be other variables influencing her behaviour. For example, the attention she receives during the treatment phase rather than the treatment itself may be causing the improvement, or it may be that a difficult classmate has left the school, thus making her school phobia less extreme. With a limited focus on the behaviour under study and a lack of control over intervening variables, it is difficult to establish whether the social work intervention is the cause of the behaviour change.

Additionally, single-system designs usually operate with a sample of one, making generalisation of the findings limited. It is difficult to draw conclusions about how the treatment may affect other clients, or how effective it may be in another setting. Finally, as Rubin and Babbie (2011) note, it is almost impossible to capture the complexity of human relationships and interventions by experimental means.

Despite the criticisms of single-system designs, we have presented them here as a tool that may be used *in conjunction with* other methods. In some situations there will be merit in assessing problem behaviours using a single-system design, but always with supporting methods such as in-depth interviews and observation studies to give added strength to the findings.

Client satisfaction surveys

Another quantitative technique that may be used to assess your practice performance is a client satisfaction survey. Client satisfaction surveys are often used to assess the level of client support for programs and program designs. Using them to assess your own practice is a simple extension of the logic of engaging clients in social work practice. Questions could be included to assess the level of satisfaction with your assessment processes, your intervention strategies, the outcomes of treatment, your interpersonal style, your methods, and so on. Additional questions could allow the client to nominate things they found helpful and things they found unhelpful. Note the caution you should exercise with regard to the results of client satisfaction surveys (which are often very positive), which we discussed in the last chapter.

File searches

Another useful quantitative method is an analysis of your client files to establish consistency of your style and treatment and the pattern of client outcomes. You may like to assess, for example, the number of client sessions, the consistency of treatment procedures, the types of intervention used, whether clients continue with treatment and any other quantitative variables listed in the files that allow you to assess your practice.

Resource assessment

The cost-effectiveness of your practice is another useful parameter of practice effectiveness. You might consider assessing the amount of resources allocated on a client-by-client basis. This might be done by costing your time and the resources consumed to give an indication of whether some treatment procedures are more cost-effective than others. In assessing the cost-effectiveness of your practice, you should also balance the dollar value with a qualitative assessment of the success of the intervention. It may be more cost-effective to see a client four times, but client outcomes may be markedly better after six sessions. It is important that cost-efficiency does not become the sole determinant of practice methods.

Qualitative methods

Semi-structured interviews

One of the most effective ways of assessing your practice is to conduct semi-structured interviews with clients and colleagues, seeking feedback on your practice methods and the effectiveness of your interventions. Qualitative interviews allow those interviewed to reflect on the issues raised and to give reflective feedback on your performance. This method is also empowering for clients in that it allows them to give feedback on their experience of treatment. In some circumstances, you may ask another worker or person to conduct the interviews so that clients can say what they think without being identified by you.

Focus groups

Another useful method is to conduct focus group discussions with groups of clients with whom you may have dealt individually or in group sessions. A focus group to discuss your practice effectiveness is a good way to allow clients to reflect on and discuss their experiences (see Chapters 7 and 8).

Supervision

Many social workers choose to evaluate practice by using structured supervision sessions with an experienced senior social worker. These regular sessions are used to reflect on practice and on cases, methods and on outcomes, and to provide some benchmarking of practice standards. Many agencies provide avenues for professional supervision of staff. Regular supervision sessions are encouraged as examples of best practice.

Observation and reflecting teams

In clinical settings, supervision involving direct observation of practice, using either one-way mirrors or videos, or with the supervisor sitting in on the interview, is common practice. Some agencies use reflecting teams of colleagues and others for this purpose. Clients can also be involved, either reflecting on the process (or the supervisor's comments) as part of the evaluation, or commenting on videos of sessions in retrospect.

If the observations are recorded systematically and written up, you have a good best-practice tool available using existing organisational processes and requiring only minor additional resources (the time to write up the feedback systematically). Of course, we recommend that these evaluation methods be conducted in the spirit of constructive criticism—otherwise you will become reluctant to subject your work to such intimate appraisal. It may also be useful to seek permission to observe others in their practice to allow you to view and learn from their work. (In organisations using peer reflecting teams, this will automatically be part of the structure of your work.)

File searches

Client files can also be assessed qualitatively. It is useful to provide qualitative comments in your files that give a summation of each case. These memos can then be used to assess your interventions across a range of clients and intervention strategies. Files can also be assessed for the type of language used to report cases, the theoretical and ideological position displayed, the effectiveness of the outcomes and the mode of interaction with the client.

Best practice strategies

Your motivation in evaluating your own practice and the effectiveness of your service should be to use the information to continually improve your practice. You should be working constantly to become a leading professional in your field and to provide the best service you can possibly achieve. Reviewing and monitoring your progress should be a constant part of your practice. In this section, we take you further and outline some of the uses of the evaluation results.

Develop quality standards

We suggest that you work towards providing a transparent set of standards for your practice and service that allows workers, clients, funders and other interested parties to be clear on what it is you are providing. This set of standards will include the type of service being provided, the amount of time given to each client, the type of intervention procedure, the resources available, and so on. A standards document can be developed in consultation with clients and staff, and can be reviewed annually. This standards document, which should include details of any complaints mechanism established in the agency, can then be presented to each client. Reference to your professional association's code of ethics should also be included.

Develop a client charter

A client charter should also be developed in consultation with client group representatives, outlining the standards clients should expect, the level of service, acceptable waiting periods, length of intervention, associated costs, resource allocation and any other relevant aspect of the service and of your practice. Consultation procedures and complaints mechanisms should also be spelt out as above.

Consult and empower

Where possible, clients should be consulted regularly about practice strategies and your practice effectiveness. They should also be included on any organisational body relating to the service.

Provide information

Information about the service and your practice procedures should be readily available to service users and to other interested stakeholders. Information should be kept up to date and be accessible. This may be done through pamphlets, the internet, service advice, annual reports, newspaper reports or other means. The information should be accessible to a culturally diverse population and to isolated groups.

Develop client-satisfaction monitoring processes

Client-satisfaction surveys, interviews and/or focus groups should be developed as standard and regular procedures for assessing practice. These should be conducted and reported on at regular intervals, and results made available to service users and other interested parties. Surveys can be included with service documentation or be available in the service location. It is also desirable to allow clients to report anonymously on their experiences, so a collection box should be provided within the organisation.

Regularly review the complaints policy

Establish a transparent, accessible and unbiased complaints mechanism that allows service users to report on service experiences. This may include a panel of professionals and client representatives from outside the service. Widely disseminate the information about your complaints mechanism and regularly review its composition, effectiveness and channels of communication.

Assess accessibility

Regularly assess your client profile to determine whether any sections of the community are denied access. Are there limited provisions for non-English-speaking clients? Is information provided in several languages? Is your office wheelchair-accessible? Is it in an area where clients are guaranteed privacy should they enter the building? Are the hours of operation suitable for potential clients? Are there strategies that should be developed to increase accessibility?

Summary

In this chapter, we have presented ideas to assist you to successfully evaluate your practice and to use the results of such evaluations to improve your practice. Your practice is critically affected by your own view of the world (your theoretical and ideological position), your professional and practice standards and methods, the context of practice, your desired outcomes and the relevant stakeholder groups (clients, professionals, agency personnel, the funding body, and so on). If you are to effectively evaluate your practice, you must be able to reflect critically on your own position and practice standards. We suggest you follow our guidelines to allow you to become a reflective practitioner, who is able to critically self-evaluate.

We have presented a variety of quantitative and qualitative methods that can be used in combination to provide effective evaluation of your practice. We suggest that you use the information gained from self-evaluation to improve your practice. With this in mind, we have outlined strategies that allow you to work towards best-practice standards. These include developing transparent standards, providing accessible information, consulting with clients and others, and regularly evaluating your performance and the service you provide. Of course, you should also actively seek out the results of relevant research done by others, and consciously and critically incorporate the findings into your practice. By attending to these strategies, you will be actively working towards best practice and establishing the foundations for a well-rounded evidence-based culture in your work.

Discussion questions

11.1   What factors influence social work practice effectiveness?
11.2   What is a reflective practitioner?
11.3   What important points should you note when evaluating practice?
11.4   Outline some of the criticisms of the scientific approach in relation to social work practice evaluation.
11.5   Note three quantitative and three qualitative methods you could use to evaluate practice.
11.6   Outline three best-practice strategies.

Exercises

11.1   Visit a social service agency and seek information on services provided. Examine the literature you receive to determine whether quality standards, monitoring processes and a complaints mechanism have been outlined. Discuss the best-practice strategies in relation to this organisation.
11.2   Go to a local health agency. Assess whether its information is provided in an accessible way for a culturally diverse population. Note whether the service is physically accessible for all clients and whether operating hours are accessible.
11.3   Pair up with a colleague or another student in class. Seek feedback on how well you perform in your role as a student/professional. Give similar feedback to your partner. What criteria did you each use to assess performance?

Further reading

Practice evaluation is an emerging field, and a number of articles and books are appearing across a range of disciplines. There is also a great deal of material on practice evaluation emerging on the internet. You should spend some time searching the library catalogues and the internet, beginning with the sites suggested at the beginning of this chapter.

12 Research in post-disaster recovery and other crisis situations

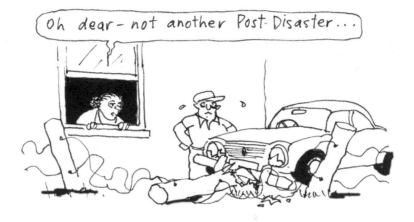

Oh dear - not another Post-Disaster...

In this third edition of the book, we have included a chapter on research in sites that have experienced disaster or crisis. Given the number of major events the world has experienced in recent times, the likelihood that there will be more and the increasing involvement of social workers in post-disaster recovery and other crisis work, we are providing this chapter as a guide to gathering data in such situations. This is a very sensitive topic, and not one to be taken lightly given the scale of disasters, the amount of trauma and the significant need for social work crisis intervention following major events experienced in recent decades. It may seem an unusual choice for a book of this nature, but we see an identified need for constructive research practice that assesses large-scale interventions as well as the practice of individuals working in these situations. We will examine rapid research interventions, and policy and program evaluations. We note that there are three potential research entry points: the immediate crisis period when intervention begins, as well as the medium- and long-term periods when assessments and evaluations of hastily implemented policy and practice can be made, thus building a body of knowledge in this emerging field. We also note that this chapter might frame the way workers respond to an unexpected local issue or even a social advocacy campaign. Essentially, the steps are similar, and following them will help ensure there is a structured approach to the social work response.

This chapter is not meant to be an appraisal of best practice in post-disaster recovery/crisis. Rather, it provides an outline of research methodologies and methods that may be used by social workers in the field. In particular, we note the need for workers to be recording policy and practice interventions in order to influence and shape socially just responses and to bring consistency and depth to the way disaster practice is conducted across the world. We can always do better, and having a body of knowledge on which to build our capacity is the most effective way to improve services and to ease trauma.

The three critical phases of crisis, medium- and long-term initiatives will be used to structure this chapter. Overlaid on these phases are the most effective ways to develop a research plan, undertake a needs assessment and evaluate programs developed to address post-disaster areas. Thus we are attempting to give shape to constructive practice in situations that may seem overwhelming.

Crisis phase

Developing a research plan

The development of a research plan for intervention in crisis situations will be dependent on your level of authority, and whether you are managing a number of staff or are a worker looking to give shape and meaning to your own individual practice. These are different levels of the same process, although for managers the task of systematising responsiveness of your team is a critical factor in your work plan.

The first stage of a research plan for social work managers in a crisis situation is to establish a reference group. This may be little more than other managers in the first instance, as you grapple with service infrastructure problems, housing and care for your team and crisis interventions on the ground. However, a critical reference group is a vital part of your ongoing management, as it gives you extended capacity and advice from a range of other professionals and local key informants. These informants can give you an understanding of the areas of critical need, the resources available and the types of services being offered by other helping organisations. Knowledge emerging from several disaster sites across the globe suggests that one of the frustrating issues for local authorities and non-government organisations (NGOs) is that there are many people looking to provide assistance, and this may not necessarily be helpful or structured in the immediate post-disaster period and therefore can actually restrict people receiving help.

Another piece of useful advice for managers is that noted by Desley Hargreaves, the head of social work services in Australia's Centrelink, the national social support agency, in an address on International Social Work Day in 2009. Desley noted that a radical and effective strategy she had adopted in the wake of the significant bushfires in Victoria in 2009 was to break down the 'silos' that existed between various government agencies and departments. A critical response management team came together from various organisations and departments, and facilitated much more effective action because of members' ability to work across the various instrumentalities they represented. Staff from these various departments and agencies worked together and were consistently able to cut through any red tape, presenting a united government voice, diffusing potential areas of inconsistent policy and facilitating immediate action for those affected.

This strategy is a useful one for those in-country workers coming together to address a major event within their own borders. It is also a potentially useful strategy for those organisations going into foreign countries to work with other governments and NGOs. A high-order reference team can assist to mobilise all agencies effectively and can also defuse inconsistent messages. At the same time, this strategy works for those who may be undertaking a social action campaign at the local or regional level.

> **The first stage is to develop a critical reference group to guide the developing response.**

The next stage of a research plan is to formulate the research questions to which you want to provide answers. These might be as basic as: What is the scale of the event, and therefore what is the most effective way to use my team in these circumstances? What is the most effective model of practice? How might these issues change as crisis becomes medium-term support and long-term planning? This stage is designed to give a structure to the developing response/campaign, and to illuminate the fact that the appropriate practice response will change over time. If you refer to Chapter 10 on action research, you will note that the process described here is similar, in that you are constantly checking and rechecking information and gathering data to refine your understanding of the issue and to fine-tune your responses or actions. With a disaster situation, events may change quickly and dramatically, and—at least in the initial stages—you will have to check information very regularly.

At the most basic level, the first question in a post-disaster recovery situation will relate to what we know about the crisis and how we might respond quickly. In the medium term, we will want to know whether our responses have been effective and how we might improve them. In the longer term, we will want to collect information and research data that will allow us to influence policy and planning, and add to the limited amount of information currently available in the area of crisis response.

Stage 2 is to develop a series of research questions that will guide the crisis, medium- and long-term responses.

Rapid Appraisal

In the initial stages of the crisis situation, you will want to access information as quickly as possible in order to make informed decisions on how best to address the situation. This section draws on the body of literature that describes Rapid Appraisal—a technique used to access data quickly and to make a rapid assessment of a situation.

Rapid Appraisal developed in the 1970s and 1980s to allow quick appraisals of (usually) developing world situations, and to assess policy and program responses. It has subsequently gained credence in public health appraisals conducted by transnational organisations such as the World Health Organization (WHO) and national government health agencies concerned to undertake rapid assessments of public health situations. Rapid Appraisal is used to gain an understanding of the community's own perceptions of their needs, to use this information to provide effective responses, and to build relationships between the community, the service providers and any external or transnational organisations coming to the situation to assist as quickly as possible. The techniques are cost-effective and timely, and therefore we would argue that this type of research is useful for those entering a disaster or crisis situation.

Rapid Appraisal uses both quantitative and qualitative sources of data. The key to successful Rapid Appraisal is the use of triangulation—using a number of methods and sources of data—to develop an informed understanding of the situation and to enhance the validity of the emerging data.

Nonetheless, it is worth noting that Rapid Appraisal is just that, and the data may be influenced unduly by a necessarily limited view. Thus it is useful to continue to check and recheck data as the situation unfolds.

Depending on the area where the crisis is underway, secondary data can provide significant information for a first-stage assessment of the area. Population and public health statistics, road maps, aerial photographs, government reports, newspapers and other accessible information can provide an understanding of both the area under study and the unfolding situation. Direct observation is also an invaluable method for scoping particular areas, noting transport and communications infrastructure damage, water and food security issues and the way people are reconstructing livelihoods.

Conducting key informant interviews is another method that can be used in the first stage to source critical local knowledge. Key informants may be national government leaders and public servants, local government personnel, aid workers, NGO representatives and other community leaders. This strategy can be problematic, of course, because these people will be caught up in supporting their community and their dominant perspective will be one of disbelief and instinctive action. Nonetheless, key informants can provide critical information on services and infrastructure, local formal and informal networks, emergency housing locations, sites for the distribution of food, clothing and financial support, likely sources of secondary data, areas where assistance may most usefully be applied, and other sources of critical information needed to allow you to work effectively.

Focus groups are also a useful method for gaining information quickly from a variety of sources, and can be used to source information from people in temporary shelters or from workers and other personnel on the ground. It is a quick way of gathering information and assessing the views of people who are critically affected on how to improve services as well as provide information on other issues such as worker support.

Immediate post-disaster narratives provide significant understanding of the ways people experience and react to disaster/crisis. It may be possible to conduct interviews with people in shelters, emergency housing, their homes or community centres to record their experiences and views, and to gain an understanding of the immediate crisis period. These stories will provide a powerful understanding of what the experience of disaster might be, people's level of trauma, and therefore what support people may need and how this might best be delivered. These immediate narratives are also a recording of an event that will provide a very useful historical record for future analysis.

Quick questionnaires are also useful ways of gathering data from people who have been affected, as well as from workers. Questionnaires can be administered on a number of occasions to the same groups of people if you are wishing to document the changing understandings and adaptations of those affected.

Another technique that can be usefully employed during the initial stages is to keep a field diary or journal where you note your observations of the evolving situation and the ways in which assistance has been developed through formal and informal channels, any barriers you are noting and any other pertinent issues that arise. These immediate reflections can be useful when you have the time to assess the full scope of your project at a later date.

Methods that can be used for Rapid Appraisal

- Secondary data
- Mapping data
- Photographs
- Key informant interviews
- Focus groups
- Quick questionnaires
- Field note diary

Rapid Appraisal will give you a great deal of information within a short timeframe. In particular, it will allow you to assess the population and health characteristics prior to the disaster or crisis, what the adaptive capacity of the population might be, what vulnerabilities exist within the population group and whether more marginalised groups live in particular areas, what the service infrastructure was prior to the event and what it might be in the immediate crisis phase, the accessibility and effectiveness of the services and supports being offered, where emergency housing is being provided, where financial and other support can be accessed, what the national, regional and local policies might be and how effective these political layers might be in a crisis, and finally, what types of transnational organisations are working in the area, how effective they are, what overlaps and gaps exist, how well-resourced they are, in what areas they might be working and what supports and infrastructure might be needed to enhance the services being provided.

Rapid Appraisal outcomes

- Population data
- Health data
- People's experiences through narrative
- Adaptive capacity of the population
- Vulnerable populations and where they are located
- Service infrastructure prior to the crisis
- Who was and is responsible for service infrastructure
- Accessibility and adequacy of services and supports
- Understanding of policy and who is responsible
- How effective local, regional and national bodies are in a crisis
- Transnational organisations—who, what, where and how?
- Required services and supports

Stage 3 is to conduct a Rapid Appraisal.

Data analysis

Analysing data collected in the immediate crisis stage of a disaster is usefully done as quickly as possible, and will involve collating all the various elements of analysis drawn from the qualitative and quantitative data collected. This will create an understanding of what has happened, who has been affected, who has responded to the emergency, how the services have been delivered, what agencies and workers have been involved, what policy drivers have shaped the response, how services might be improved, what people are saying they might need and how this might be delivered. At this point, you essentially are creating the story of the disaster and mapping the responses. There may be several audiences for these data, and therefore a variety of ways the data may be reported. For example, you might be writing a quick report for your agency/department in order that essential information is shared and understood. You may be writing a report for government in order that additional resources and responses are provided. You may be writing a report for the reference group that will alert them to gaps and overlaps in services. A more analytical reporting may take place at a later date when you have time to produce an in-depth report on the event. Data will also be used to guide social work interventions, which will include providing advice and support to the public, arranging emergency housing, providing food, clothing and financial support, and debriefing workers.

Medium-term stage

Developing a research plan

In the medium term, potential research projects will be quite different, and are more likely to expand to include community members in participatory action research and workers in debriefing projects. The types of question to which you will be seeking answers will not be focused so much on the event as on the sequelae. You will be more interested in how effective the response has been, what the needs of the community might be, what policy drivers are needed and whether the services and practice models have been effective. During this phase, you will be working to optimise the response, to bring forth the narratives of people who have been involved in some way, and this will include both community members and workers, to ensure that organisations continue to work cooperatively and effectively and that, as crisis services withdraw, adequate supports remain.

During this phase, you should also be seeking information on groups that may have been overlooked in relief support. There is significant research emerging from post-disaster recovery sites indicating that, for example, women are often overlooked in terms of financial relief, disaster information dissemination and appointments to decision-making positions. Alarmingly, there is an increasing understanding from sites as diverse as New Orleans, Haiti, Bangladesh and the Pacific Islands that their safety is often compromised in emergency shelters/housing. There is also research that suggests young girls are being trafficked out of relief shelters and that children's safety is undermined when they have lost their parents and other family members. Undertaking research at this point will allow you to assess not only how effectively support is being offered, but also whether it is actually compromising the resilience and survival of particular groups.

In this phase, it is useful to establish a community reference group that will allow you to assess the issues emerging as a result of post-disaster support, and to engage and mobilise particular groups. Your community reference group should include representatives of women's organisations as well as mainstream organisations, representatives of marginalised groups, community leaders and service provider representatives. This reference group will provide a greater level of community participation in the evolving research agenda, and provide some support for the community to direct ongoing actions.

> **The first stage is to develop a community reference group to give community guidance and ownership to ongoing developments.**

Evolving the research questions during this stage of recovery will encompass negotiations with the community reference group and your own assessment of service gaps and overlaps. At this stage, you may wish to examine ongoing community needs, effectiveness of information dissemination practices, gaps in service provision, ongoing housing and other service needs, reconstruction, levels of community engagement, policy needs and ongoing support needs once the crisis has passed. If you refer to Chapter 8 on assessing community needs and strengths, you will find useful information on how you might conduct an assessment of needs within your community. At the medium-term stage, you may also want to debrief workers, assess practices they have used and their effectiveness, assess service gaps and problematic service delivery, assess working conditions and care provided to workers, and look at any other factors that may have affected worker effectiveness. It is very important at this stage of the recovery process that you are aware of the impacts of trauma and long working hours—often in poor conditions—on workers.

> **Stage 2 involves developing research questions so that data will guide ongoing service provision and support.**

Participatory action research

As you move into the medium-term response, your research will be much more participatory. Chapter 10 on action research will guide you in understanding this type of research and its origins more fully. In the context of post-disaster and crisis work, it is useful to note Denzin and Lincoln's (2005) understanding of participatory action research. They note that it is *participatory*; it is *practical* in that it is focused on immediate issues; it is *critical* to helping people recover; it is *reflective* in that it assists people to understand their situation in order to create change; it is *transformative* in that it seeks to transform people and practices in positive ways; and, most importantly, it is *emancipatory*, in that it seeks to assist people to positively adapt. In post-disaster recovery, these issues are vitally important to ensuring that people respond and adapt in positive ways—and making them active agents of change is a helpful way of re-establishing individual and community resilience.

Methods that might be used are similar to those listed above. However, you are likely to have more time and assistance to complete the work, and you will have community members assisting you to source adequate and reliable information. Gauging the level of community functioning at this point can be achieved using similar techniques to those described above. A first stage is to collect and analyse secondary data—maps, aerial photographs of cleared sites, newspaper reports, crisis analyses from organisations that have been working in the field, government and NGO reports on the crisis and its aftermath, reports on infrastructure restoration, statistical information from governments and other sources, reports on government and private organisations and NGOs in the field and those who are pulling out, and of course observation. This information will allow you to assess how the situation has evolved, what assistance has been provided and by whom, and what policy has been developed and why.

Other methods that can usefully be used at this stage include key informant interviews with government, private and NGO organisations working in the field, and with policy-makers who have implemented policies to address the situation. Key informants might also include workers from various organisations and from various geographical areas involved in the crisis, community leaders, women's group leaders, those in charge of temporary shelters and other accommodation, those involved in providing and restoring infrastructure and other social work managers in the field. You might also consider interviewing key informants from various organisations/countries that have sent workers to the disaster site to gain an understanding of how they are viewing the support and actions from a distance.

More direct methods can be used to obtain data from those deeply involved in the crisis and its aftermath. This is where advice from your community reference group will be invaluable in providing contacts and an informed understanding of how supports have been experienced. Interviews, focus groups and/or questionnaires can be used to gather information at the community level on what factors are shaping people's adaptations, how food and water security is being achieved, what strategies people are adopting to secure their livelihood in the face of changed circumstances, what further supports might be required and what problems have arisen in communities. This information can be used to report on positive and negative adaptations, and will provide very useful assistance in developing policy and programs to assist positive adaptations and defray negative adaptations. It will also expose factors that may be affecting marginalised people and the more vulnerable in the community.

Assessing the impact of the disaster on workers is a vital part of this stage of research. Workers are often brought into a situation for short periods of time, have poor housing conditions, work under conditions of extreme stress for long periods, are trying to respond to a diversity of critical situations, have limited resources, may need to work with interpreters, work long hours, and may suffer post-traumatic stress disorder. Assessing the conditions and situation of workers at this point may help to protect them, and to provide supports and debriefing.

It also allows you to assess what practice models have been effective, what insights can be given to practice, and what policies are useful or required to ensure more effective practice. Was counselling with individuals helpful? Was family therapy and/or group work useful and in what situations? What organisational resources were most effective? Was a strengths-based approach appropriate? How did workers empower individuals and communities? What vulnerable groups were less accessible and why? In accessing this information, questionnaires can provide a broad range of information quickly. However, as with community members, it is useful to triangulate data-gathering techniques in order to source an in-depth understanding of the situation and of insights that can be offered by individuals. Thus, while a questionnaire is a good idea, so too is taking a purposive sample of your respondents and conducting in-depth qualitative interviews. These interviews will offer insights and suggestions that are unlikely to emerge through a formatted quantitative questionnaire. These insights will bring the voices from the field and give a richness to your data and your understanding. The participation of those most affected also guides an evolving response and allows people to have an input into the way policies and practices will assist recovery.

Methods that can be used during the medium-term stage

- Secondary data
- Observation
- Key informant interviews
- Interviews with community members
- Focus groups
- Questionnaires

Collecting data during this phase of the disaster recovery will allow you to understand the way people have responded to the crisis, what methods of support have been helpful, what limitations or difficulties are being experienced and how policy and practice can be reshaped to ensure a more constructive outcome. It is also helpful to document the evolving response in order to build our knowledge base of understanding of post-disaster recovery.

What participatory action research will provide

- An understanding of individual and community strategies/adaptations in post-disaster situations
- Services and support information
- An understanding of what organisations are involved, what they are doing and how various organisations have, and are, working together
- Information about policies and practices, and ways in which these could be improved
- Information on workers, their practices, limitations and supports for good practice

---

Data analysis

At this point of the process, information is vital to ensure both reconstruction efforts and individual and community support are facilitated. Data collection and analysis will be a time-limited activity, and will be undertaken for a variety of different reporting styles. Participatory action research project information will also be shared in order to ensure the community is engaged and active in shaping its future. The community reference group will assist with targeting research reports effectively and will also be involved in shaping an ongoing research agenda. Data may be presented in the form of presentations to community groups, organisations and governments, as well as short reports on service needs, vulnerable groups, policy advice and worker supports and practice. At this stage, the chief aim may be advocacy in order to secure more funding, targeted support and policy formulation. You may also be seeking to raise awareness of the responses to the crisis and to share information with your organisation and community reference group. It is also helpful at this stage to write your research into a fuller report and consider writing journal articles. The aim here is to inform the wider community and to advise on good social work practice and policy.

Long-term phase

Development of a research plan

In the longer term, you will have the luxury of reflecting on the crisis, the post-disaster and recovery phase, those who were most vulnerable, policy requirements and social work best-practice models in crisis work. At some point in the reconstruction period, there will be formal points where governments and transnational organisations will hold formal hearings and/or call for submissions in order to collect information on the crisis, what worked and how it might have been better addressed. Adding a social work perspective to these formal processes is a very helpful way of informing the wider community on social work best practice, policy shortcomings that restricted effective support, vulnerable groups, reconstruction support, better targeting and so on. Often this phase is termed a *vulnerability assessment*, and enables an assessment not only of the current crisis, but also of how vulnerable certain groups might be to future disasters.

Quite apart from the formal proceedings that might be conducted in the wider community and within your organisation, it might be helpful to develop a research plan for a project that assesses the particular event with which you were engaged in order to develop an in-depth analysis of post-disaster recovery processes, effective policy and practice, ways that workers might be better supported in a crisis situation and a vulnerability assessment for future reference. At this point, you will have the luxury of time and reflection. You may also have data collected during the earlier stages of the disaster at the crisis point and the medium-term point. This will assist you to develop a funding proposal. Seeking external funding from government sources, NGOs or philanthropic bodies, or funding from within your organisation, will allow you to conduct a useful analysis of the social work response to the crisis. There is a lack of understanding and knowledge about social work practice in disaster situations, and thus we would urge you to consider this further step if you have knowledge and expertise to share.

Stage 1 might be to consider sources of funding in order to develop a larger study on social work in post-disaster recovery.

Questions you might usefully address at this point are more in depth and theoretical. They may include an examination of post-disaster cross-organisational responses in the crisis and medium term; an examination of social work responses in various organisations and ways that workers cooperated; an examination of policy enablers and barriers that restricted or enhanced practice; an examination of how various groups responded and which groups were vulnerable in the post-disaster period and why; an examination of effective and creative practice in disaster situations; an examination of worker responses to crisis work; an examination of how vulnerable certain groups are to future disasters; or even an examination of the way your organisations responded and worked in the field, and might work more effectively in the future. The important point to consider is that this stage allows you to develop an in-depth understanding for public dissemination, for improving our responsiveness and for noting how vulnerable populations might best be assisted. Workers often forget that this work is relatively new, that organisations and governments are struggling to develop knowledge to inform quick action in future emergencies, that vulnerable people suffer and that each new crisis brings its own unique demands.

Stage 2 is to develop an informed and theoretically focused question or set of questions that will enhance our professional understanding of crisis work.

In-depth theoretical analysis

This stage of research is a more individual or organisational one, and thus the use of a reference group is an option you may or may not find useful. It is sometimes helpful if you have been funded by an external organisation to meet regularly with a small reference group that includes stakeholders from the funding body, representatives from your organisation and representatives from the site of the disaster, if possible. This group can guide your research and provide advice and support when needed.

Vulnerability assessment

A vulnerability assessment describes the way we might analyse vulnerability of people to disaster, food and water insecurity, poverty and sustainability. These assessments might be conducted to compare the vulnerability of different countries, or within countries to determine development priorities, or within regions to target and assist vulnerable groups. Vulnerability refers to the degree of exposure to risk as well as the person's/group's capacity to adapt to the event. Indicators of vulnerability might include the diversity of livelihood strategies, education levels, income, land ownership, ability to diversify and so on. By contrast, resilience refers to the capacity of the person or group to adapt in a positive and sustainable way to the stressors they have experienced. The more resilient they are, the more likely the person or community is to adapt.

Assessing vulnerability and resilience requires that data be collected on the level of threat, the likely biophysical impacts, the socio-economic impacts and the adaptation strategies adopted. This can be done using a top-down approach whereby potential climate events are assessed, along with the level of vulnerability of the affected population and the likely adaptations. It can also be done from a bottom-up approach, beginning with a vulnerable population/community and assessing people's susceptibility to threat, their current adaptations, their likely future exposure to threat and their likely adaptations based on their level of risk and resilience. A reference group can include stakeholder representatives from local communities, aid organisations, government departments and so on.

> **Stage 3 may involve the establishment of a reference group if desirable.**

Your research at this point will involve an analysis of theories that have guided post-disaster recovery and vulnerability, and your need to examine research literature in this field is paramount. A literature review will necessarily encompass research articles from other sites and circumstances, reports from government and NGOs on previous actions, an analysis of practice theory and social policy, and a more in-depth understanding of crisis work, social work case studies and any other relevant material that will give you a detailed theoretical understanding to guide your evolving research.

This stage will also involve the collection of new data from secondary data sources, including maps, in-country reviews, government and NGO reports, research papers, population and health statistics, analyses of services and infrastructure and new community formations.

Original data may also be collected in this stage from a variety of sources and using a variety of methods. Because of the nature of the crisis and its aftermath, and the research question you have formulated, you may be interested in conducting in-depth interviews with key informants from government, NGOs, community groups and so on in order to gain an in-depth understanding of how significant people involved in the crisis felt about the emergency, the response and the reconstruction effort. This type of qualitative data is very helpful for exploring the ways in which critical people feel the process might have been enhanced, the ways organisations might have more effectively worked together, how policy might have been more responsive and so on.

Additional data can be obtained by selecting case study sites and collecting data at the community and household level. Methods used might include focus groups, in-depth interviews, questionnaires and observation studies. Contacting workers for their insights and with the luxury of time to explore their understanding is also very useful at this point for expanding our understanding of effective practice. In essence, what did workers think was most effective and why, how were human rights protected and enhanced, and how were socially just outcomes achieved? Methods might include focus groups, in-depth interviews and questionnaires.

Methods that can be used during the long-term stage

- In-depth literature search
- Mapping and climate science data
- Secondary data analysis
- Key informant interviews
- Focus groups
- In-depth interviews
- Questionnaires

This information will give you insights into the way governments and other organisations organised the relief and reconstruction, the way critical policy-makers in governments and NGOs responded and why, how people and communities responded to the crisis and how they viewed the supports provided, and how workers felt about their experiences, and the practices and policies that were effective.

What in-depth analysis will provide

- Insights from government organisations and NGOs
- Understandings from people and communities about the disaster and the response

- A detailed understanding of workers' insights into their experiences
- A detailed understanding of what types of practice and policy were most effective

Data analysis

This stage allows more time for data analysis and for linking data findings with established theory and practice. A more in-depth and critical analysis is possible, and this data can both inform policy at transnational, national and organisational levels, and enable best-practice models to be developed for future scenarios. Importantly, the data from these in-depth studies adds to our as yet sparse body of knowledge in this area. Thus it should be thick and detailed, and there may be a number of outputs—including a research report, articles, book chapters and potentially a book on social work practice in crisis situations. There are significant possibilities for publishing, and for informing policy-makers and other workers about the research you have undertaken and how it builds capacity and knowledge.

Summary

In this chapter, we have visited a new area of research practice: that of understanding the nature of disasters and effective social work responses. We have outlined three stages where research plans may be quite different and used for quite diverse purposes. The first is the immediate crisis period, when the objective is to obtain information on the situation as quickly as possible in order to formulate a useful and adequate social work response. The medium term offers the possibility of reflecting on the situation, those most vulnerable and how services might have been better targeted. It is also a period when it is possible to evaluate practice and improve models of practice and service delivery. The long term offers the possibility of reviewing the crisis, the response, the ways in which social workers assisted, and what policies and practices were most effective. We believe this chapter provides a way of shaping social work responses at a time of crisis. Without a formal plan at each stage of the process, social workers are likely to operate in a reactive and haphazard way. Organisations have a responsibility to support workers in these circumstances, and the more we know about effective practice and the best ways in which we might support our workers, the more effective we will be. Importantly, by documenting our interventions we add to the knowledge base and become central players in crises that are impacting across the world. We look forward to seeing more social workers publishing in this challenging area.

Discussion questions

12.1 What are the three stages we have suggested as useful points for researching practice in a post-disaster situation?

12.2 Are there other ways we might have structured this?

12.3 What are the different types of questions you might ask at each stage?

12.4 What outputs might be produced at each stage?

12.5 What are the reasons for these particular outputs?

Exercise

Examine a disaster situation. Read what you can about the social work response.

12.1 Where were social workers located?

12.2 What work did they do?

12.3 How effective were they?

12.4 Were they central to the recovery effort?

12.5 Who might you speak to in order to find out further information on social work in this crisis?

Further reading

Denzin, N.K. and Lincoln, Y.S. (eds) 2011, *The Sage Handbook of Qualitative Research*, 4th edn, Sage, Thousand Oaks, CA.

13 *Other methods*

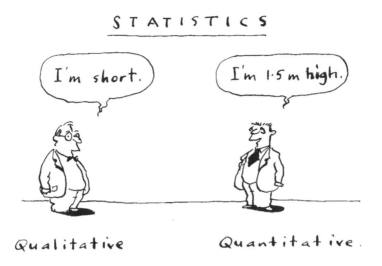

In previous chapters, we have addressed the most common types of social work methods you may use in your role as a researcher. This chapter will outline some further methods that will be very useful for you to have in your research toolkit. When you are conducting a piece of research, it is important to use the most appropriate method to gather the data you need. Often your choice will be circumscribed by the funds available to you as well as by other resources such as time, help from other staff, access to computer equipment and access to the data source. Your choice of method is made on the basis of a careful weighing up of all options. Study the methods in this chapter carefully, and reflect on their usefulness to you. They may allow you to be more creative and in some cases, as with secondary analysis, may save you valuable time and resources.

Secondary analysis

Secondary analysis is the process of using data that have already been collected for some other purpose to provide answers to your research question. When secondary analysis is used to examine an organisation's records, it becomes a powerful tool to help practitioners to reflect systematically on their practice. As a practitioner, you will be aware of many types of data available in a practice setting. For example, imagine that you are working in a community health centre as part of a regional health service. You will have client files of your own and those of other workers, detailed medical records from the other services under the regional health umbrella and, presumably, historical records.

With growing demands for accountability and evidence-based practice, researching these rich sources of data is becoming increasingly important. Giles et al. (2011, p. 2) comment that 'the reflective practitioner of the past ... is now becoming the reflective practitioner researcher'. Secondary analysis of clinical and other agency records is termed 'clinical data mining' (CDM). Giles et al. (2011) argue that CDM is complementary to evidence-based practice (see Chapter 11), and is another research methodology on the continuum of research methodologies, with its own strengths and weaknesses. Whereas evidence-based practice tends to be researcher driven, CDM is practitioner driven. This is the localised research you do to find out about the impacts of and patterns in what is happening as a result of your agency's interventions. To be effective, it is important to have organisational support and infrastructure to develop ways to identify and collect the right data, and to help practitioners with the more sophisticated methods of data analysis available.

Of course, there are public domain sources as well, and no doubt you are familiar with many of them. These would include the national Census data, material produced by federal, state and local government authorities, and reports published by non-government welfare agencies. This type of material is increasingly available in online formats, and will be useful for any study undertaken—even at the local level. For example, suppose that you wish to study culturally and linguistically diverse (CALD) people and their access to your community health centre. It would be useful to know the breakdown of your local area's population by language spoken at home, or country of birth—statistics readily obtainable from Census material. When studying the Census data (which will be available online or through the local library), note also the proportions of different ethnic groups. Imagine that the ethnic population of your area is 30 per cent and (to simplify) that one-third of these are from Asian countries and two-thirds from Southern European areas. Now examine the records kept at your community centre. If fewer than 30 per cent of those using the service are from a non-English-speaking background, then you have a problem. If, for example, only 2 per cent of clients are Asian immigrants and 5 per cent are Southern Europeans, you have a serious problem. What you should note from this example is that you have conducted a research project without having gathered any original data!

Why do we conduct secondary analysis?

Giles et al. (2011) note that CDM is used for practice knowledge-building, clinical decision-making and reflective practice. They provide a useful summary of the purposes of CDM (Giles et al. 2011, p. 8):

- refine and enhance practice wisdom
- describe and evaluate practice
- promote evidence-informed practice
- identify best practices
- promote evidence-informed reflective practice by the practitioner
- promote team-building and pride in professionalism.

Governments in the global North (also called the 'West') are increasingly collecting large data sets that researchers can access to answer questions about patterns of medical conditions, poverty and other social conditions, levels of support and service available, the distribution of welfare and other services. When secondary analysis of these kinds of broader data sets is carried out, it can address the same range of research purposes that are served by more direct research methods.

Types of research using secondary analysis

Secondary analysis can be used to conduct an exploratory study, a descriptive study or even an explanatory study. Exploratory studies are about exploring possibilities and generating ideas for further research. You may, for example, explore your records to assess client composition. This exploration may reveal that women make up more than 50 per cent of the agency's client load and that these women are clustered in the 25–45 years age bracket. This exploratory study may generate a hypothesis that males are less likely to seek help. Remember, this has not been *proved* by your exploration. You would need to conduct a further study to *test* such a hypothesis. Exploratory studies are good ways of generating hypotheses in research areas where you have some interest.

Secondary analysis is an excellent source of descriptive material in that records may be assessed to provide a descriptive profile of the client source. Similarly, secondary analysis can provide explanatory material that supports a hypothesis concerning causal links between variables.

Secondary analysis

- Secondary analysis is the process of using data that have already been collected for some other purpose to provide answers to your research question.
- Secondary analysis can be used for:
  - Exploratory studies
  - Descriptive studies
  - Explanatory studies.
- Sources of secondary data:
  - Agency records
  - Client files
  - Census records
  - Other public domain material
  - Data collected for other research

Problems with secondary analysis

While secondary analysis is an excellent way of conducting research, you should be aware of some serious pitfalls associated with such data. First, think back to the examination of the CALD composition of the community health centre's clients. If your centre is in an area that has a high transient population, you may be using an unreliable source of data. Because Censuses are conducted only once every five years (ten years in some countries), and it takes up to two years for the data to be analysed and disseminated to the public, you may be using material that is dated and no longer relevant to your area. Be aware that the data you use for secondary analysis may be seriously out of date.

Further, you must also be aware that the original data you are using for secondary analysis were obtained for a particular purpose. It may be that this purpose undermines the data's validity. For example, in research conducted on Australian farm women, Margaret Alston discovered that historical Census material would indicate that no women worked in agriculture or mining in the nineteenth century. This was perplexing, as she knew from other historical records such as diaries and newspapers that women were working in these areas. All was revealed when she discovered through further sources, including parliamentary records, that a decision was made in the 1890s to discard the records of women in these fields because politicians of the time wished to present a face to the world that

showed Australia was a *developed* nation. The idea of womei
the fields would have destroyed this image! Consequently, histo
do not record this information, and do not give an accurate p
work of women (Alston 1995). If you are unaware of the cont... ... which
the data were recorded, you may accept records with serious errors as true
recordings. Be aware that secondary analysis data must be seen *in context*.

You should also note that records may be unreliable because people
may record what they think *should* be recorded, not necessarily what *is*.
In her investigation of farm women, Margaret Alston realised that many
men who filled out Census records under-reported the farm contributions
of their wives. This appeared, in most cases, to be an unconscious factor
shaped by their limited definition of farm work. Women took farm work
to be a broader range of activities, including bookwork, travelling to buy
parts and supplies, providing meals for staff, and so on. Be conscious of
the fact that those who contributed the original data may hold a different
interpretation of reality to the one you may hold.

You should also remember that data may be inconsistent because of
problems with the original recording. If you are using agency records, for
example, different staff may record similar cases in a different way; they
may also be under pressure as a result of overwork and lack of time, and
therefore inconsistently record their own cases. Be aware that recording
may be inconsistent.

Additionally, you should note that some records may be missing or may
have been destroyed, and that consequently you might not have a reliable
source of data. For all these reasons, you should carefully assess the source
of your data and consider how reliable and valid it is. Relying on flawed
data will ensure that your results are also flawed. A useful way to get around
this problem may be to use other sources of data as well, to ensure that your
results are valid.

Problems with secondary analysis

- Data may be dated.
- Data must be seen in the context of the time in which they were
  recorded.
- Data may present a sanitised version because of different interpre-
  tations.
- Data may be inconsistently recorded.
- Some data may be missing.

Using the internet in social work research

Before leaving the topic of secondary sources, we must mention the use of the internet as a valuable resource for doing social research. The recent explosion in information and technology through the development of the online databases and information portals has led to a treasure trove of new resources for social researchers. A major challenge, however, is learning to navigate your way through this treasure trove and working out what is valuable and what is not.

All the problems we have discussed in relation to using secondary sources apply to using online data. An important skill for every researcher these days is to be a critical consumer and navigator of the World Wide Web. The internet itself provides excellent resources in how to evaluate information on the web. Many university libraries also have online tutorials on evaluating web-based material.

While the internet is increasingly being used as a medium for social research, with online surveys becoming more popular, be wary of using results from such research, or this medium as a research tool, too freely. Remember that only people with access to the internet at home or work will be likely to respond to such surveys. The focus of social work research is usually aimed at people who are disadvantaged, and who therefore are more likely than other groups to be excluded from participating in internet studies.

On the other hand, libraries are increasingly providing free online full-text versions of journal articles and research reports. Complete books are now online, both commercially and through libraries. Library catalogues and databases are often available to you through your home computer, and offer a marvellous resource that was unthinkable only a few years ago.

Another valuable use of the internet is as a source of types of questions, questionnaires, data sets and codebooks that are related to the topic in which you are interested. There are also sites that offer help in just about every aspect of doing research. Research texts increasingly offer guidance for web-based surveys. For example, in their book *Internet, Mail and Mixed-Mode Surveys*, Dillman, Smyth and Christian (2009) provide step-by-step guides to using the internet for surveys, including pro formas for emails and examples of web surveys. For an example of an internet resource for research methods, try <http://www.socialresearchmethods.net/kb/index.php>.

Using the internet in social research
- Learn to evaluate web-based material critically.
- Be aware of the limitations of using the internet as a primary research tool in social work research (e.g. for surveys).
- Take full advantage of the internet's rich resources in teaching how to undertake research.
- Learn to access the array of resources reporting existing research, including databases and library catalogues, questionnaires and databanks of questions, datasets and tools for interrogating them.

Content analysis

Another research method that is very useful is content analysis: the analysis of some form of communication—written, audio or visual—for trends or patterns, and the style and techniques used. Like secondary analysis, content analysis examines existing material, and does not necessarily require the researcher to collect original data. Content analysis is useful for examining not only what is included and how it is presented, but also what is excluded. For example, content analysis of women's magazines from the 1950s would provide an interesting idea of the issues that were seen to be relevant for women at the time. While there may be much on household tips, dress-making and cooking tips, there would probably be few articles on juggling work and family, coping with stress or dealing with sexual harassment in the workplace. Consequently, when conducting a content analysis study, be very conscious of what is not there as well as what is, and analyse what the message means for the recipient. It may be interesting for us, as social workers, to conduct a comparative content analysis of historical social work records with more modern records. Such a study would tell us much about the types of interventions used or the methods of assessment, as well as about the way records were kept.

Content analysis
Content analysis is the analysis of some form of communication for trends or patterns.

How to conduct a content analysis

When conducting a content analysis study, bear in mind that you may be interested not only in a quantitative analysis of the material, but also in a qualitative assessment of the way the material is presented, its style and the values represented. A content analysis study should include a series of well-planned steps. First, you must isolate your sample. If you are studying social work records in your agency, you might decide to compare a sample of records from the first year of operation with a sample from the current year. You note that the social work service began in 1968. You therefore choose to sample all records from February to June 1968 and compare the material with records from February to June 2002. Bear in mind that the timeframe is arbitrary, and depends largely on the amount of material available. In a large agency, a week of records may be as much as you can handle. Alternatively, you may choose a random sample of records, a systematic sample or some other form of sampling method that may be appropriate. Refer to Chapter 5 for types of sampling method.

Your next step is to decide on the categories to be employed in your analysis. This might be based on the type of content in the documents you are studying or on certain values expressed in the material. Whatever the categories you choose, they should be exhaustive and mutually exclusive. With the social work records study, you might choose to divide records into categories associated with assessment procedures and intervention strategies. Alternatively, you may be more interested in the values expressed in the reports, or some other form of categorisation.

The third step is to determine what it is you wish to measure. This may be based on the number of times a word or a theme appears, or on the amount of space or time given to a certain category. Finally, you must determine how you will record your analysis—in a database, in a frequency table or in some other systematic way.

Once your data are collected, you must carefully analyse the material to determine what conclusions you should draw. For example, your social work records study may have revealed that the historical records indicate that methods of assessment and intervention were very conservative and that the thrust of the intervention strategy was to change the client. Modern records may reveal more diverse types of interventions and a more critical evaluation of the social system. Of course, they may reveal nothing of the sort! What such a study will do, however, is provide a very interesting comparative analysis.

Conducting a content analysis

- Determine your sample.
- Decide on categories to be employed.
- Determine what it is you are measuring.
- Decide on the recording technique.
- Analyse data.
- Draw conclusions.

Case study 13.1: An analysis of sports reporting in rural media

In 1996, Margaret Alston conducted an analysis of media representations of women's sport in rural New South Wales. The study was funded by the New South Wales Department for Women, and its aim was to determine whether media bias existed in sports representation. Three rural areas of differing sizes were selected for the study. All media—newspapers, radio and television—were investigated. Alston was concerned to gain a comprehensive picture of both winter and summer sports coverage and to look at quantitative as well as qualitative measures of presentation.

Because of the amount of media material avaliable, Alston decided to sample one month of newspapers in winter and one in summer, as well as two weeks of radio and television in both summer and winter. The quantitative categories selected were female only, male only, mixed sport, horses and dogs. Alston determined that this would be measured in the newspapers by the number of articles and the space in square centimetres, and by the number and size of photographs. For radio and television, the same categories were used and these were measured in seconds of airtime devoted to each category. The qualitative measures were the style of language used and (for the newspapers) whether photographs were active or passive shots (that is, whether those photographed were actively engaged in sport or posed for the camera).

A database was set up on computer, which allowed the research assistant to enter extraordinary amounts of data. For example, there were over 4500 entries for newspapers alone. Once entered in the database, the program allowed data to be manipulated, counted and analysed very easily and efficiently.

Not surprisingly, the data revealed that media bias in sports reporting was widespread and overwhelming. Newspaper coverage of women's sport was only 5 per cent of total sports coverage, while for television it was 13 per cent and for radio 7 per cent. Female sport received far less coverage than horses and only slightly more than dogs. Qualitative analysis revealed that the language used to report male sport was often aggressive, with terms such as 'battle' and 'strong' common, while female sports stories were often colourless and banal. Female sports photographs were also much more likely to be posed while male photographs were more often action shots. By using content analysis, this study was able to reveal the full extent of media bias against women's sport and the nature of the forms of bias. Subsidiary methods such as interviews with sports administrators and female athletes demonstrated the full implications of this bias, such as a resulting lack of sponsorship, a lack of priority given to talent-development opportunities for girls, less motivation to succeed and a dearth of female role models in sport.

Source: Alston (1996).

Observations

A particularly important method for social workers is observation. Observation allows us to overcome some of the limitation inherent in other methods. For instance, a survey of school children may reveal that none of them admits to being a schoolyard bully. While this may be true, it may also be that respondents do not admit to being bullies because it is not socially desirable behaviour. A study using observation techniques, with the researcher spending time in the playground observing the behaviour of children, may reveal quite different information.

Observation, quite simply, is the process of *watching* behaviour. It may be structured or unstructured, and it may involve the researcher being a participant or a non-participant in the behaviour being observed.

Observation
- Structured
- Unstructured
- Participant
- Non-participant

Structured observation

Structured observation is a method of systematically observing certain predefined behaviours and using a predetermined set of observation categories. These observations may be noted by the research participants themselves (for example, a client suffering depression may keep a diary of the number of times they are distressed) or by the researcher. Taking the schoolyard example, a researcher may observe the playground activities and note each time unnecessary physical and verbal force is used.

Structured observation is employed in quantitative studies where precise and quantifiable measurements are sought. In such cases, the problem is carefully defined, the observation site is determined and the observation categories are clearly developed. Those categories may include actions, attitudes, modes of speech or any other element that is a key factor in the research study. Because of the nature of the research design, structured observation studies are chiefly used in explanatory research.

Structured observation

- Quantitative
- Carefully planned
- Behaviour type observed and carefully defined
- Categories developed
- Time period determined
- Observation study completed
- Used mainly in explanatory research

Unstructured observation

Unstructured observation is a more qualitative method because there is no careful definition of the behaviour to be studied. The researcher observes behaviour and events in an endeavour to *explore* the situation under investigation. There is no careful plan and no organised categories of observation units. An example of an unstructured observation study may be one where the observer spends time in an institutional setting (for example, a nursing home) observing the way the organisation operates, the interactions between staff and residents, and other elements of the institution. The researcher may have no stated research objective other than to observe the effect of institutional life on residents. After a while, the observer may note patterns of behaviour or operations that affect the health and wellbeing of residents. This may be medication regimes, policies relating to the time residents are woken each morning, the way meals are delivered or other factors. Unstructured observation allows the researcher to 'soak up' the environment and to make observations that are free from any preconceptions about the situation. In a study using unstructured observation, the researcher may record incidents, impressions, dialogue and other important points about the research situation. Because of the research design, unstructured observation is more likely to be used in exploratory or descriptive studies.

Unstructured observation

- Qualitative
- Flexible research plan
- No preconceived ideas about what behaviour is to be observed
- Categories developed during the study
- Time period determined
- Observation study completed
- Used mainly in exploratory or descriptive research

Participant observation

The extent of the involvement of the researcher in the study situation must be assessed before research begins in an observation study. The researcher may choose to be a participant observer in the study or be a non-participant observer.

A *participant observer* becomes a part of the research situation. They participate in all activities and interact with those being researched. There are serious ethical dilemmas that must be considered before undertaking such a study. Some of the more famous participant observation studies—such as Whyte's (1955) study of street-corner gangs—collected rich data because they *did not* disclose to the observed that behaviour was being researched. Nowadays, such studies are viewed as ethically untenable, and generally are not conducted. Participant observers must note that disclosing their research activities will necessarily influence the behaviour being observed. Subjects will be less likely to disclose sensitive and critical information, and they may be inclined to change their behaviour to conform to what is seen to be socially desirable.

The participant observer must decide what data to record, how they will do this given that they are participating in the situation, and how these data are to be analysed. Participant observation studies may be quantitative or qualitative, depending on the research objectives. Such a study may be useful if you are evaluating the effects of a new social work program. You may choose to become a participant in the program to assess the issues from a client's perspective. By contrast, a non-participant study is one where the researcher is not participating in the behaviour or situation being examined.

Participant observation

- Researcher is part of the study situation.
- Ethical considerations require disclosure.
- Must assess effect on research situation of disclosure.
- May be quantitative or qualitative.
- Must decide what is to be recorded.
- Time period is determined.
- Note that the presence of the participant observer may influence the behaviour being studied.
- The observation study is completed.

Research design in observation studies

As with any piece of research, you should give careful thought to your research plan, noting that this will depend on whether you choose to use a quantitative or qualitative research framework, and on whether you are a participant or a non-participant. Give some attention to defining your research problem. Determine the level of your participation and whether your observation will be structured or unstructured. Decide on the sample, bearing in mind that it will include the observation site or event, the people to be observed and the duration of the observation period. Before you begin your study, you must decide how you will gain entry to the situation. It may be very difficult to become a participant observer in certain closed situations such as an institutional setting. Finally, you must decide how the data are to be analysed and reported.

While observation studies provide valuable information that may be unavailable through other means, you should note the limitations of these methods. By definition, they are time-consuming and cannot be used for large groups or for different time periods. Further, findings may be influenced by the participation or presence of the researcher, and there is no guarantee that the data are valid. Nevertheless, observation studies are useful for providing information about behaviour in a natural setting, and allow the researcher to observe and record a wide range of information.

Research design in observation studies

- Define the problem.
- Choose the sample, including site, event, people to be observed and timeframe.
- Determine the level of researcher participation.
- Determine whether observation is structured or unstructured.
- Decide what is to be recorded.
- Analyse and report results.
- Note the advantages and limitations of the method.

Case studies

Case study research is research focused on a single case, issue, group, organisation or event. It is quite different from the single system design discussed in the previous chapter. In contrast to other methods, case study research does not seek patterns of behaviour by comparative analysis of a number of subjects. Rather, it examines one case—usually defined as a typical case—in order to fully investigate and thoroughly analyse the details that may be lost in a larger study. Case study research is particularly important in social work settings because it allows a typical case, client, event, group or other phenomenon to be studied in order to reveal information that will aid the analysis of, and afford insights into, the wider target group. The information will assist in the development of an appropriate intervention strategy.

Imagine that one of your clients is a carer of an HIV/AIDS patient. This may be a new client group for you, one about which you know little. By investigating the situation, tensions and pressures placed on your client, your case study research will give you a great deal of information about the wider population of carers of HIV/AIDS patients.

Case study research is also useful when you wish to study a particular group (for example, you may have established a group of sexual assault survivors), an organisation (such as a branch office) or an event (such as a social action campaign). Such case studies will yield rich data about the wider population or social system; therefore, this type of research should not be dismissed as insignificant research.

Case studies may be used in quantitative research as a means of clarifying the research hypothesis and as a form of pre-test. In qualitative studies, case study research is an important exploratory method. Feminist researchers view case study research as a very important way of exploring the experiences of different groups of women in different situations and cultures. As Reinharz (1992, p. 174) states:

> The case study is a tool of feminist research that is used to document history and generate theory. It defies the social science convention of seeking generalisations by looking instead for specificity, exceptions and completeness. Some feminist researchers have found that social science's emphasis on generalisations [has] obscured phenomena important to particular groups, including women. These case studies are essential for putting women on the map of social life.

When conducting a case study, you need to determine what it is you wish to investigate, what particular characteristics of the case study are important, and what it is you wish to achieve. Choose your case carefully, as it must represent a typical or special example, and decide how the data will be gathered and analysed. Finally, give some thought to the reporting of the case and how best to disseminate your insights and discoveries.

The advantages of case study research include the fact that data are often readily available, that it allows an examination of complex situations which may render other methods unsuitable and that it may require less resourcing. The limitations include a lack of quantification and a lack of ability to generalise.

Case study
- Studies a single case, group, organisation or event.
- Does not seek generalisations or comparisons.
- May be used in qualitative or quantitative research.
- Particularly important in feminist research.
- A case study design includes an outline of the problem, how the case will be chosen (sampling), data-collection and analysis techniques, and the way the study will be reported.

Summary

This chapter has presented a range of methods that will be useful for social work researchers. Methods presented here include secondary analysis, content analysis, observation and case study research. We have also discussed some critical points about using the internet in social work research. Each of these methods has its own particular advantages and limitations. The method you choose will ultimately be determined by the type of data you are seeking, the resources at your disposal (including time), your access to the situation and the nature of the research subjects. By balancing these factors, you will be able to determine what is the most appropriate method to address your research problem.

Remember that with any piece of research you should consider the value of triangulation—using more than one method to provide comprehensive data. Each of the methods described in this chapter, while important in its own right, can be used in conjunction with other methods to increase the validity and reliability of the data, and to add weight to the conclusions drawn from the study.

Discussion questions

13.1   What is secondary analysis?

13.2   What sources of data are available for secondary analysis in a social work setting?

13.3   What are the advantages and limitations of secondary analysis?

13.4   List some of the ways the internet can be used in social work research. What cautions apply?

13.5   What is content analysis?

13.6   How would you conduct a content analysis study?

13.7   Outline the different types of observation studies.

13.8   What are the advantages and limitations of observation studies?

13.9   Why is case study research important?

13.10 What are the advantages and limitations of case study research?

13.11 How would you undertake a piece of case study research in your work or study setting?

Exercises

13.1   Go to the library or access Census data online and study the Census records for your area. List the ethnic and age breakdown of your community and the five dominant occupations for men and women. What have you learned about your community and what do you think might be its welfare service needs?

13.2   Examine the front page of your local newspaper for a one-week period. How many stories featured women and how many featured men? What does your analysis suggest?

13.3   Spend some time in the waiting room of the accident and emergency section of your local hospital conducting an unstructured observation study. What have you learned?

13.4   Spend time with a work colleague or fellow student assessing how they balance their work/study activities with their family life. What does your case study tell you about the issues facing workers/students in your organisation?

13.5   Visit the website <http://www.socialresearchmethods.net/kb/index. php>. Explore some of the links, including the one on unobtrusive research methods. Try the search page, with its links to other parts of the website.

Further reading

Babbie, E. 2010, *The Practice of Social Research*, 12th edn, Wadsworth, Belmont, CA. See Chapter 11, 'Unobtrusive research'.

Berg, B.L. 2007, *Qualitative Methods for the Social Sciences*, 7th edn, Pearson, New York. See chapters on content analysis and unobtrusive methods.

Dillman, D.A, Smyth, J.D. and Christian, L.M. 2009, *Internet, Mail and Mixed-Mode Surveys*, John Wiley & Sons, Hoboken, NJ. This book discusses when internet surveys are useful and when mailed surveys or interviews are preferable. It contains good examples of how to undertake internet surveys.

Dudley, J. 2011, *Research Methods for Social Work: Being Producers and Consumers of Research*, 2nd edn, Allyn and Bacon, Boston, MA. Chapter 10, 'Constructing observational studies', examines participant observation and non-participatory unstructured observation studies, with social work examples.

Engel, R.J. and Schutt, R.K. 2009, *The Practice of Research in Social Work*, 2nd edn, Sage, Thousand Oaks, CA. Chapter 9, 'Qualitative methods', deals with case studies and various forms of observation.

Giles, R., Epstein, I. and Vertigan, A. (eds) 2011, *Clinical Data Mining in an Allied Health Organization: A Real World Experience*, Sydney University Press, Sydney. The introduction, by Ros Giles, Anne Vertigan, Irwin Epstein and David Rhodes, provides a comprehensive overview of clinical data mining (CDM). Chapter 3, 'Tackling solastalgia: Improving pathways to care for farming families', by Phoebe Begg and Sarah Thompson, offers an excellent case study of how CDM can help practitioners document the impacts of their practice, change practice and improve service provision.

Hardwick, L. and Worsley, A. 2011, *Doing Social Work Research*, Sage, London. Chapter 7, 'Observation, narrative and other approaches', contains a good discussion with exemplars for recording data from structured and unstructured observations.

Morris, T. 2006, *Social Work Research Methods*, Sage, Thousand Oaks, CA. Chapter 19, 'The function of technology at each step of the way', contains an excellent discussion of the uses of technology at each stage of the research process.

Reinharz, S. 1992, *Feminist Methods in Social Research*, Oxford University Press, New York. See Chapter 8, 'Feminist content analysis', and Chapter 9, 'Feminist case studies'.

PART IV

Statistical analysis

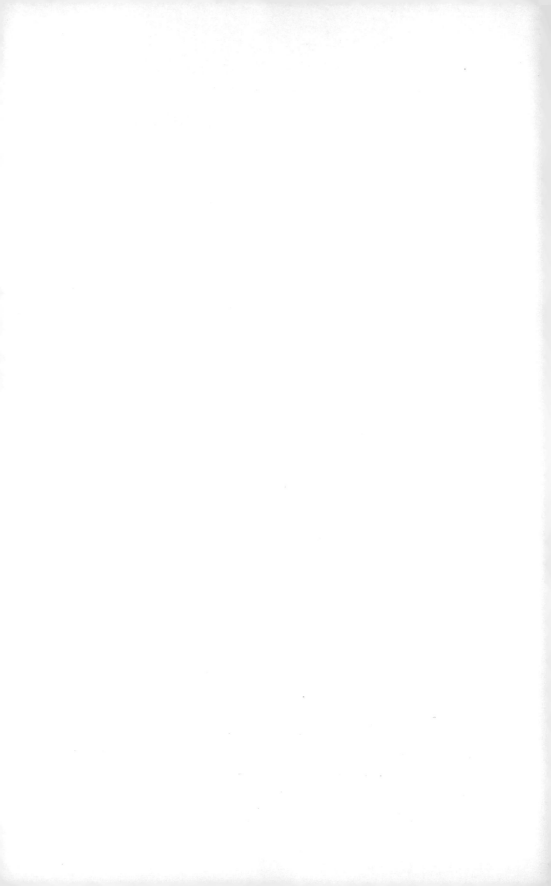

14 *Producing results: Qualitative research*

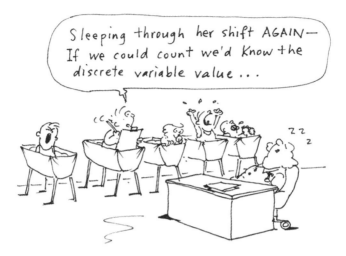

In this and the following three chapters, we discuss how to analyse the information you gather (data), in order to address the questions that generated your research project. In this chapter, we introduce the key aspects relating to qualitative data analysis. Chapters 15, 16 and 17 discuss data analysis for quantitative research.

Traditionally, the thought of data analysis has struck terror into the hearts of many research students in the social sciences, with many having visions of attempting to calculate statistics from difficult mathematical equations. However, this first chapter on qualitative data analysis deals with analysis that traditionally does not rely on mathematics at all. Even in quantitative analysis, nightmares about mathematics are now a thing of the past. Computers make calculations the easy part of research. In these chapters, we discuss the basic principles of organising your data so that computers can perform the statistical analysis you need. We also introduce you to some of the basic principles of data analysis as a preparation for the procedures that you will need to understand for your own research. The aim is to demonstrate the links between research questions, design and data analysis, and to provide a framework for thinking through fundamental approaches to data analysis as you plan a research project. Remember that the goal of research is to find answers to research questions and to develop theory. Whether we do this through qualitative or quantitative means or a combination of methods depends on establishing the most comprehensive ways of addressing the research question. You should therefore familiarise yourself with both methodologies and think creatively about their uses in undertaking your own research.

In this first chapter on qualitative data analysis, we discuss how qualitative researchers deal with the data they collect, and the careful processes that are undertaken to analyse this data. To keep things simple, we will explore the main principles of qualitative analysis using illustrations from one approach only: Corbin and Strauss's (2008) grounded theory approach to qualitative data analysis, a method based on Strauss and Corbin's earlier editions (1990 and 1997) and Strauss and Glaser's original work (e.g. see Glaser 1978, 1992; Glaser and Strauss 1967; Strauss 1990). This approach has been chosen because Corbin and Strauss give a clear explanation of what qualitative researchers actually do with their data, and because Corbin has developed useful guidelines for each stage of data analysis. This approach encompasses many of the principles of data analysis used in other types of qualitative research—although the emphases are different—and so serves as a useful introduction to qualitative analysis generally (Reissman 2008; Sarantakos 2005). The chapter concludes with a detailed example of qualitative analysis that illustrates the usefulness of data-analysis programs.

Differences between qualitative and quantitative analysis

Qualitative data analysis is different from quantitative analysis in several fundamental ways. First, as noted above, it does not rely on mathematics or numbers in the same way as quantitative analysis. Sometimes qualitative researchers count numbers of themes, or the numbers of people for whom certain themes apply, and sometimes they use computer packages in a similar way to quantitative researchers for certain aspects of their work. They may also describe their sample using quantitative terms (for example, 56 women and 24 men, five under 40 and ten aged 40 or over). In the main, however, qualitative researchers analyse their data using logic and theoretical and methodological principles, rather than by applying statistical formulae or quantification.

Thus qualitative data analysis is about interpretation rather than mathematics. It is about finding the meanings that people ascribe to their experiences. Corbin and Strauss (2008) describe qualitative analysis as using the same kinds of problem-solving and other common modes of thinking that occur in everyday life, except at a more self-conscious and scientifically rigorous level than usually occurs. As they do not emphasise figures or calculations, qualitative researchers mainly use text and explanation to present their data, instead of the charts and graphs that are typical of quantitative research results.

Second, there is not the same agreement on how to perform data analysis that exists in quantitative approaches (Reissman 2008; Grinnell and Unrau 2010; Corbin and Strauss 2008). Whereas quantitative researchers have well-documented, structured rules and procedures for data analysis (see Chapters 15 and 16), the procedures used by qualitative researchers are not as explicit and are more subjective. In fact, qualitative researchers argue that it is one of the strengths of qualitative research that it does *not* have a set of rules for data analysis. For example, Corbin and Strauss (2008) maintain that standardised sets of rules would only stifle and constrain qualitative researchers in their efforts to develop new theories. They point out that qualitative researchers work in such different contexts, with different aims, methods, gifts and talents, that it is impossible as well as undesirable to have strict rules of data analysis. They stress that their method of qualitative data analysis is meant to provide a guideline or framework only, rather than a set of rules such as quantitative researchers would provide, and that researchers should view qualitative analysis as an art as well as a science.

A third major difference between qualitative and quantitative data analysis is that qualitative data analysis usually occurs simultaneously with the data-collection phase, in a continuous, cyclical process. This requires that researchers be flexible in moving between and among tasks and steps in a non-linear process to produce rich and meaningful understandings of the data. Padgett (2008) and Corbin and Strauss (2008) refer to the process of moving from inductive analysis to deductive and back to inductive, with Padgett describing it as 'constant comparative analysis'. Indeed, Corbin and Strauss (2008) emphasise that data analysis can begin with the first interview or piece of evidence that is gathered, a process that encourages the researcher to think analytically rather than descriptively, and so move on to theorising without becoming lost in a mass of complex data. In quantitative analysis, by contrast, the data-collection phase occurs first, and data analysis only begins when the last interview or questionnaire has been coded and entered into the computer.

A fourth difference between qualitative and quantitative research, already alluded to, is that qualitative researchers may use a variety of methods as the study progresses. For example, a qualitative researcher may use information that is analysed from documents, as well as interviews that evolve as the researcher obtains more insights into the issue being researched. The researcher may also hold small-group meetings to clarify the emerging issues. In this way, the researcher builds up the data, creating a rich understanding of the study area. Whether such different methods are used will depend on the context of the study, the relevance of various sources as they are discovered and the hypotheses that evolve.

If a particular study does not yield useful information as planned, there is little the quantitative researcher can do but report the results as they occur, whereas in qualitative research the researcher is free to pursue alternative directions and use different methods of analysis according to their usefulness. As we have noted, this variety of methods makes standardised techniques for qualitative data analysis difficult. But we are able to give guidelines about the process. What is rigorous in qualitative data analysis, however, is the approach to thinking analytically and creatively about complex social phenomena. Essentially, there is no substitute for experience where qualitative data analysis is concerned.

These differences between qualitative and quantitative data analysis mean that they have different *strengths* and *weaknesses*. This was alluded to in our earlier discussion of reliability and validity (Chapter 3), in which it was noted that qualitative researchers prides themselves on the validity of their data, but that criticisms have been levelled with regard to the reliability of the data (or consistency or ability to be replicated). In contrast, the findings of some quantitative studies have been criticised as not being valid in the real world, or for simplifying complex issues to the point where they are not relevant. The strengths of quantitative studies include that they are relatively easy to replicate (that is, their reliability is easy to establish) and that they generally involve sophisticated comparisons of variables. Qualitative studies, on the other hand—because they often study a single situation in depth—have a corresponding weakness in their ability to compare variables in different conditions or to make claims about causality. However, because qualitative studies take into account the context in which the research is conducted and researchers have the flexibility to check and recheck their findings in the field (since data analysis occurs simultaneously with data collection), they claim validity.

Four differences between qualitative and quantitative data analysis
- Qualitative analysis relies on interpretation and logic whereas quantitative analysis relies on statistics (qualitative researchers present their

analyses using text and argument, whereas quantitative researchers use graphs and tables).

- Qualitative analysis has no set rules—rather, there are flexible guidelines—whereas quantitative analysis follows agreed upon standardised procedures and rules.
- Qualitative analysis occurs simultaneously with data collection, whereas quantitative analysis occurs only after data collection is finished.
- Qualitative analysis may vary its methods depending on the situation, whereas methods of quantitative analysis are determined in advance as part of the study design.

The process of qualitative data analysis

Before outlining Corbin and Strauss's 'grounded theory' approach to qualitative data analysis in detail, we will discuss the general assumptions behind, and steps involved in, the process of data analysis that all researchers from qualitative perspectives follow in some form. This may seem slightly contradictory, having just asserted that qualitative researchers do not follow standardised rules of data analysis. Nonetheless, despite there being no agreement on specific rules of analysis, there is agreement on the processes that qualitative researchers undertake to analyse their data, even if these are expressed in different ways by different researchers.

Several assumptions underlie most processes of qualitative data analysis. First, remember from earlier chapters that qualitative researchers are interested in the complexities of social reality. Their methods of data analysis, therefore, attempt to capture the meanings and relationships involved in these complexities.

Another assumption often made is that the experiences of both the researcher and the researched can be taken into account when collecting and analysing the data. Corbin and Strauss (2008) note that both researcher and researched construct meaning together in the generation of their data. For example, in the study of postnatal depression described in Chapter 3, the researchers consulted the participants about the questions to be asked and reported back their initial results for discussion and analysis. In Chapter 1, we discussed how qualitative researchers often see themselves and their experiences as an important part of the research process, because they reject notions of objectivity. Instead of being separate from the research process, qualitative researchers may analyse their own interactions with the issues and/or people they are researching as a critical part of the analysis. The researcher's own experience and skills—or 'experiential data'—are drawn from the researcher's personal, research and literature-reading experiences. Corbin and Strauss refer to this as being sensitive to the nuances of the data by drawing on our knowledge and experience: 'Background knowledge and experience not only enable us to be more sensitive to concepts in data, they also enable us to see connections between concepts.' (2008, p. 34) Explicitly mining this source of data leads to much better theory-building, which is the ultimate task of qualitative researchers. However, Corbin and Strauss warn that experience should not be used as primary data, but rather as something to be drawn on in sensitising the researcher to nuances of their data.

In earlier chapters, we described the process of qualitative research as being 'inductive'. By this we meant that the hypotheses and theory coming from the research are generated from the data itself (in the cyclical process described above), and are thus 'grounded' in the data that the researcher has gathered. In Chapter 2, the analogy of a climbing pyramid was used to describe how qualitative researchers begin at the bottom rungs— the broadest base of the pyramid—before gradually climbing up to higher levels of abstraction. This is the opposite to the route taken by quantitative researchers, who begin at the top of the pyramid, with concepts, dimensions, indicators, variables and hypotheses worked out before the data are collected.

Corbin and Strauss (2008) and Padgett (2008) make the following important point about inductive and deductive activities in the research process: all researchers are involved in both inductive and deductive thinking in a cyclical manner. The difference between qualitative and quantitative research is the starting point of the process.

Sarantakos (2005) identifies three general stages in qualitative data analysis, which describe what is going on during induction, deduction and verification. Again, it is emphasised that these stages occur cyclically. Sarantakos (2005) terms the first stage *data reduction*. This is the stage where data are coded, summarised and categorised in order to identify important aspects of the issue being researched. Data reduction also helps the researcher decide what further data to collect, how and who to sample next, and what methods of analysis to use and, finally, to arrive at conclusions. All these activities involve induction, and sometimes deduction as well. The important goal of data reduction is to identify the main themes emerging from the research by categorising the information as it is collected. In some forms of qualitative research, data collection, data reduction and data analysis are almost indistinguishable (Sarantakos 2005).

The second stage of qualitative data analysis, according to Sarantakos (2005), is *data organisation*. This is the process of assembling the information around certain themes and points, and presenting the results—usually in text. The third phase is *interpretation*. This involves identifying patterns, trends and explanations that lead to conclusions, which can be tested through more data collection, reduction, organisation and interpretation. Further data collection, reduction, organisation and interpretation occur until the categories or themes that are being researched are 'saturated'— that is, there are no more new insights or information being generated.

Aspects of qualitative data analysis

- Qualitative data analysis aims to capture the richness and complexity of lived experience.
- Qualitative data analysis includes the experiences of the researcher, both before and during the research (experiential data).
- Qualitative data analysis consists of three general stages, which follow one another in a continuous cycle: *data reduction, data organisation* and *interpretation*.

Qualitative data analysis: The grounded theory approach

Strauss and Glaser first published their book *Discovery of Grounded Theory* in 1967. In 1998, Strauss and Corbin (1998) published their second edition of *Basics of Qualitative Research*. Juliet Corbin continued this series following the death of Anselm Strauss, publishing a further edition of *Basics of Qualitative Research* in 2008 (Corbin and Strauss 2008). We draw on these works to outline their understanding of a grounded theory approach to data analysis. This discussion illustrates the rigorous thinking that goes into analysing qualitative data, and the processes involved in transforming this data into 'grounded theory'. You will see that Strauss and Corbin's (1998) and Corbin's and Strauss's (2008) approach involves the three activities (data reduction, organisation and interpretation) described above. Throughout the whole process, induction, deduction and verification are occurring continuously.

Briefly, Corbin and Strauss's (2008) method of data analysis involves *data collection, data coding* and *memoing*. The researcher goes back and forth between each of these phases, which together make up the 'coding paradigm'. *Data collection* is the finding/gathering of information for the researcher to analyse. *Data coding* is a general term used by Corbin and Strauss to mean conceptualising data: careful examination and thinking about the data, often in conjunction with experiential insights, which leads to asking generative questions. Generative questions make comparisons and distinctions between the information collected and stimulate the line of inquiry in profitable directions. Corbin and Strauss use the term *coding* to refer to any product of this sort of analysis that creates categories, as well as exploring the relationships between them. Three types of coding are discussed below.

Memos are separate analytical notes that the researcher makes to help them think theoretically about their findings; these record theoretical questions, concepts, hypotheses, summaries of codes, insights, clues for further data collection, and so on. Memos keep track of coding results, stimulate further coding and integrate theory.

Corbin and Strauss (2008) note that qualitative researchers from a grounded theory perspective use the coding paradigm in a very different way from other qualitative researchers. Whereas more positivist qualitative researchers move forward in a linear way from data collection through to coding and hypothesising, and then collect new data to verify their hypotheses, grounded theory researchers move back and forth between data collection, coding and memoing from very early in the process, and continue to do so throughout the project. The developing theory is grounded in the data because it develops through intensive and systematic analysis of data, sometimes sentence by sentence or phrase by phrase (Glaser 1978, cited in Strauss 1990, p. 22, and reflected in subsequent editions including Corbin and Strauss 2008). Data collection quickly leads to coding, which may soon lead to memoing, either of which will guide the researcher to more data collection, or more coding and memoing, or even to reinspection and analysis of old data that has already been analysed. A grounded theory approach allows the researcher to return to old data at any point in the research process, even when the researcher is writing the last page of their final report!

The process by which researchers collect more data as a result of their coding and memoing activities is termed *theoretical sampling*. This is sampling of people, situations, events or activities that is guided by the need to compare ideas or answer questions in the process of developing theory. This type of sampling is very different from sampling in quantitative research because it is driven by the emerging theory. The basic question behind theoretical sampling is: 'What groups or subgroups of populations, events, activities (to find varying dimensions, strategies, etc.) does one turn to next in data collection? And for what theoretical purpose?' (Glaser 1978, cited in Strauss 1990, pp. 38–9, and reproduced in many works since as a standard definition of theoretical sampling). It is useful when sampling theoretically to look at the deviant or atypical cases—or what might be referred to as the 'outriders'. In assessing these cases, you are better able to illuminate the norms emerging from your data.

The early phases of data analysis in this approach are more open than the later ones, although it may take long periods of data collection, coding and memoing before the researcher decides on which categories and concepts are the most important (the most important categories are termed *core categories*). As theoretical sampling guides the collection of more data, memos become more theoretical and 'integrative', and core categories emerge. Once core categories have been established, the researcher concentrates on relating other categories to them, gradually making the developing theory more 'dense'. Additional categories and properties related to the core categories will continue to be 'discovered' throughout this process. As the research proceeds, memos become more elaborate and conceptual, making links and integrating earlier ideas so that the entire theory can be written up in the final report. Corbin and Strauss (2008) emphasise that each research project will be unpredictable in terms of the way the steps of data collection, analysis (coding) and interpretation (memoing) evolve. However, there are several essential operations you should note when undertaking qualitative analysis from a grounded theory perspective.

Managing data

Padgett (2008) and Miles and Huberman (2002) refer to qualitative data analysis as a hierarchical typology of abstraction where the researcher moves from the raw data (field notes, documents transcripts and memos) to coded transcripts and analytical memos to a conceptual map of the emerging theory. To achieve the transition between stages cleanly, you need to deal with your data in a systematic way. The guidelines in the box are the result of our experience managing large amounts of qualitative data.

Guidelines for managing qualitative data

- The main advice we can give is to begin early!
- Organise and store your data for maximum efficiency and retrieval.

- Copy digital recordings and transcribe any taped interview material as soon as is practical so that this precious material is not lost or corrupted. If this process is delayed, copy the recordings on to your computer and on to another separate drive immediately and keep them in separate locations. You should try to have the transcribing done as you go to minimise the delay in analysis and to keep abreast of the costs.
- Mark each recording, document, field note and memo with the date, time, place and source of information.
- Once you have had your recorded material transcribed, make backup copies of your files and again keep copies in separate places. When formatting your file, leave a wide margin on the left-hand side of the paper, to allow you to make notations as you read.
- Read and reread your transcript, marking preliminary codes in the margins. After reading several transcripts, write your codes on a large sheet of paper, noting linkages between codes and sub-codes. Note that this beginning schema will change several times during the course of your analysis before you are completely satisfied with the emerging theory.
- During your analysis, write memos noting the linkages between codes, questions that arise, ideas for theoretical sampling and any other issue that is significant.

As the conceptual framework becomes clearer, you will note that some data is more relevant than others and it is okay to focus on the more relevant material.

A final piece of advice is to use a computer program to store and retrieve your material. Several programs are available, including INVIVO and Ethnograph. These programs allow ease of data management and can assist you to organise and conceptualise your data. If you are conducting a large project, the purchase of one of these programs is very worthwhile.

Data collection

We have already seen how qualitative data can be collected from a range of sources, including interviews, group meetings, documents and field observations. Beginning the data analysis as early as the first, second or third interview or day of observation helps prevent the richness of the data from becoming overwhelming. This is because early analysis guides the direction of the next interviews or observation by providing analytic questions and hypotheses about categories and their relationships. As the analysis of new data develops, so the guidance of the analysis becomes more explicit.

Just as coding and memoing begin early in the process of data collection and continue throughout the life of the project, so data collection continues because coding and memoing raise fresh questions that need to be addressed through either gathering new data or re-examining old data. Theory-guided data collection (theoretical sampling) often also leads to new methods of data collection—for example, a series of directed interviews to supplement the more casual ones already done during fieldwork.

Coding

Strauss's (1990, p. 27) comment is often quoted as a basic premise of qualitative data analysis: 'The excellence of the research rests in large part on the excellence of the coding.' The ability to code well and easily is one of the keys to successful qualitative data analysis. Coding involves much more than simple description—it is important that it become analytical as quickly as possible. One of the most difficult aspects of qualitative data analysis is learning to move from the data to the more abstract level of theory. To assist researchers to code data in a way that is relevant and helpful in forming categories, Strauss (1990), Strauss and Corbin (1998) and Corbin and Strauss (2008) suggest the following paradigm of what to look for in the data when coding:

* conditions
* interaction among actors
* strategies and tactics
* consequences.

Conditions become easy to recognise when the researcher looks for cues in words such as 'because', 'since' and 'as'. Similarly, *consequences* can be revealed by phrases such as 'because of that', 'the result was' and 'in consequence'. *Strategies and tactics* are usually easy to discover and observe, and *interactions* among actors consist of all other interactions that are not strategies or tactics. While this paradigm may be useful to you in analysing your data, the most important thing you should be looking for are the emerging *themes*—the issues that are important to the people from whom the data is collected.

As the data collection and analysis progress, so coding changes as concepts are developed. Corbin and Strauss (2008) identify three types of coding that occur at different phases in the research: *open coding*, *axial coding* and *selective coding*. Other authors may use different terms to describe this process, but most refer to the original labels identified by Strauss and Corbin (1998) and Corbin and Strauss (2008).

Open coding

Open or first-level coding is the initial type of coding that is done early in the research. It is the unrestricted coding of data that aims to produce provisional concepts and dimensions that seem to fit the data. In turn, these will result in many more questions and provisional answers about conditions, strategies, interactions and consequences. As the researcher proceeds through the data, the process snowballs, with more information raising new questions that in turn lead to the search for more information. From this description, it can be seen that the skill and training of the researcher in 'opening up' the data to tentative interpretation are a crucial part of the process.

At this early stage, Corbin and Strauss (2008) reassure us, it does not matter whether the codes are 'right' or not, as further inquiry will soon establish which categories are more or less useful in describing what is happening in the data. Thus codes are modified, and even discarded, as data collection and coding continue. Because this process of modification and elaboration is central to the analysis, it is important not to become committed to particular codes too early. Be careful not to be swayed by pre-existing theoretical understandings—remain open to all possibilities. Although it may seem as though codes are proliferating in the early stages, this slows down and some codes are eliminated as the data are checked for verification (that is, checking that the code really does fit). Gradually the code becomes saturated and is placed in relationship to other codes. The important function of open coding is to help the researcher move quickly to an analytic level by 'fracturing the data', or breaking it apart so that the exciting process of developing grounded theory can begin.

There are two main types of code: *in vivo* and *constructed*, or sociological, codes. *In vivo* codes come directly from the language of the people being studied, and are usually vivid in imagery as well as being analytically useful. They are terms or descriptions that explain the basic problems or processes faced by the people being researched and can lead to associated theoretical codes. For example, in Strauss's (1990) study of people–machine interactions in hospitals, people often used the term 'monitoring'. This is an *in vivo* code that describes a set of behaviours by patients and nurses. It implies various conditions under which the monitoring is done, the consequences of monitoring or not monitoring, and so on (that is, the items in the coding paradigm above).

Constructed or sociological codes, on the other hand, are codes formulated by the researcher that are based on the researcher's own knowledge as well as the data being studied. Constructed codes can add more sociological meaning to the analysis than *in vivo* codes because they go beyond local meanings to broader concerns, and because they are constructed systematically.

Strauss's (1990) original work in this area represents a classic contribution and is often drawn on by writers on qualitative data analysis. He offers several guidelines for open coding, which are summarised as shown in the box.

Guidelines for open coding of qualitative data

- Look for *in vivo* codes.
- Give each code a provisional name (whether *in vivo* or constructed) without worrying too much about whether it is right—this can be modified later.
- Move quickly to dimensions that seem relevant to given words, phrases, etc.
- Concentrate on finding comparative cases in order to explore the dimensions.
- From the beginning, continually ask a series of questions of the data, including:
  – To what study are these data pertinent?
  – What category does this incident indicate?
  – What is actually happening in the data? (What's the main story here and why?)
- Analyse the data minutely (line by line or phrase by phrase) until the category seems saturated. Ask many questions about words, phrases, sentences and actions in the line-by-line analysis as you go.
- Pay attention to the coding paradigm: conditions, interactions, strategies and consequences.
- Frequently interrupt the coding to write a theoretical memo.
- Do not assume the relevance of traditional variables such as age, race or sex until they emerge in the data.

Source: Strauss (1990, pp. 29–31).

Once a particular code seems to be relatively saturated, the researcher may move more quickly through the data, noting repetitions and scanning the pages for something new. At that point, the minute examinations begin again. Thus the intense form of open coding occurs at various stages throughout the analysis. Saturation is achieved when your data fit into established codes and no new codes emerge. It is wise to reflect upon your coding at this point before moving to the next level to ensure that your analysis reflects the data. Have you missed anything? Does your interpretation cover all the major ideas presented by those interviewed? Is there a need for further theoretical sampling?

Axial coding

The next stage, axial or second-level coding, is an important, particular aspect of open coding that occurs in the later stages of the open coding process and is different from the looser kinds of open coding that occurred earlier. (Other kinds of open coding can also alternate with axial coding.) Axial coding occurs once the researcher decides to code more intensively and concertedly around one category at a time (hence its name, as the analysis revolves around the axis of one category). It is more abstract, and involves interpretation on the part of the researcher. Look for relationships between codes and themes. Link codes and work towards a higher level of abstraction. Axial coding increases in intensity as the researcher moves towards developing core categories, and precedes selective coding. It also runs parallel to the increasing number of relationships being specified among categories (although not all this coding will be done as intensively as axial coding).

Selective coding

Once the researcher has decided on the core categories that are central to the research, they can move into selective coding. Selective coding means that the researcher codes systematically only for the core codes and those codes that are related to them. The core code, once decided upon, becomes the guide to further theoretical sampling and data collection. Thus selective coding is different from open coding but occurs within the context developed while doing open coding. Selective coding becomes increasingly dominant as the analysis progresses. During selective coding, analytic memos become more focused and theory becomes integrated.

In summary, Strauss's original seven rules for coding data are still relevant today (see box).

Seven rules of thumb for coding data

- Do not merely describe or summarise the phrases of the data—discover genuine categories and name them (at least provisionally).
- Relate categories as specifically and variably as possible to the four items in the coding paradigm (conditions, consequences, strategies and interactions).
- Relate categories to sub-categories, all to each other—that is, make a systematically dense analysis.
- Do all of the above on the basis of specific data. Frequently reference this data by page, quote or precis.
- Underline, for ease of scanning and sorting later.
- Once you have decided on the core category or categories, relate all categories and sub-categories to the core—that is, move from open coding through axial to selective coding so that the analysis becomes integrated.
- Later, minor or unrelated categories and hypotheses can be discarded as more or less irrelevant. Otherwise, the researcher must attempt to specifically relate them to the major core of their analysis.

Source: Strauss (1990, p. 81).

Core categories

During qualitative data analysis, the researcher is constantly searching for the 'main story', concern or theme that accounts for most of the variation in the patterns of behaviour being observed/talked about. Corbin and Strauss write that the researcher should repeatedly ask themselves 'What is the main story here?' as a kind of motto question throughout the research, to remind themselves that what they are searching for is the *core category* (or categories—there can be more than one). They also advocate that researchers should begin to label potential core categories as early as possible.

A core category is related to most other categories and their properties (see, for example, Hallberg 2006). It is the key category around which theory generation occurs by making the grounded theory *dense* and *saturated* as relationships between the core category and sub-categories are discovered. Theoretical sampling further saturates the categories because they are related to many others and recur often in the data: 'The core category must be proven over and over again by its prevalent relationship to other categories.' (Glaser 1978, cited in Strauss 1990, p. 35) The more data there are supporting the core categories, the more the researcher can be sure of having chosen the core categories accurately. Core categories should integrate theory and have explanatory power if the research is to be successful. To facilitate the process of theory-building around core categories, there are some pictorial strategies that you can use. We are not alone in suggesting you make some form of graphical representation of your data (e.g. see Slone 2009). Try drawing a diagram of your codes and the way they fit together, count the number of times core categories occur, look for missing links and, importantly, note contradictory evidence.

Criteria for selecting core categories

- The core category must be the most central category, and should be related to as many other categories and their properties as possible.
- It must appear frequently in the data (that is, the indicators pointing to the concept of the core category must appear frequently). Thus it is seen as a stable pattern.
- It relates easily to other categories.
- It has clear implications for a more general theory.
- As the details of the core category are worked out, so the theory is developed.
- It allows for building in maximum variation to the analysis, since the researcher is coding in terms of its dimensions, properties, conditions, consequences and so on.

Source: Strauss (1990, p. 36).

Memos

Memos are analytic notes that are kept separately from coding notes, and that are made throughout the research project. As the project progresses, so different types of memos are written. Early in the research there may be initial orienting memos, preliminary memos and 'memo sparks'. Later on, memos deal with initial discoveries, new categories, distinguishing between two or more categories, and other relationships between categories. As the research progresses, so memos become more elaborate, analytic and theoretically dense. They may include integrative diagrams as well as recording theoretical questions, hypotheses, summary of codes, further directions, and so on. Memos provide a way of keeping track of coding and of the researcher's thoughts. They are the major means of integrating theory in grounded theory analysis.

Strauss provides many rules for writing memos, some of which are described in the box.

Rules for writing memos
- Keep memos and data separate.
- Record the date of the memo.
- Write down memos as ideas occur, even if it means interrupting coding.
- Include references and important sources.
- Don't force memo-writing (though writing a code can assist memo-writing if you are stuck).
- Label memos according to the codes to which the memo relates.
- Modify memos as research develops. (Strauss notes that the data is more precious than the theory. If the theory doesn't fit, it should be modified to fit the data.)
- Keep a list of codes handy to check that you have not missed any relationships.
- When writing memos, talk about the codes as they are theoretically coded, not individual people (this helps maintain the level of analysis as relationships among concepts).
- Write ideas up one at a time.
- Use diagrams in memos to explain ideas.
- Mark memos 'saturated' when the categories are saturated.
- Always be flexible in your techniques for writing memos.
- Keep multiple copies.

Source: Strauss (1990); Strauss and Corbin (1998); Corbin and Strauss (2008).

In order to ensure the credibility of your findings and theory development, document everything you do during analysis, ask a colleague to assess your data to see whether they arrive at the same results and/or check the results with the research participants to see whether they agree with your analysis. Additionally, you might consider further theoretical sampling with people with markedly different views to balance any bias, and ensure that you carefully assess atypical cases. In these ways, you act to ensure the validity of your findings.

Use of computers in qualitative data analysis

The process of qualitative data analysis has become far more manageable with the increasing sophistication of qualitative data analysis software. Two packages that we would recommend are INVIVO and Ethnograph. Both allow for large amounts of data to be managed more effectively by enabling sorting and coding. What used to be an arduous chore, involving massive amounts of interviews and observations recorded on paper, has now become streamlined. You should take the time to learn to use one of these packages. It will be time well spent. It is particularly important to consider purchasing a program if the project is large and you are likely to use the program again.

Summary

In this chapter, we have considered the differences between qualitative and quantitative data analysis and examined in detail the processes of qualitative data analysis involved in Corbin and Strauss's grounded theory approach, and have paid due attention to the detailed advice given by Anselm Strauss, considered one of the critical theorists in this area. We have seen how qualitative data analysis requires rigorous interaction with the data in order to develop new theory, which at all stages in the process is 'grounded' in data through a continuous, cyclical process between data collection, coding (analysis) and memoing (interpretation). Three types of coding have been discussed, and handy hints for coding and memoing have been provided.

In Chapter 1, some criticisms of qualitative research as being too microscopic and focused only on interaction rather than larger social/political or structural issues were raised. Corbin and Strauss (2008) answer such criticisms by maintaining that proper coding can encompass both interactional (micro) and structural (macro) analysis, and even link the two theoretically, although this takes much time and thought. In their edited book *Grounded Theory in Practice* (1997), and their 2008 edition of *Basics of Qualitative Research*, they provide detailed examples of the way grounded theory researchers develop detailed codes leading to theoretical explanations. Analysis of close-in connections between contextual conditions and interactions can be widened to coding that analyses the impact of broader institutions, social and political forces on individual experience. The ultimate balance between the relative focus on macro- and micro-level analysis will be up to the individual researcher and research project. Thus qualitative data analysis is an exciting prospect with potential applications across a wide range of research activities, not just those micro interactional studies that traditionally have been seen as the appropriate place for qualitative analysis.

Discussion questions

14.1 What are some differences in the ways qualitative and quantitative researchers analyse their data?

14.2 Describe the different ways qualitative and quantitative researchers use induction, deduction and hypothesising, and develop indicators, dimensions and concepts.

14.3 What are three general stages in qualitative research, according to Sarantakos (2005)?

14.4 What does Strauss (1990) mean by the terms data collection, coding and memoing?

14.5 What are the four aspects that should be looked for when coding data to develop categories?

14.6 Describe the differences between open coding, axial coding and selective coding. What are their purposes and when do they occur in the research process?

14.7 What is theoretical sampling?

14.8 What is the role of core categories in qualitative data analysis?

Exercises

14.1 There are a number of books and journal articles presenting the findings of qualitative research. Locate one such study in your library—preferably by a researcher who used the grounded theory approach. What are the core categories in the study? How was the grounded theory developed? How do the researchers present their results? How do they verify their conclusions?

14.2 Select another piece of qualitative research from a sociological journal. How explicit are the authors about their methods of data analysis? Was a computer program used? How are the results presented? Could you replicate this study? Comment on the validity of the findings.

Further reading

Corbin, Juliet M. and Strauss, Anselm 2008, *Basics of Qualitative Research: Techniques and Procedures for Developing Grounded Theory*, Sage, Thousand Oaks, CA.

Grinnell, Richard M. and Unrau, Yvonne A. (eds) 2010, *Social Work Research and Evaluation*, 9th edn, Oxford University Press, New York.

Huberman, M.A. and Miles, M.B. 2002, *The Qualitative Researcher's Companion*, Sage, Thousand Oaks, CA.

Padgett, D.K. (2008), *Qualitative Methods in Social Work Research*, 2nd edn, Sage, Thousand Oaks, CA.

Reissman, Catherine Kohler 2008, *Narrative Methods for the Human Sciences*, Sage, Thousand Oaks, CA.

Sarantakos, Sotirios 2005, *Social Research*, Palgrave Macmillan, Melbourne.

15 Producing results: Quantitative research

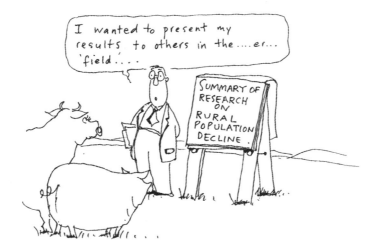

In the previous chapter, we saw that there were four major differences between qualitative and quantitative data analysis. First, unlike qualitative research, quantitative research has clearly defined rules about how to go about data analysis. Second, quantitative data analysis involves mathematics and statistics. Third, quantitative research usually follows a single method of data analysis that has been worked out in advance as part of the design of the study. Finally, data analysis occurs after all the data have been collected in quantitative research.

Noting that many studies will incorporate both quantitative and qualitative methods, some of the differences in data analysis mean that in these days of computer analysis, quantitative data analysis can be relatively easy, even though it involves the use of statistics. In this chapter we set out some fundamental principles of data analysis for quantitative research as well as a guide to coding your results for computer entry. Examples from the SPSS program for data analysis are used. This is because SPSS is the most common program used in universities and large welfare organisations. There are many other programs which are easy to use.

Factors affecting quantitative data analysis

Four factors determine the type of quantitative data analysis to be used (de Vaus 2002). These are the number of variables, the level of measurement, the purpose of the statistics (whether descriptive or inferential) and ethical responsibilities.

The number of variables

The first factor is the *number of variables* being analysed. This depends on the types of research question the study addresses. Data analysis involving one variable at a time is termed *univariate analysis*; data analysis involving two variables is called *bivariate analysis*; and data analysis involving three or more variables is known as *multivariate analysis*.

Often the reporting of quantitative results begins with descriptions of the sample and results using univariate statistics to paint a general picture. Following this general description, more complex statistics are performed to investigate relationships between two or more variables.

Examples of questions involving different numbers of variables

- *Univariate*—one variable
  ('How many?', 'What type?')

- *Bivariate*—two variables
  ('Does living in the country or city affect the sort of service provided to income-support agency clients on their initial visit?')

- *Multivariate*—more than two variables
  ('Does age affect the different experiences people from the country or city have when they visit an income-support agency for the first time?')

Level of measurement

The second factor that must be taken into account when planning quantitative data analysis is the *level of measurement* of the variables being analysed. Review Chapter 3 for definitions of *nominal, ordinal, interval* and *ratio* levels of measurement.

Choosing the appropriate level of measurement for each variable depends on several factors. In general, it is best to measure variables at the highest level of measurement possible. Higher levels of measurement provide more information, and allow more powerful statistical techniques to be used. In addition, it is always possible to reduce the level of measurement after data is collected (for example, from interval to ordinal), but it is mostly not possible to increase the level of measurement once you have collected data at a lower level.

On the other hand, asking for too much detail (too high a level of measurement) may lead to inaccurate or untruthful replies. For example, if you asked how often people attended an income-support agency during the last two years (interval level), they may be unable to give an exact number of times and either make up an answer or not answer the question at all. However, they may respond with reasonable accuracy to an ordinal range of responses ('at least weekly', 'approximately once per fortnight', 'between fortnightly and monthly', 'three or four times a year', 'twice a year', 'once only'). From this brief example, it can be seen that deciding on the appropriate level of measurement for each variable is an art in itself—one that requires consideration of a range of issues.

Descriptive and inferential statistics

The third factor in deciding which types of data analysis should be performed is whether the researcher wants to use the data for *descriptive* or *inferential* purposes. *Descriptive statistics* are those that summarise the patterns of information or data obtained from the sample. *Inferential statistics* tell us whether the patterns found in the sample we have studied are likely to be found in the general population from which the sample was drawn. That is, can the information that we have discovered from analysing the results from our sample (descriptive statistics) be generalised to the wider population? Inferential statistics are used when we have a random sample from the population. They rely on assumptions drawn from probability theory, which in turn assume that each element in the sample has an equal chance of being selected.

Ethical responsibilities

Ethics are critical in data analysis. While most people would agree with Dudley (2010, p. 243) that 'it is absolutely necessary to be as thorough, accurate and honest as possible' in analysing our data, it is also very easy to distort the underlying patterns and mislead people about the results (de Vaus 2002, p. 209).

One source of misleading or unethical data analysis is sloppy coding. Data that have been entered into a spreadsheet or statistical program need to be carefully checked for accuracy before they are analysed. Incorrect data can lead to incorrect results and misleading conclusions. Of course, data can also be deliberately manipulated or distorted in myriad ways to mislead people. Distortions can be made by omitting unpalatable findings from reports, or by leaving out responses to questions that don't produce the desired results. There are plenty of examples of researchers who have intentionally fabricated results as well. De Vaus (2002, p. 209) argues that replicating results is one of the chief safeguards against falsification. However, this is not always possible—especially in small-scale studies. Needless to say, being vigilant about the ethical standards of your data analysis is essential in good research.

The rest of the chapter provides an introduction to computer coding and data entry, showing how quantitative data are entered into a computer for analysis. We also show how variables at different levels of measurement are coded.

Four factors that determine how data are analysed
- The number of variables to be analysed (univariate, bivariate or multivariate analysis)
- The level of measurement of the variables (nominal, ordinal, interval or ratio)
- Whether descriptive or inferential statistics are required
- Ethical responsibilities

Source: De Vaus (2002).

Coding, data entry and computer packages

Coding at different levels of measurement

You should note that the unit around which you code is the variable. Answers addressing each variable are coded for each possible response. In earlier chapters, we introduced the idea of coding results for data entry into a computer by using numbers as codes. With interval and ratio data, coding is relatively simple because the code is usually the same as the answer and can be entered directly into the computer. Variables in which the code numbers refer to actual numbers are termed *numeric* variables in computer packages such as SPSS.

Ordinal level data is coded according to each response—for example, small, medium, large, with 1 representing small, 2 medium and 3 large. With nominal data, coding becomes more complex, especially with open-ended questions. We have discussed how the nominal variable 'gender' has two categories, which may be coded 1 for female and 2 for male, and that these numbers differentiate categories but do *not* imply 'greater or less than'.

Coding open-ended questions (nominal level)

Coding open-ended questions often means that you have to group answers into categories. How you do this depends on the purpose of your question. When coding open-ended questions, you can code for more than one answer to each question. You will need to check the manual of the program you are using for specific instructions on how to do this. Variables in which the code numbers refer to words, not numbers, are termed *alphanumeric* or *string* variables in computer packages such as SPSS.

A handy hint for coding nominal data is to use coding systems that have been devised by large research organisations (such as the Australian Bureau of Statistics). Coding schemes for information such as 'occupation', 'qualifications' and 'type of household' are already available from these organisations at different levels of specificity. It saves a lot of work (and reduces error) if you use a coding system that has been tried and tested by others. This will also allow you to compare your results with other large studies and Census findings. However, this is not essential. If you are devising your own code, you should remember to ensure that your response categories are mutually exclusive, exhaustive and unidimensional (see Chapter 7).

Missing data

Whether you are coding nominal, ordinal, interval or ratio data, it is important to code all answers, even when the respondent did not answer some questions. It is also important to be able to distinguish non-responses, or refusals to answer particular questions, from 'no' and 'don't know'. We suggest a different code for each of these answers. When codes are classified as 'missing data', they are not included in the statistics calculated by the computer, but the numbers of 'missing cases' are recorded in the results. It is important to use the same missing data categories for each research project so that you do not become confused. What has worked for us has been to use 7 (or 77 or 777, depending on how the variable is coded) for 'don't know' (some questionnaires do not provide this option and respondents may write this over the question), 8 for 'not applicable' and 9 for 'no answer' where an answer is not given. The missing data can then be included as part of your data entry and programs such as SPSS will ignore them when calculating statistics and frequencies.

Principles of entering your results

Codebooks

Before beginning to enter your data into the computer, you need to work out your coding scheme. A codebook, also called a coding frame, records everything you need to enter the data from your survey or interview into a computer for analysis. Computer packages such as SPSS generate codebooks for you once you have set up your electronic data file. However, it is also useful to create your own codebook for yourself and data entry assistants as a way of thinking through what needs to be entered into the computer.

Some codes can be established before you collect your data. If you include these codes on the questionnaire or interview schedule itself, it makes data entry much easier and reduces the possibility of error. Coding for closed-ended questions, scaled questions and questions with a numeric (number) answer can be included in the research instrument in this way. Examples are provided below. However, other codes—such as answers to open-ended questions—will be developed from the data itself. In both cases, you need to plan how many answers you will record, and how many categories of response are possible for each answer. Codebooks are especially important if there is more than one person entering data or if there are open-ended questions.

What to include in your codebook
- The question asked
- The name for the variable that is used in the program
- The type of data used for that variable (numeric, alphanumeric— often called string variables)
- The first and last columns in which the variable is located
- The valid codes for each variable
- The 'missing data' codes for each variable
- Any special coding instructions

Source: De Vaus (2002, p. 158).

An example of coding for statistical analysis

Coding variables—and creating a data file

We will use parts of questions from Chapter 7 to show how data are coded into a data file in a statistical program such as SPSS. The data from all the questions for each person you interview, or who fills out a questionnaire, becomes a case—which is a separate line in the data file for each respondent. Each case contains all the information from one respondent, coded into numbers and set out according to each variable. The variables are listed in columns across the data file, as shown in the example below.

Note that *Questions 1, 3* and *4* are variables at the nominal level of measurement. *Question 2* is at the ordinal level of measurement. All the questions are closed ended except *Question 4*, which is open-ended. Thus the codes for the first three questions could have been worked out in advance, as we know what the range of answers will be.

In Table 15.1, the names of the five respondents and their answers to the four questions are summarised. This table shows how five respondents (cases) answered five questions (variables). Listed under each question heading is the short name (variable name—usually restricted to eight characters) that will be listed in the computer to name each variable. SPSS also allows you to enter a longer variable label, which will provide a more detailed heading in results tables. Note that two variable names are listed for Question 4. This is because we have decided to allow two answers from each respondent to be entered for this question. We have also given each person an identity code (ID), which will also be entered into the computer to make sure we know which answers belong to which respondent.

There are two ways of looking at Table 15.1. First, it is possible to obtain a holistic 'snapshot' of each respondent by looking across the rows (or record). For example, J. Smith is a sole parent who thought that the staff listened reasonably carefully but was not given information about his or her right to appeal and found the staff's behaviour formal and rushed. T. Black, on the other hand, is also a sole parent who felt less listened to by staff than J. Smith, but was given information about his or her right to appeal decisions. T. Black also found staff to be rushed and further reported that they did not seem to be interested in him or her.

The other way of looking at this table, instead of looking across the rows for each individual respondent, is to compare the answers down the columns, thus gaining a picture of the range of answers for different variables. For example, we can see from column 2 that we have answers from two sole parents, and one of each from the following groups: disability support payment, unemployment benefit and young homeless. Similarly, people's experience of whether staff listened carefully to them (column 3) ranged from 1 (did not listen carefully) to 5 (listened carefully), with three

Figure 15.1 Examples of closed-ended questions, scaled questions and an open-ended question showing coding embedded in questionnaire

ID   □□□   1–3

1   Please tick the box which describes the social security payments you were receiving when you first visited the office of the Department of Social Security:

Sole parent pension	□□	01	
Young homeless allowance	□□	02	4–5
Aged pension	□□	03	
Disability support payment	□□	04	
Special benefit	□□	05	
Unemployment benefit	□□	06	
Other	□□	07	
Not receiving payments at the time	□□	08	

2   Please indicate how you felt about your first interview with departmental staff by circling a rating out of 5 for the following statements. On the scales, 1 = strongly disagree and 5 = strongly agree.

From my first interview at the Department of Social Security I would say:

a. staff listened carefully to what I had to say.

1_____2_____3_____4_____5   6
strongly   neutral   strongly
disagree   agree

b. staff acted as though I was lying.

1_____2_____3_____ 4_____5   7
strongly   neutral   strongly
disagree   agree

3   Were you told of your right to appeal decisions made by the department during your first interview?

Yes   1   8
No   2

4   Please describe how the staff behaved towards you during your first interview at the Department of Social Security

_____

_____

Table 15.1 Answers to the questions from Figure 15.1 in table form

Respondent (ID)	Type payment (PAY)	Staff listen (ATTIT1)	No believe (ATTIT2)	Info re appeal (APPEAL)	Staff behaviour (BEH1, BEH2)
J. Smith (001)	Sole parent	3	4	No	Formal, rushed
P. Collins (002)	Disability support	5	1	Yes	Friendly, took time for me
M. Chapman (003)	Young homeless	1	5	No	Rude
A. Jones (004)	Unemployment	5	3	Yes	OK, friendly
T. Black (005)	Sole parent	2	4	Yes	In a hurry, didn't seem interested in my questions

people being somewhere in the middle. As we shall see in the following chapter, these sorts of 'pictures' or summaries of the data are exactly what descriptive univariate statistics provide, but on a larger scale involving all the cases in our sample.

Developing a data file

We now move to the second stage of our coding demonstration, by transforming the same information that appeared in words and numbers in Table 15.1 into numerical computer codes for each variable. When these numerical codes are entered into a computer, together they are termed a *data file*.

The first step in transforming data into a data file is to create a codebook, as discussed above. In your codebook, you should record for each variable the aspects identified by de Vaus (2002) listed above. These days this information is usually entered directly into the computer. In SPSS, you enter this in the 'variable view' window. There are easy to follow instructions for each step of the way.

An illustration of a codebook entry for the first variable in Table 15.1 (type of payment) appears in Example 15.1. This information will all be entered as part of the program file or equivalent. This variable could be precoded on the questionnaire, as it is a closed-ended question from which respondents choose one of the options. Note that two columns are given for each answer. This is because it is possible that there may be more than ten answers, once the responses to 'other' are considered.

Example 15.1: Codebook entry for Question 1

Question 1: What social security payments were you receiving when you first visited the office?

Variable name:	PAY	
Variable label:	Type of social security payment	
Value labels:		
	No payment	00
	Sole parent	01
	Young homeless	02
	Aged pension	03
	Disability support	04
	Special benefit	05
	Unemployment	06
	Other	**
*** codes for other*:		
Veteran's payment, Carer's pension, etc.		07
		08
Missing values:		
	Don't know	77
	Not applicable	88
	No response	99

Note that there is a choice marked 'Other' in this question. The coder can choose whether to just consider all answers of 'other' as a single category, or whether instead to record the details of each other sort of 'other' payment separately. The answers to 'Other' can then be coded as for other open-ended questions, within the existing structure of the closed question.

This exercise is repeated for each variable until all have been entered into the codebook and you have a comprehensive record of the coding you are putting into the computer. The page for Question 2 may look like Example 15.2.

Example 15.2: Codebook entry for Question 2

Question 2a: Scale rating (1–5) about agreement with whether staff listened carefully to what I had to say.

Variable name:	ATTIT1	
Variable label:	Staff listened carefully	

Value labels:	Strongly disagree	1
		2
	Neutral	3
		4
	Strongly agree	5
Missing values:		
	Don't know	7
	Not applicable	8
	No response	9

The codebook entry for the third question (Example 15.3) would be even simpler because there are only two values for this variable. (Having only two values, this variable is called a dichotomous variable. Dichotomous variables have special properties for statistical purposes.) Note that when deciding on different codes, we recommend that you use similar codes for each variable, which makes coding easier to remember. For example, 'yes' could always be coded 1. Similarly, the codes for missing values are easiest if they are always similar across different questions (for example, 'don't know' as 7 or 77 or 777, depending on how many columns you use).

Example 15.3: Codebook entry for Question 3

Question 3: Were you told of your right to appeal decisions made by the agency during your first interview?

Variable name:	APPEAL	
Variable label:	Whether notified about appeal process	
Value labels:		
	No	0
	Yes	1
Missing values:		
	Don't know	7
	Not applicable	8
	No response	9

The coding for open-ended questions is more complicated, depending on the range of answers that are received. Note that because we will code both the variables BEH1 and BEH2 with the same value labels, we can include them both in the same entry in the codebook, as demonstrated in Example 15.4. (Remember that we are allowing ourselves the opportunity to record two answers to this question. The codes will be the same in both variables so that we can add them up later.) When coding multiple variables as one entry in your codebook, make sure that you have allowed sufficient space for, or the ability to distinguish between, each variable.

If the person has given more than two answers, you will need to decide how to deal with this and record it in the codebook so that all coders follow the same rule for each survey or questionnaire (see Example 15.4). There is no right or wrong approach to this situation; what is important is to be consistent. In the example, we have decided to use the first two answers the person gives.

Example 15.4: Codebook entry for Question 4

Question 4: Please describe how the staff behaved towards you during your first interview at the Department of Social Security.

Variable name:	BEH1, BEH2	
Variable label:	Perceived staff behaviour at first interview	
**Value labels:		
	No comment	00
	Formal	01
	Rushed, hurried	02
	Friendly	03
	Took time for me	04
	Rude	05
	Okay	06
	Uninterested	07
Missing values:		
	Don't know	07
	Not applicable	08
	No response	09

***Note:* If more than two options are listed, code the first two only.

Coding open-ended questions requires skill and careful thought. Even in this simple example, it can be seen that there are some similarities in these five respondents' comments about staff behaviour, and some subtle differences that may or may not be important to code. At this early stage, with only five responses, it is best to code the answers in as much detail as possible, and wait until more cases have been examined before deciding how to recode open-ended questions into smaller numbers of categories.

Entering your data into the computer

Having decided on your coding frame program file for these four questions, you are now ready to enter the information into a computer. Different packages, and even different versions of the same packages, use different methods for entering the results of your study. However, the basic principles we have described—labelling each variable with a variable name, then coding all possible values for each variable including non-responses and other missing data (that is, listing value labels for each variable)—are general principles that apply to most databases and statistics packages.

When research results are entered into a computer, they are entered as a data file. The answers from each person (respondent) are systematically recorded so that the computer can count, collate and compare different answers to the same question (univariate analysis), or the way different answers vary for different people between different questions (bivariate and multivariate analysis).

In order for the computer to do this, each respondent's answers are recorded across a line of columns. The same questions are answered for each respondent in the same order, and the computer is told which columns refer to which variables.

Thus researchers must enter into the computer the name of each variable (giving it a label called a variable name). They must also enter all the different codes or answers/values for each of these variables in the appropriate columns or spaces provided for each respondent.

Figure 15.2 Example of data file (with variables labelled)

ID	PAY	ATT1	ATT2	APPL	BEH1	BEH2
001	01	3		0	01	02
002	04	5		1	03	04
003	02	1		0	05	00
004	06	3		1	06	03
005	01	2		1	02	07

Using the codes that we identified above, the data file (called data view in SPSS) is what the computer reads to analyse the data as given in the example. See whether you can relate the information from this data file to the information that was listed in words in Table 15.1, using the codebook examples to decode the numbers.

Entering into SPSS

Note that when you are entering your own results, some packages are more user-friendly, and will provide prompts for each variable. SPSS for Windows is very easy to use. A useful reference to keep on your shelf is Pallant's *SPSS Survival Manual*, 4th edn (2011). This book provides easy-to-follow directions to allow you to deal with common data analysis issues.

Summary

In this chapter, we have presented four factors that determine the types of quantitative data analysis you will perform. We then discussed how to code your results at different levels of measurement ready for computer analysis, showing how to develop a codebook and from that a data file.

For more detailed instructions on how to enter data and set up a statistics package, you will need to consult the manual of the package that is available to you, and probably seek the assistance of someone who has experience with that particular package. The principles of data entry, and the thinking behind those principles presented here, however, are generally applicable to all computer packages.

Discussion questions

15.1   What are the four factors affecting quantitative data analysis?
15.2   List whether the following questions require univariate, bivariate or multivariate analysis:
  (a) Are people from culturally and linguistically diverse backgrounds given the same information as native English speakers by income-support agency staff?
  (b) What type of social security payments do you receive?
  (c) Do younger people have more satisfactory experiences than older people when they visit an income-support agency?
  (d) What factors affect the experiences people have when they visit an income-support agency?
15.3   Consider these two questions:
  1 How old are you? Please write your age in years in the space provided.

2 Please indicate your age by ticking the box which shows the range within which your age falls:

Under 15 years	☐	46–55 years	☐
16–25 years	☐	56–65 years	☐
26–35 years	☐	66 years and over	☐
36–45 years	☐		

    (a) Are the questions open or closed ended?
    (b) At what level of measurement are the two questions located?
    (c) Which question do you think is preferable and why?
15.4 What is the difference between descriptive and inferential statistics?

Exercises

Create a codebook and write a data file for three hypothetical respondents in answer to the following questions:
15.1 In what area do you live? (Please write your postcode only.)
15.2 Do you think this area needs an after-school leisure centre?
    Yes
    No
    Maybe
    Don't know
15.3 If you have children, please answer these questions:
    (a) How many children under the age of 12 live in your house?
    (b) Are your children interested in:
       • aerobics?
       • pottery?
       • creative writing?
       • computer games?
    (c) Would they use an after-school leisure centre if it was properly supervised and these kinds of activities were provided?
    (d) What other after-school activities might your children want to do at an after-school leisure centre?

Further reading

Babbie, E. 2011, *The Basics of Social Research*, 5th edn, Wadsworth, Belmont, CA. Chapter 14, 'Quantitative data analysis', introduces quantification of data and codebook construction and data entry.

David, M. and Sutton, C. 2011, *Social Research: An Introduction*, 2nd edn, Sage, Thousand Oaks, CA. Chapters 16 and 23 cover quantitative coding in good detail.

de Vaus, D.A. 2002, *Surveys in Social Research*, 5th edn, Allen & Unwin, Sydney. See Chapter 9, 'Coding', which is particularly good on coding multiple responses to open-ended questions, and Chapter 10 on preparing data for analysis, which extends the discussion in this chapter to recoding, creating new variables and standardising variables.

Engel, R.J. and Schutt, R.K. 2009, *The Practice of Research in Social Work*, 2nd edn, Sage, Thousand Oaks, CA. See Chapter 12, 'Quantitative data analysis'.

Pallant, J. (2011), *SPSS Survival Manual*, 4th edn, Allen & Unwin, Sydney. Parts 1 and 2 deal with creating a codebook, creating a data file, and cleaning and screening data. This is an excellent step-by-step guide to SPSS for all users.

16 Statistics for social workers: Analysis of a single variable

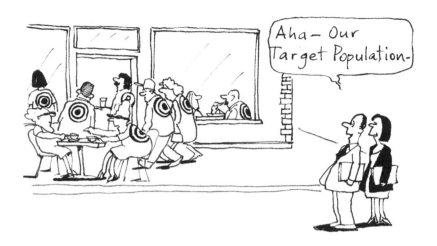

Having examined coding procedures, we now introduce you to a range of statistical techniques and tests that social workers are most likely to use in their research. It is important for you to understand the four factors introduced in the previous chapter—level of measurement, number of variables, whether statistics are intended to be inferential or descriptive, and consideration of the ethical implications surrounding your chosen data-analysis strategy—as these are significant elements in any data analysis. Our aim in this chapter is to introduce the main concepts in quantitative analysis, so that you know how to analyse your data and the possibilities that such analysis offers you as a researcher. We want to help you think through what data analysis you will perform in your own research, and to enable you to critically examine the analysis reported in other studies.

Statistical analyses used properly provide powerful arguments for many of the issues you face in your everyday work life. In this chapter, we describe complex statistical processes in plain English. We have assumed that you are interested in the logic of the processes and how you can use the results in your own research to improve the quality of your conclusions, rather than complex mathematical proofs. Sometimes, therefore, we will present formulae without the mathematical explanations that are beyond the scope of this book.

In particular, this chapter introduces you to the following factors in statistical analysis:

- continuous and discrete variables
- frequency distributions
- describing a distribution (central tendency, dispersion, taking into account levels of measurement)
- the normal distribution.

In order to explain statistics and what they mean in relation to the population about which you want to know more (termed the *target population*), we have invented a fictitious example. Our example uses small numbers so that we can demonstrate with simple calculations the logic of statistics and how they estimate what is actually going on in the target population.

In our example, Lucy Liu is a social worker at a hospital. She works in an outreach service provided for mothers after discharge from hospital following the birth of their child. She works part time, and her caseload consists of 20 babies. For the purposes of this example, the target population may be Lucy Liu's caseload of new babies, or more likely it would be all the new babies in the hospital's catchment area.

As we saw in Chapter 5, we often have a target population in mind but it is very difficult to collect a random sample from this population. Instead, we may decide to select our random sample from a sub-set of the target population that we consider to be typical in some way. This sub-set is called the *sampled population*. In our example, the sampled population is Lucy Liu's caseload. We must remember that any conclusions we draw from our research are actually only statistically valid for mothers and babies in Lucy's caseload, although we may feel comfortable about extending our conclusions to all children in the local area.

Continuous and discrete variables

A variable is called *discrete* if the set of possible values it can take is a discrete number of values or categories (the value of the variable is often called a score). The number of times a baby wakes during the night is a discrete variable—each value of the variable is a whole number, representing the number of times a baby woke on a particular night. If the baby woke five times, we say the variable has a value or score of five. Other examples include eye colour, gender and number of siblings. A *dichotomous* variable is a discrete variable with only two categories, such as gender (female or male). Remember that when variables have categories as their values (for example, female and male) we usually assign each category with a numeric value for ease of processing (female = 1, male = 2). In this case the numeric values are labels only and do not indicate order in themselves.

A variable is called *continuous* if it takes any numerical value in a given interval. This means it does not just have whole number values like 3 or 4, but can take on intermediate values like 3.345 . . ., for example. We could say that the 'length of time a baby is awake' is a continuous variable because, in theory, we could say the baby was awake 3.356 minutes.

The distinction between variables is important because, like levels of measurement, it guides the selection of appropriate statistical techniques.

Statistics with one variable: univariate analysis

Frequency distributions

One of the most common ways of presenting descriptive statistics (that is, data that describes or summarises your findings) is through the use of frequency distributions. Frequency distributions allow us to record the frequency of each value of the variable being reviewed.

In our fictitious example, Lucy has noticed that one of the most pressing concerns for mothers is the number of times babies wake during the night. She has decided to ask the mothers in her caseload to keep records to allow her to record patterns of waking behaviour. The first step in constructing a frequency table is to record the *raw data*. Table 16.1 shows the number of times each child woke on a particular night in Lucy Liu's caseload.

Table 16.1 Lucy Liu's caseload sample: Number of times children woke, Wednesday/Thursday, 23–24 March

Name	Number of times child woke during night
Rosie	3
Tom	4
Nick	1
Peter	2
Meredith	3
Mary	2
Jessica	1

Name	Number of times child woke during night
Wendy	5
John	2
David	3
Steven	7
Susan	5
Sarah	3
Philip	1
Trent	9
Daniel	0
Kate	3
Dominique	0
Alison	2
Dylan	1
Total: 20 children	57

We can summarise the information recorded by the raw data to make it more comprehensible. The simplest way to summarise raw data is in a frequency distribution that shows, in our case, the number of children who woke the same number of times. Table 16.2 shows the frequency distribution of the number of times children in Lucy Liu's caseload woke on a particular night. We call it a population frequency distribution because Lucy Liu's caseload is the population in which we are interested and from which we will take a sample later.

Table 16.2 Population frequency distribution: Number of times children woke, Wednesday/Thursday 23–24 March

Name	Number of times awake	Frequency
Daniel + Dominique	0	2
Nick + Jessica + Philip + Dylan	1	4
Peter + Mary + John + Alison	2	4
Rosie + Meredith + David + Sarah + Kate	3	5
Tom	4	1
Wendy + Susan	5	2
Steven	6	0
Steven	7	1
	8	0
Trent	9	1
Total 20 children		Total 20

Cumulative frequency distribution

A *cumulative frequency distribution* can be constructed when the data is measured at an ordinal or higher level of measurement. It allows frequencies to be summed down the column, giving a 'rolling count'. From Table 16.3, for example, we can see that ten babies woke up to twice during the night.

Table 16.3 Cumulative frequency distribution: Number of times awake

Name	No. of times awake	Frequency	Cumulative frequency
Daniel + Dominique	0	2	2
Nick + Jessica + Philip + Dylan	1	4	6
Peter + Mary + John + Alison	2	4	10
Rosie + Meredith + David + Sarah + Kate	3 .	5	15
Tom	4	1	16
Wendy + Susan	5	2	18
	6	0	18
Steven	7	1	19
	8	0	19
Trent	9	1	20

Percentage frequency distributions

A *percentage frequency distribution* adds percentage values to your data. The frequency percentage column in Table 16.4 indicates for each entry the percentage of the whole group or sample represented by that particular piece of data. Thus we can see that 25 per cent of the group woke three times. The cumulative percentage data column, which is added as you go down the column, allows us to ascertain that, for example, 50 per cent woke up not more than twice. Note that cumulative percentage columns always end with 100 as their total.

Table 16.4 Percentage frequency distribution: Number of times awake

Name	No. of times awake	Frequency	Frequency %	Cumulative frequency	Cumulative %
Daniel + Dominique	0	2	10	2	10
Nick + Jessica + Philip + Dylan	1	4	20	6	30
Peter + Mary + John + Alison	2	4	20	10	50
Rosie + Meredith + David + Sarah + Kate	3	5	25	15	75

Name	No. of times awake	Frequency	Frequency %	Cumulative frequency	Cumulative %
Tom	4	1	5	16	80
Wendy + Susan	5	2	10	18	90
	6	0	0	18	90
Steven	7	1	5	19	95
	8	0	0	19	95
Trent	9	1	5	20	100
Total		20	100	20	100

Grouped frequency distribution

When dealing with interval and ratio level data, where there may be a large number of possible scores, it is often simpler to divide the range of possible values into equally spaced intervals and to calculate the frequency with which the scores fall within each interval. It may be necessary to have a final open-ended interval to include all remaining possibilities. Grouping the data in this way often makes patterns more obvious. When deciding which groupings to use, it is important to reduce the number of values to a small number while still maintaining some level of measurement precision. If the values are spread evenly, then groupings should also be evenly spread. Table 16.5 shows a grouped frequency distribution for the 20 cases in our example. Note the way that the categories have been grouped so that they are of equal size, include all cases and do not overlap.

Table 16.5 Grouped frequency distribution table: Number of times awake

Number of times awake	Frequency
0–3	15
4–7	4
> 7	1

Representation of frequency distributions

The simplest representation of a frequency distribution is a table. If we examine Table 16.2 above, we see that all the different possible values for the variable (number of times awake) are listed in the second column. When you construct frequency distributions for ordinal and interval/ratio data, it is most important to arrange the possible values of the variable in numerical order (as in the tables above). The next column (called the frequency column) shows the frequency with which the variable has this value. Other optional columns can then be added. Sometimes researchers work solely in percentages and leave out the raw frequency column altogether, because it is much easier to see patterns in the data when it is represented in this way.

Note that if you are writing up a frequency distribution table from a sample instead of from the whole population, you must include a line underneath the table recording the number of cases in the sample for which a score was not recorded. This is called 'missing data' (see Table 16.6 on p. 313). For example, if one of the families in Lucy Liu's caseload was away on the night the data was collected and did not record the data, there would be one missing case, which would be noted beneath the table. This is important information to include as it may affect the validity or reliability of any conclusions drawn. De Vaus (2002, p. 214) provides a handy list of the information that must be included in frequency tables (see box).

Information that should be included in a frequency table

- Table number and title
- Labels for the categories of the variable
- Column headings to indicate what the numbers in the column represent
- The total number on which the percentages are based
- The number of missing cases
- The source of the data (particularly important if the data are from a different source than your own survey, such as Census data for comparison with your findings)
- Sometimes footnotes are needed that provide the actual question or working definitions on which the table is based.

Source: De Vaus (2002, p. 214).

Graphical representations of data

Sometimes a graphical representation provides a more concise and more easily interpreted representation of data than a frequency distribution table. While graphs reduce the detail available to the reader, they may be more readily accessible to a non-research savvy audience. There are several types of graph and a range of pictorial representations of data. In this section, we provide a description of the most common.

Histograms and bar charts

Histograms and bar charts have two axes that intersect at right angles. One axis (usually the horizontal one) is divided into intervals, representing the various possible values of the variable. The other axis (usually the vertical one) is divided into intervals, representing frequencies. Histograms depict the data graphically with vertical bars adjacent to each other, as shown in Figure 16.1. Bar charts are very similar to histograms except that the bars are separated (Figure 16.2). Bar charts can be used for nominal level data to show different variables.

Figure 16.1 Histogram

Frequencies of payment type

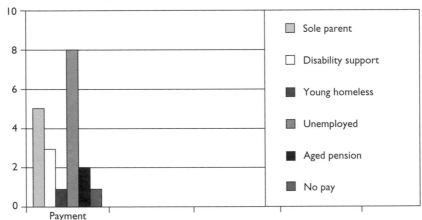

Figure 16.2 Bar chart

Frequencies of payment type

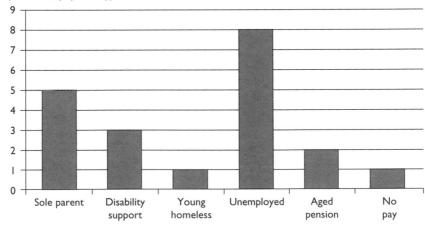

Pie charts

Pie charts are circular charts divided into slices. Each slice represents a possible score, and its size is proportional to the occurrence of that score in the sample (see Figure 16.3).

Figure 16.3 Pie chart

Frequencies of payment type

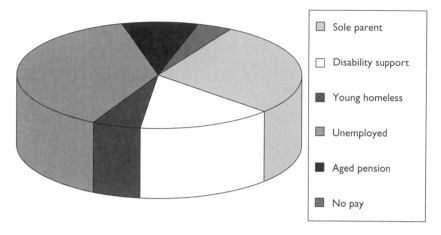

- Sole parent
- Disability support
- Young homeless
- Unemployed
- Aged pension
- No pay

Pictographs

Pictographs are an exciting way to summarise data and are often used in newspapers. Figure 16.4 is an example of a detailed pictograph.

Figure 16.4 Pictograph

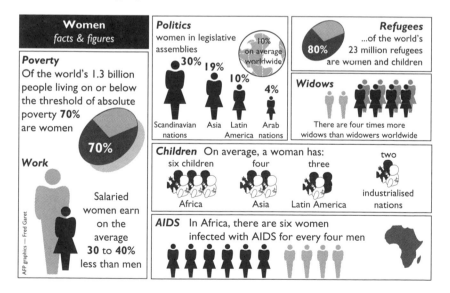

Frequency polygons and curves

The frequency polygon is another type of graph that is useful when dealing with ratio or interval level variables that can be regarded as continuous (age, height, salary, and so on). Frequency polygons can be drawn from histograms by joining the mid-point of each bar to create a polygon (Figure 16.5). Polygons show the shape of the data very well.

Figure 16.5 Frequency polygon—ages of students in social work research methods on-campus class

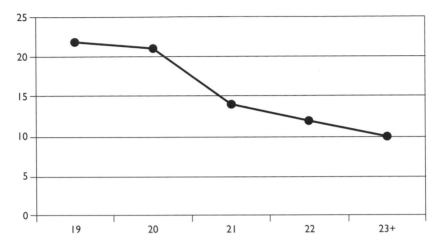

For other methods of visually presenting data, see Weinbach and Grinnell (2010, Chapter 2) or de Vaus (2002, Chapter 13).

Summarising frequency distributions: Descriptive statistics
In social research, it is rare to have a whole population to use for statistics. Instead, we use a sample—in quantitative statistics we use a random sample. Sample statistics estimate the statistics for the whole population. As we saw in Chapter 5, they are more or less accurate depending on how well the sample reflects or represents the population. To illustrate how statistics from samples estimate the values found in the population, a random sample was taken from Lucy Liu's caseload, with replacement as the population of this caseload is so small (see Chapter 5). Table 16.6 shows the frequency distribution of this random sample of seven cases.

While frequency distributions display the range of answers to questions, descriptive statistics go further in providing critical information about data. This is particularly important when we want to understand how much variation there is in our data. Two descriptive statistics are particularly useful in this context. They are the statistics that tell us:

• the most typical response, called *measures of central tendency*
• the spread or variation of responses, called *measures of dispersion*.

Table 16.6 Sample frequency distribution: Random sample of number of times awake

Number of times awake	Frequency	Frequency %	Cumulative frequency	Cumulative frequency %
0	1	14.3	1	14.3
1	1	14.3	2	28.6
2	2	28.6	4	57.3
3	1	14.3	5	71.6
4	0	0	5	71.6
5	1	14.3	6	85.9
7	1	14.3	7	100.0
Total	7			

Note: No. of missing cases = 0

There are several different ways of measuring central tendency and dispersion. The most common measures of central tendency are the *mode, median* and *mean*.

Measures of central tendency

The mode

The mode is the only measure of central tendency for nominal data. It can, however, be calculated for all types of data if required. It is the score that occurs most often in the sampled population. In Table 16.2, for example, the mode from the sampled population is waking three times in the night. However, the mode in our sample is twice per night (Table 16.6)—a close estimate of the actual population mode. Note that the mode does not tell us anything about how typical this most common category is, or about the shape of the frequency distribution.

The median

The median can be calculated for ordinal, ratio and interval data. It is the usual measure of central tendency for ordinal level variables. If the scores for each member of the sample population are arranged in numerical order, then the median value is the middle value. We estimate this by finding the middle value for our sample. When there is an even number of scores, as in the following example, then the median is the average of the two central scores:

1, 2, 2, 3, **4, 6,** 7, 8, 10, 11

In this case, the median is calculated by averaging 4 and 6. Thus 5 is the median of this grouping even though 5 is not one of the scores listed.

If there are an uneven number of scores then the median is the central number:

1, 3, 5, 8, **9**, 12, 14, 16, 18

In this case the median is 9.

You will note that in Table 16.2 there are 20 babies; therefore the median is the score between the 10th and 11th subjects. Note that as the score for the 10th is waking two times, and the score for the 11th is waking three times. Therefore the median for this group is waking 2.5 times.

An easy way to estimate the median is to use the cumulative percentage column in your frequency distribution table. The median is found in the 50th percentile (or the point where 50 per cent of cases fall). In Table 16.4, for example, the median waking is two times—an approximation of the median that was more precisely calculated above. In the sample, the median is also two waking times (Table 16.6).

The mean

The mean can be calculated for interval and ratio level variables only, and is the most commonly used statistic for these levels. The mean is the arithmetic average value of the variable over the sampled population. To calculate the mean, we add up the scores for all the members of the sample and then divide by the sample size. You will note from Table 16.1 that the babies woke a total of 57 times. As there are 20 babies, the mean number of times the babies in the sampled population woke is 57/20 = 2.85 times. For the sample, the mean is 20/7 = 2.9 times (Table 16.6).

Sometimes a random sample of a population will contain 'outliers'. These are values of the variable that are quite extreme in that they have a very low frequency in the sampled population. If such outliers appear in your sample, they will distort your sample statistics, particularly if the sample is small.

In many cases that you will uncover during the course of your research career, you will have good reason to suspect that the variable you are measuring is 'normally distributed' over the population (see below for a description of the normal distribution). In such a case, if you feel that 'outliers' have distorted your estimate of the mean, the median of the sample may be a better estimate of central tendency as it is unaffected by extreme scores. This is because the mean, mode and median of a normally distributed population are equal.

> ### Measures of central tendency
> - **Mode:** the score that occurs most frequently. The only measure of central tendency for nominal data.
> - **Median:** the value of the middle when scores are arranged in order. Used for ordinal and higher level data.
> - **Mean:** the arithmetic average value of the variable over the sampled population. Calculated by dividing the sum of all the scores by the sample size. Used for interval and ratio level data. Can be distorted by 'outliers'.

Measures of dispersion

While measures of central tendency can give a great deal of information about the distribution of scores, measures of dispersion are used if we wish to understand the degree of variability, or how widely our scores are dispersed.

Variation ratio

The variation ratio is defined as the fraction of members of the population outside the mode of the variable's distribution. For example, the variation ratio of the population in our example is 15/20 = 0.75. If we estimate this using our sample, the variation ratio is 5/7 = 0.71. The higher the variation ratio, the more poorly the mode describes the distribution. In our example, the mode only describes 25 per cent of the population. When we took a random sample, our estimate for the mode was wrong. The higher the variation ratio, the more likely it is that the estimated mode in your sample will be wrong.

The variation ratio is the only measure of dispersion for nominal data.

Range

The range is the difference between the highest and lowest value of the variable. In our example of the number of times the babies woke during the night, in Table 16.3 we can see that the highest number is 9 and the lowest is 0, so the range is 9–0 = 9. The range, like the mean, can easily be distorted if there are 'outliers', extreme scores at either end.

Decile and interquartile ranges

Both the decile range and the interquartile range are ways of assessing the effectiveness of the median as the summary measure of the distribution. Both measures avoid the distorting effect of extreme cases by 'dropping off' the cases at the edges of scores. The decile range shows the range of the middle 80 per cent of the cases, while the interquartile range shows the range of the middle 50 per cent of cases. They are calculated from the cumulative percentage columns by dropping the top and bottom 10 per cent of cases (for the decile range) or the top and bottom 25 per cent of cases (for the interquartile range). You can see how this will give you a measure of dispersion that is uncontaminated by outliers. Decile and interquartile range are the usual measures of dispersion for ordinal level variables. In our example, the interquartile range of the population is 1–3 times awake (we drop off the top and bottom 25 per cent), and the decile range is 1–5 (we drop off the top and bottom 10 per cent). (You should check this at Table 16.4.) If we use our sample, we would estimate that the interquartile range is 1–5, as is the decile range (Table 16.6).

Variance and standard deviation

The standard deviation and variance are the most frequently used measures of dispersion for interval and ratio level frequencies. When used in conjunction with the mean, they tell us a lot about the spread of the distribution without having to use the raw figures. Like the mean, the standard deviation takes all values into consideration when it is calculated. In fact, in the case of a normally distributed variable (see below), the distribution is completely defined if we know the mean and the standard deviation.

The variance is the average square distance from the mean of all the scores in the sampled population.

For a population size of N and where μ represents the mean of the set of scores, the variance σ^2 can be calculated using the formula:

$$\sigma^2 = \Sigma(X-\mu)^2/N$$

Why average square distance, you may ask—why not just average distance? The reason for this is that the distance from the mean may be positive or negative; if we average these values, negative and positive values will cancel each other out.

When we have a sample, the estimate we use for the population variance is not what we might expect. Instead of dividing by n (the number in the sample), we divide by n−1. Why do we do this? It can be shown mathematically that dividing by (n−1) gives us an unbiased estimate of the population variance. If we divide by n, we get an estimate that tends to always be less than the real value.

The sample variance s^2 for a sample of size n uses the following formula:

$$s^2 = \Sigma(X - \overline{X})^2 / (n - 1)$$

The standard deviation of the distribution is the square root of the variance. This is useful because standard deviation is measured in the same units as the values of variables (in our example, number of times waking per night).

The standard deviation of the distribution is the square root of the variance. Therefore standard deviation or σ is calculated using the following formula:

$$\sigma = \sqrt{\Sigma(X - \alpha)^2 / N}$$

or in the case of a sample:

$$s = \sqrt{\Sigma(X - \overline{X})^2 / (n - 1)}$$

where s is the standard deviation of the sample, $\overline{X}$ is the sample mean and n the number of cases in the sample.

Table 16.7 shows an example of variance and standard deviation using our example of waking babies and using the scores listed in Table 16.6. Remember that the average number of times awake ($\overline{X}$) calculated above is 20/7 = 2.9.

Table 16.7 Calculating the variance and standard deviation

	No. of times awake (X)	No. of times awake minus the mean (X − $\overline{X}$)	No. of times awake minus the mean squared (X − $\overline{X}^2$)
	0	−2.9	8.41
	1	−1.9	3.61
	2	−0.9	0.81
	2	−0.9	0.81
	3	0.1	0.01
	5	2.1	4.41
	7	4.1	16.81
Total	20		34.87
$\overline{X}$	20/7= 2.9		
s^2			34.87/6 = 5.81

Variance is $\Sigma (X - \overline{X})^2/(n-1)$ 34.87/6 = 5.81

To calculate the standard deviation of a population you must list scores, determine the mean, subtract the mean from the score, square the result, add the sum of this column, divide this sum by the number of cases to calculate variance and determine the square root of the variance to calculate standard deviation.

The standard deviation allows us to determine how widely our scores are spread. A small standard deviation indicates a small variation in scores while a large standard deviation reflects wide variation.

To illustrate in a different way, let us take two samples of social workers working for a department of community services. One sample works in the city and the other in a rural area. The workers are asked to list the number of cases of child abuse seen in a single week.

Sample A: City workers

6, 9, 1, 13, 16

Note there are five cases, so n = 5 and the mean is calculated by summing the scores and dividing by n.

6 + 9 + 1 + 13 + 16 = 45 Mean = 45/5 = 9

Sample B: Country workers

1, 3, 2, 7, 2

Again we sum the scores and divide by n (5) to calculate the mean.

Mean = 15/5 = 3

Tables 16.8 and 16.9 are calculations of the standard deviations of the two groups.

Table 16.8 Calculating the standard deviation of the city workers' cases

No. of cases (X)	Mean	No. of cases minus the mean ($X - \bar{X}$)	No. of cases minus the mean squared ($X - \bar{X}$)²
6	9	−3	9
9	9	0	0
1	9	−8	64
13	9	4	16
16	9	7	49
			Total $\Sigma(X - \bar{X})^2$ = 138

Table 16.9 Calculating the standard deviation of the country workers' cases

No. of cases (X)	Mean	No. of cases minus the mean $(X - \bar{X})$	No. of cases minus the mean squared $(X - \bar{X})^2$
1	3	−2	4
3	3	0	0
2	3	−1	1
7	3	4	16
2	3	−1	1
			Total $\Sigma(X - \bar{X})^2 = 22$

Variance = 22/4 = 5.5

Standard deviation = $\sqrt{}$ variance = 2.35

We can deduce from these two examples that there is greater variation in the city workers' scores and that the country workers' scores are grouped more closely together.

It is most unlikely that you will have to perform these calculations these days, given that most advanced calculators and statistical packages will do it for you; however, it is important to understand variance and standard deviation and what, together with the mean, they tell us about the distribution.

Measures of dispersion

- **Variation ratio:** the fraction of the members of the population who are outside the mode. The higher the variation ratio, the more poorly the mode describes the distribution. Variation ratio is the only measure of dispersion for nominal data.
- **Range:** the difference between the highest and lowest value of the variable. Can be distorted by 'outliers'.
- **Decile range:** shows the range of the middle 80 per cent of the cases.
- **Interquartile range:** shows the range of the middle 50 per cent of cases. Both measures are designed to reduce the distortion produced by 'outliers'. Used for ordinal level data.
- **Variance and standard deviation:** the most frequently used measures of dispersion for interval and ratio data. Standard deviation allows us to determine how widely our scores are spread. The smaller the value of the standard deviation, the better the mean describes the distribution.

The normal distribution

Much of your future research will deal with data that are approximately 'normally' distributed over the population. What does this mean? Essentially, it means that the values of the variables are spread across a range of scores in a particular pattern in a way that sees them cluster around a common mean, mode and median. If we draw the pattern, we will see the bell-shaped curve. The distributions of many continuous variables can be described as normal distributions. If the distribution of a particular variable is 'normal', its probability curve is an example of a 'normal curve'. A normal curve can be described simply by a mathematical formula that uses the mean and the variance. This means we can know a great deal about our data once we have good estimates of the mean and variance.

Three normal curves are shown in Figure 16.6. The probability curves of normally distributed variables all have a typical bell shape, and in fact the normal curve is often called the bell curve. The first thing to note is that the mean, mode and median are all the same for each curve (0 for one, 2 for the second and 0 for the third). Second, when you compare the curves, you can see that the larger the standard deviation is, the greater the spread of the curve.

Figure 16.6 Examples of normal curves

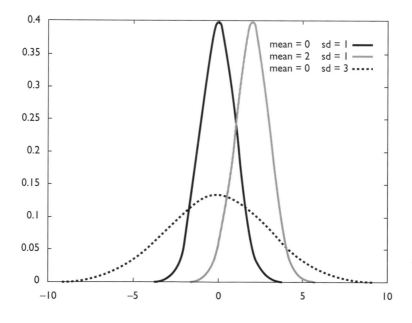

There are some other important properties that you should note. Once we know that a variable has a normal distribution, the standard deviation becomes a powerful tool. In the case of a normal curve, the area under the curve between plus or minus 1 standard deviation from the mean is 0.68. That is, the probability of X having a value within plus or minus 1 standard deviation from the mean is 0.68. This means that 68 per cent of scores lie within plus or minus 1 standard deviation of the mean (See Figure 16.7).

For example, if the average age of people in a nation is 25 years and the standard deviation is 8 years, then 68 per cent of people in that country will be aged between 17 and 33 years. In a similar way, 95 per cent of scores lie between plus or minus 2 standard deviations from the mean and 99.74 per cent lie between plus or minus 3 standard deviations from the mean.

Figure 16.7 The area under the normal curve

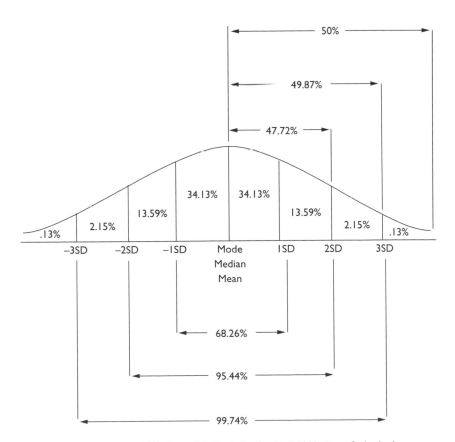

Source: R.W. Weinbach & R.M. Grinnell Jr, Statistics for Social Workers, 3rd edn, Longman, New York, 1995.

In our example of a nation, 95 per cent of people would be aged between 9 and 41 years (25 plus or minus 2 × 8) and 99.74 per cent would be between 1 and 49 years (25 plus or minus 3 × 8). So if we can get good estimates for mean and variance, we can speak meaningfully about the spread of the data.

The importance of normal distributions in statistics: The sampling distribution of the mean

We have created a population of 5000 imaginary students studying history. The students' scores were normally distributed, with a mean of 50 (a bare pass) and a standard deviation of 11.2. From these examination scores, we took a number of simple random samples—three samples of 30 students and three samples of 100 students. The means and standard deviations of the samples are shown in Table 16.10.

Table 16.10 Means and standard deviations of samples from history students: Sample sizes 30 and 100

30 students	Sample 1 (30)	Sample 2 (30)	Sample 3 (30)
Mean	47.3	50.7	49.6
Standard deviation	12.4	13.2	12.2

100 students	Sample 4 (100)	Sample 5 (100)	Sample 6 (100)
Mean	48.85	50.25	50.40
Standard deviation	10.129	12.52	10.99

From Table 16.10, we can see that each time we take a sample, we get different estimates for the mean and the standard deviation which are close to, but not the same as, the actual mean of the population (50 marks) and the actual standard deviation (11.2 marks).

Further, we can see that the sample means are closer to the actual population mean in the larger samples (samples 4, 5 and 6). If we had taken every possible sample of size 30, calculated all the sample means and drawn a relative frequency curve of the sample means, we would have seen that these means were distributed approximately normally, with a mean of 50. When we do the same for the larger samples of 100, the sample means will again approximate a normal curve but with a much smaller standard deviation.

Figure 16.8 shows relative frequency curves for the sample mean for samples of size 30 and 100. The graph for the sample of 100 is very tall and thin (a very small standard deviation), showing that the probability that our estimate of the mean will be near the population mean is very high.

Figure 16.8   Relative frequency curves for sample means size 30 and 100

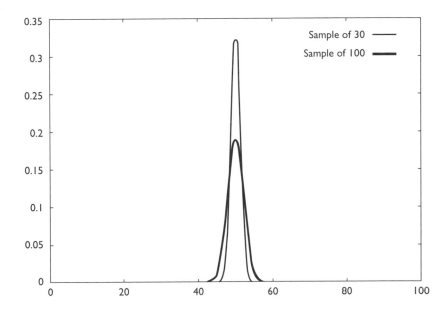

In summary, there are three important points to be learned from this example, which are graphically depicted in Figure 16.8:

- The distribution of the sample means is normal (and this will happen even if the original population from which the sample is taken is not normally distributed, or skewed in some way).
- The mean of the sample means is equal to the population mean from which the samples were drawn (notice how the peak of each curve is at 50).
- The distribution of sample means is less dispersed as sample size increases (the sample of 100 is taller and thinner).

If the distribution of sample means is less dispersed as sample size increases, it follows that the mean of any single sample is likely to be closer to the mean of the population as sample size increases. This is why we advised you in Chapter 5 to take as large a sample as you can.

Together, these three points illustrate a most important theorem in statistics, the *central limit theorem* (see box).

Central limit theorem

If random samples of a certain size n are drawn from any population (regardless of its distribution or shape), as n becomes larger the distribution of the sample means approaches normality.

   This theorem can also be used to show that for a large population and sample, it is often safe to assume that the variable is distributed normally.

Standard error

We have seen that when we take all the possible samples of size n, the sample means have an approximately normal distribution. If we take the mean of all these sample means, we get the mean of the population. The standard deviation of all these sample means gives us an estimate of the spread of the error that we would encounter if we estimated the mean from just one sample of size n (which is what you would normally do in research). This standard deviation is called the *standard error*, and indicates the potential error in the sample statistics by comparison with the population statistics. It can be shown that the standard error is $\sigma/\sqrt{n}$ (where σ is the standard deviation and n the sample size). In our example with a sample size of 30, the standard error is $11.2/\sqrt{30} = 2.04$. In the case of our sample of size 100 the standard error is $11.2/\sqrt{100} = 1.12$. This suggests that the greater the sample size, the closer it will come to approximating the population statistics.

Standard error

For a sample of size n and a population with mean μ and standard deviation σ, the standard error of the sample mean E is given by the formula:

   $$E = \sigma/\sqrt{n}$$

In our second set of samples, we used a sample size of 100. We could see that our estimates for the mean were closer to the actual population mean in these larger samples. This is confirmed by the standard error—that is, $(11.2/\sqrt{100} = 11.2/10 = 1.12)$, which is much smaller than the standard error for a sample size of 30 (2.04). This is demonstrated in the graphs of distributions of sample means for different sample sizes (Figure 16.8). Thus larger samples give more accurate estimates of the actual population mean.

The standard error is inversely proportional to the sample size, and hence we see what common sense already tells us: that our sample mean will be much more likely to be close to the population mean if we use a large sample.

Standard error is also used to calculate sampling error. As the sample mean is itself a variable from a normal distribution, we know that 95 per cent of the time it will have a value within two standard deviations (2 × standard error) of its mean, which is in fact the population mean. So we can be 95 per cent confident that our sample mean is an accurate estimate of the population mean to within two standard errors. Thus, when you read tables that tell you the sample sizes required for various sampling errors at the 95 per cent confidence level, the sampling error reported is in fact two standard errors. We discuss the concept of confidence intervals in more detail below.

Converting scores to Z-scores

The standard deviation has another important function. It can be used to tell us where an individual is situated in relation to the group. Sometimes we might wish to compare the values of interval or ratio level variables taken from different samples or populations. If we know the means and standard deviations of the sample scores, we can do this by calculating a standard score, or Z-score.

The Z-score transforms our original variable into a new variable, which is distributed normally and has a mean of 0 and a standard variable of 1. This distribution is very well tabulated. We can convert any normal distribution to the Z or standard distribution and then use tables to look up probabilities of individual Z-scores. This means that we can reduce two (or more) quite different normal distributions to the same distribution and compare them.

The Z-score will tell us the number of standard deviations away from the population mean that the score is located. The Z-score is calculated by taking the mean from the raw score and dividing by the standard deviation.

Calculating the Z-score

$$Z\text{-score} = \frac{\text{raw score} - \text{mean}}{\text{standard deviation}}$$

Example

Imagine you wish to contrast the results of two students in two different subjects to see which student did better. Imagine that Ruth scored 65 in her Social Work Theory subject and Emma scored 51 in Social Policy. You cannot be entirely sure that Ruth is the better student because the grades reflect the students' work on different subject material. However, if we can calculate the Z-scores for each student in relation to the rest of the students taking each subject, we can calculate how each fared relative to their group, and this allows us to compare the two students.

Suppose that the mean for the Social Work Theory group is 70 and the standard deviation 10. Ruth's Z-score is therefore:

$$Z = \frac{65-70}{10} = -\tfrac{1}{2} = -0.5$$

Ruth's score therefore falls 0.5 standard deviations *below* the mean for her group.

On the other hand the mean for the Social Policy group was 50 and the standard deviation is 5. Emma's Z-score is therefore:

$$Z = \frac{51-50}{5} = -\tfrac{1}{5} = -0.2$$

This tells us that Emma's score is 0.2 standard deviations *above* the mean.

In relation to the two groups of students, Emma's score of 51 is thus a better score.

How to use tables of the standard normal distribution (Z-scores)

To determine the percentage of the population that fell below the Z-score, we look up a table of areas under the normal curve, such as Table 16.11.

In examining where Emma's score (0.2) falls, and describing what this information tells us, we have taken one cell from Table 16.11, as shown in Table 16.12. Emma's score lies in row 0.2 and column 0.00. We can see that 7.93 per cent is the percentage of values of the random variable Z which will fall in the interval between 0 and 0.2 + 0.00 = 0.20. If you prefer, 7.93 is the percentage of the total area under the normal curve between 0 and 0.20. The table only gives the value between 0 and 0.20 because the standard normal curve is symmetrical about 0, so we can immediately say that the percentage

Table 16.11 Percentage areas under the normal curve

Z	.00	.01	.02	.03	.04	.05	.06	.07	.08	.09
0.0	00.00	00.40	00.80	01.20	01.60	01.99	02.39	02.79	03.19	03.59
0.1	03.98	04.38	04.78	05.17	05.57	05.96	06.36	06.75	07.14	07.53
0.2	07.93	08.32	08.71	09.10	09.48	09.87	10.26	10.64	11.03	11.41
0.3	11.79	12.17	12.55	12.93	13.31	13.68	14.06	14.43	14.80	15.17
0.4	15.54	15.91	16.28	16.64	17.00	17.36	17.72	18.08	18.44	18.79
0.5	19.15	19.50	19.85	20.19	20.54	20.88	21.23	21.57	21.90	22.24
0.6	22.57	22.91	23.24	23.57	23.89	24.22	24.54	24.86	25.17	25.49
0.7	25.80	26.11	26.42	26.73	27.04	27.34	27.64	27.94	28.23	28.52
0.8	28.81	29.10	29.39	29.67	29.95	30.23	30.51	30.78	31.06	31.33
0.9	31.59	31.86	32.12	32.38	32.64	32.90	33.15	33.40	33.65	33.89
1.0	34.13	34.38	34.61	34.85	35.08	35.31	35.54	35.77	35.99	36.21
1.1	36.43	36.65	36.86	37.08	37.29	37.49	37.70	37.90	38.10	38.30
1.2	38.49	38.69	38.88	39.07	39.25	39.44	39.62	39.80	39.97	40.15
1.3	40.32	40.49	40.66	40.82	40.99	41.15	41.31	41.47	41.62	41.77
1.4	41.92	42.07	42.22	42.36	42.51	42.65	42.79	42.92	43.06	43.19
1.5	43.32	43.45	43.57	43.70	43.83	43.94	44.06	44.18	44.29	44.41
1.6	44.52	44.63	44.74	44.84	44.95	45.05	45.15	45.25	45.35	45.45
1.7	45.54	45.64	45.73	45.82	45.91	45.99	46.08	46.16	46.25	46.33
1.8	46.41	46.49	46.56	46.64	46.71	46.78	46.86	46.93	46.99	47.06
1.9	47.13	47.19	47.26	47.32	47.38	47.44	47.50	47.56	47.61	47.67
2.0	47.72	47.78	47.83	47.88	47.93	47.98	48.03	48.08	48.12	48.17
2.1	48.21	48.26	48.30	48.34	48.38	48.42	48.46	48.50	48.54	48.57
2.2	48.61	48.64	48.68	48.71	48.75	48.78	48.81	48.84	48.87	48.90
2.3	48.93	48.96	48.98	49.01	49.04	49.06	49.09	49.11	49.13	49.16
2.4	49.18	49.20	49.22	49.25	49.27	49.29	49.31	49.32	49.34	49.36
2.5	49.38	49.40	49.41	49.43	49.45	49.46	49.48	49.49	49.51	49.52
2.6	49.53	49.55	49.56	49.57	49.59	49.60	49.61	49.62	49.63	49.64
2.7	49.65	49.66	49.67	49.68	49.69	49.70	49.71	49.72	49.73	49.74
2.8	49.74	49.75	49.76	49.77	49.77	49.78	49.79	49.79	49.80	49.81
2.9	49.81	49.82	49.82	49.83	49.84	49.84	49.85	49.85	49.86	49.86
3.0	49.87									
3.5	49.98									
4.0	49.997									
5.0	49.99997									

Source: From Weinbach and Grinnell (2010). The original data for Table 16.11 came from Pearson (1930). The adaptation of these data is taken from Lindquist (1938).

of values of Z lying between -0.20 and $+0.20$ is $7.93 \times 2 = 15.86$ per cent. We also know that 50 per cent of values of Z are less than 0, so we can now say that $50 + 7.93 = 57.93$ per cent of values of Z are less than 0.20.

Table 16.12 Extract of percentage areas under the standard normal curve between 0 and Z (from Table 16.11)

Z	.00	.01	.02	.03	.04	.05	.06	.07	.08	.09
0.0										
0.1										
0.2	07.93									
0.3										
0.4										
0.5	19.15									

We can see from this example that 57.93 per cent of Emma's class scored lower than she did.

We can also see where Ruth's score falls. Remember that Ruth scored −0.5, and therefore is in the bottom half of her class. If we look at the table we can see that the area equating to 0.5 is 19.15. Because Ruth's score is negative, we take 19.15 from 50 to determine where she came in her group, that is, 50 − 19.15 = 30.85 per cent. We can deduce from this that only 30.85 per cent of the class scored below Ruth's score.

Confidence intervals

We have seen how statistics from samples give us an estimate of population parameters. We hope they are close, but we need to know how likely it is, or how confident we can be, that the result from our sample reflects the actual statistic in the population. The confidence interval specifies a range of values within which the actual population mean lies.

Once we know our sample mean and standard deviation, and using the fact that 95 per cent of scores from a normal distribution lie within two standard deviations of the mean, we can calculate a *confidence interval*. This confidence interval tells us the range within which we can be 95 per cent confident that the actual population mean lies. The range of scores is called the *confidence interval* and the degree of certainty we have that the population percentage will fall within that range (in this case 95 per cent) is called the *confidence level*.

While we will not explain how to calculate confidence intervals because computer packages do this for us, it is important to know how to read and interpret them. For example, take Sample 1 from Table 16.10. The mean of the sample was 47.3. We can calculate the 95 per cent confidence interval using Z-scores and our knowledge that 95 per cent of normal scores lie within two standard deviations of the mean $(-2 < Z < +2)$. When calculated, the 95 per cent confidence interval for Sample 1 is 43.22 − 51.38.

This means that we are 95 per cent confident that the population mean lies between 43.22 and 51.38. In fact we know that the population mean is 50, which does lie within our 95 per cent confidence interval.

We return to the topic of confidence intervals and confidence levels in the following chapter when we discuss statistical tests of significance.

Normal distribution and Z-scores

A 'normal' distribution is a bell-shaped, symmetrical curve with special properties:

- The mean, median and mode all fall at the same point.
- Sixty-eight per cent of its area falls within one standard deviation from the mean and nearly all its area falls within 99.74 per cent.
- If a variable is normally distributed and we know the mean and variance, we can know a lot about the spread of the data.
- The central limit theorem is used to show that, for a large population and sample, it is often safe to assume that the variable is distributed normally.
- Using the properties of the normal distribution, standard deviation can be used to tell us where an individual is situated in relation to the group. By converting a raw score to a Z-score (which is the score expressed in standard deviation units), we can compare different scores from different groups with different means (see the example of Ruth and Emma above).
- Standard error is used to calculate sampling error. Sampling error is used to determine confidence levels.
- Once we know the sample mean and standard deviation, we can calculate a *confidence interval*, which is the range within which we could expect the population parameter (e.g. mean) to fall based on the sample statistic. A *confidence level* is the estimate of the probability that the true population parameter will fall within that range.

Summary

In this chapter we have introduced you to statistics you will need to analyse results using one variable. We have covered:

- some basic analytical concepts
- continuous and discrete variables
- frequency distributions

- describing a distribution (central tendency, dispersion, taking into account levels of measurement)
- the normal distribution.

Discussion questions

16.1 What is a cumulative percentage column and when would you include one? What is its use?

16.2 What are the differences between a histogram, bar chart, pie chart and pictograph?

16.3 What is the measure of central tendency for nominal data?

16.4 What is a measure of dispersion for ordinal data?

16.5 If the mean, the median and the mode all fall at the one point in a distribution, what shape will it be?

16.6 If Susan scores 70 in an exam in which the mean is 60 and the standard deviation 20, and Sally scores 60 in an exam in which the mean is 45 and the standard deviation 15, who has done better relatively?

Exercises

Locate a quantitative study researching a topic that is relevant to you. Answer the following questions:

16.1 List the main variables from this study and their levels of measurement.

16.2 How are the variables described? What graphical and other means are used to summarise the findings?

16.3 Are the measures of central tendency and dispersion appropriate?

Further reading

De Vaus, D.A. 2002, *Surveys in Social Research*, 5th edn, Allen & Unwin, Sydney. Part IV, 'Analysing survey data', provides a clear and detailed account of the statistics in this chapter.

Pallant, J. 2011, *SPSS Survival Manual: A Step-by-step Guide to Data Analysis Using the SPSS Program*, 4th edn, Allen & Unwin, Sydney. Parts 3, 4 and 5 offer excellent explanations of the statistics covered in this chapter, with step-by-step guides to using SPSS for the data analysis.

Weinbach, R.W. and Grinnell, R.M. 2010, *Statistics for Social Workers*, 8th edn, Allyn & Bacon, Boston, MA. See Chapters 1–4.

17 Statistics for social workers: Two or more variables

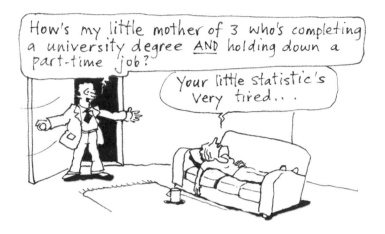

Having examined statistical analysis involved with one variable, we turn to what to do with two or more variables. Statistical comparison of two variables is called bivariate analysis. It is a very common problem in research to need to determine whether there is or is not an association between two variables and, if there is, to explore the nature of that relationship. The first task is to examine the two variables to see whether there appear to be patterns or associations between them. One way to do this is to draw up cross-tabulations.

Cross-tabulations

Cross-tabulations are tables showing the relationship between two variables. Table 17.1 shows the cross-tabulation between the two variables in the example in Chapter 7—the relationship between location (whether people live in the country or city) and their experience of staff treatment (good, satisfactory or bad) at income-support agency offices. This table is called a 'three by two' table, indicating that there are three rows and two columns. For the purposes of illustration, we have increased our hypothetical sample to 300 people, 150 from the country and 150 from the city.

Table 17.1 Experience at income-support agency offices by location (observed frequencies: raw scores)

Experience at agency office	Location		
	Rural	City	Total
Good	33	57	90
Satisfactory	74	61	135
Bad	43	32	75
Total	150	150	300

Note that the table has a title and a number. Both the columns and rows are labelled. The independent variable (location) is across the top of the table in columns, and the categories of the dependent variable are in the rows. The box at the intersection of a column and row is called a *cell*. Cells contain the number of cases from the sample that have the values of both the row and column at which they intersect. Thus 33 people from the country had a good experience at agency offices, while 43 rural people had a bad experience. The end row and end column are called marginals, and show the totals for each row and column. We can see that there were 150 people each from the country and the city: 90 of them felt the service was good, 135 felt it was satisfactory, and 75 had a bad experience. This makes 300 people in all, as shown in the bottom right-hand marginal cell.

From Table 17.1, it appears that people in the city could be more satisfied overall with their experiences at an agency office than people in the country, but it is difficult to tell. An easier way is to use percentages. Technically, there are three kinds of percentage that we could calculate, each of which provides different information. These are:

- percentages across the rows
- percentages down the columns
- percentage of each cell compared to the total of all the cells.

If you are not sure which percentages are being used in a table, work out which way they add to 100. This information should be in the table (as marginals), but sometimes it is omitted.

In this example, we are interested in the effect the independent variable has on the dependent variable (that is, whether living in the country or city affects the experiences people have when they visit an agency office), so it makes sense to examine how sub-groups of the independent variable vary in terms of the dependent variable. In this example, because the independent variable is across the top of the table, we calculate percentages down the columns, so that we can see how the dependent variable changes with the independent variable (Table 17.2).

Table 17.2 Experience at income-support agency offices by location (percentages)

Experience at agency office	Location	
	Rural	City
Good	22	38
Satisfactory	49	41
Bad	29	21
Total	100	100
	(n=150)	(n=150)

From Table 17.2, we can see that 22 per cent of rural dwellers felt that their experience at the agency office was good, compared with 38 per cent of city people. On the other hand, 29 per cent of rural people had bad experiences compared with 21 per cent of city dwellers. In these statements, we are comparing the percentages for each category of the independent variable (location) across the categories of the dependent variable (experience visiting an agency office).

From this brief glance at the percentages, it does appear that country people are less satisfied than city people with their treatment when they visit an income-support agency office. To find out whether these differences are significant, we need to perform statistical tests. Firstly, however, de Vaus (2002) summarises the steps in detecting association between two variables in a table. These are important for you to learn and to understand.

Steps in detecting relationships in cross-tabulations

1 Determine which variable is to be treated as independent.
2 Choose appropriate cell percentages:
   (a)   column percentages if the independent variable is across the top
   (b)   row percentages if the independent variable is on the side
3 Compare percentages for each sub-group of the independent variable within one category of the dependent variable at a time.
4 If the independent variable is across the top, use column percentages and compare these across the table. Any difference between these reflects some association.

> 5 If the independent variable is on the side, use row percentages and compare these down the table. Any difference between these reflects some association.
>
> *Source:* De Vaus (2002, p. 245).

Tables are only useful as ways of presenting information when there are relatively few cells. They are most useful when variables have a maximum of six or seven categories each (de Vaus 2002). If variables have too many categories, it may be possible to collapse some of the categories. This can be done for nominal, ordinal and interval level variables.

Note that Table 17.2 is fairly simple to read (compared with one, say, that includes all the different percentages possible, as well as raw frequencies in each cell). It contains all the important information in skeleton form, from which it is possible to calculate any other information as needed (such as raw figures or row percentages). Presented in this way, it also gives us an indication of the answer to our question—that is, whether living in the country or the city affects the experiences people have when they visit an income-support agency office. De Vaus (2002) provides a useful summary of what information to include in cross-tabulations so that they are simple and clear to read, yet any other calculations can be made from the skeleton information provided in the table.

> **Information to include in bivariate tables**
> - Include table number and title (dependent variable by independent variable)—for example, 'Table 17.2: Experience at income-support agency'.
> - Clearly label each variable and each category of each variable.
> - Use '%' to head percentage columns.
> - Define variables in footnotes to avoid lengthy titles. Footnote how many were in the 'missing data' category (don't know, refusals, no answers).
> - If the independent variable is across the top (as has become the convention), use column percentages only.
> - Place a 100 per cent figure beneath the column to show that percentages have been used.
> - Place the column marginal frequency beneath each column (this shows the numbers on which the percentages are based, and enables the re-calculation of cell frequencies and the grand total).
>
> *Source:* De Vaus (2002, p. 249).

Testing for statistical significance

In this section, we introduce you to some key concepts in testing for statistical significance, provide an overview of the tests from which you can choose and then discuss in more detail the logic behind the more common tests.

Statistical significance

When investigating a relationship between two or more variables, we are looking for evidence that the relationship is clear and not just the effect of chance. Usually we only undertake one study of a research question, drawing only one sample. We need to be reasonably clear that any detected relationship cannot be dismissed as simply the result of sampling error, and that the patterns we can see in the variables taken from our sample actually occur in the population from which the sample came.

Remember Chapter 3 and our discussion of the null hypothesis, which assumes that there is no relationship between variables? This is the implicit assumption on which research is based. If we find, contrary to the null hypothesis, that there is a relationship between the variables in our sample, we are faced with two possibilities: either we have drawn a poor sample that does not reflect the trends in the population (sampling error) or there actually is a relationship between the variables in the population from which we took our sample, and we have some evidence on which to reject the null hypothesis. Tests of statistical significance give us a way of working out which is the correct explanation for our findings.

When testing for significance, we choose what risk we are willing to take that the relationship we observe between the variables in our sample has been caused by sampling error. This risk (probability) is called the *level of significance* of the test, and is a figure ranging from 0 to 1 (usually represented as p). For example, if we get a p of 0.05, we know that in five out of 100 samples, the results in our sample would be due to sampling error. The closer the p value is to 0, the more likely it is that the results are *not* due to sampling error. Thus the lower the significance level, the more confident we can be that the results in our sample are due to real differences in the population.

In most research reports significance levels are represented as 'p'. When you read research reports and articles you will no doubt come across this type of statistical shorthand. Consider the following statement that reflects the way much statistical evidence is reported.

The average number of cases of child abuse dealt with by city social workers in the Department of Community Services is twelve and for country workers it is five. This difference is statistically significant at the 0.05 level (which could also be written as $p < 0.05$).

The writer is suggesting that the probability that these results could have occurred through sampling error is five in 100, so is reasonably confident that there is in fact a relationship between location and number of child abuse cases.

Having understood what level of significance level (or p) means, we now have to choose an appropriate level for our research. In other words, at what level do we reject the original assumption that there is no relationship between the variables (or null hypothesis)? Social researchers, by convention, usually choose either the 0.05 or 0.01 significance levels. There are problems with both of these levels. These are best discussed in the context of Type 1 and Type 2 errors.

Type 1 and Type 2 errors

If we are too easy on ourselves and choose too large a level of significance, we run the risk of rejecting the null hypothesis when in fact our results are due to sampling error. This is called a Type 1 error. With the standard 0.05 significance level, five in 100 chances that our results are due to sampling error could be too many to risk, and mean that we conclude there is a relationship between variables when in fact there is not. De Vaus (2002) writes that this type of error is most likely with large samples. Thus he recommends that it is best to use the 0.01 level of significance with larger samples.

On the other hand, if we are too tough and choose too small a significance level, we might not reject the null hypothesis, assuming our results are due to sampling error when in fact they do represent a relationship between variables that occurs in the population. This is called a Type 2 error. Selecting the 0.01 level means that we could mistakenly conclude that there is no relationship, when in fact there is.

All the statistical tests in the following discussion are tests of significance, or p, for the sample results we obtain. The art (and danger) of choosing the level of significance with which we are happy, and interpreting our results accordingly, is balancing the risks of Type 1 errors against those of Type 2 errors. Much of this assessment depends on the type of study we are doing. For example, if our study involves risks to health—for example, comparing the effects of different types of treatments for alcohol abuse—we would choose much smaller levels of significance than for another study—say, on the preferences of holiday-makers.

For a fuller discussion of the logic of testing for statistical significance, and avoiding Type 1 and Type 2 errors, see Weinbach and Grinnell

(2010, Chapter 5), de Vaus (2002, Chapter 13) or Engel and Schutt (2010a, Chapter 11).

Two other important concepts to understand before discussing statistical tests are the notions of one- and two-tailed hypotheses.

One-tailed and two-tailed research hypotheses

When formulating a research hypothesis, we specify a relationship between two (or more) variables. Sometimes we nominate the direction of the relationship. This is called a *one-tailed hypothesis*. An example of such an hypothesis might be:

> Clients are more likely to have a positive experience in rural income-support
> agency offices.

When we do not specify the direction of the relationship (thus, in our example, we are not saying if the experience is positive or negative), we have a *two-tailed research hypothesis*. An example might be:

> Clients are likely to have a different experience in rural income-support
> agency offices.

Selecting the right statistical test

The credibility of a research project will stand or fall on the selection of the most appropriate statistical test. There are many statistical tests we can use; choosing the right one requires serious thought. Weinbach and Grinnell (2010, pp. 126–9) note that there are five factors that should guide your choice of a statistical test. These are:

- the sampling method used
- the distribution of the variables within the population
- the level of measurement of the independent and dependent variable
- the amount of statistical power that is desirable
- the robustness of the tests being considered.

There are two main types of statistical test: *parametric* and *non-parametric*. *Parametric* tests are more powerful. They require that a random sample be drawn, that the variables are normally distributed within the population, and that at least one variable is at the interval or ratio level of measurement. Parametric tests are used when the probability distribution of the variable is known. Weinbach and Grinnell (2010) suggest that if the mean and standard deviation describe a study's findings fairly well (which means that the variables are normally distributed within the sample), then parametric statistics *may* be appropriate for examining the relationships between variables within the study.

Non-parametric tests are generally less powerful than parametric tests but can be used in studies where the conditions for parametric tests cannot be met. For example, if variables are at nominal or ordinal level, or if samples have been drawn from different populations or are very small, non-parametric tests may be the most appropriate. Sometimes the lesser power of non-parametric tests can be compensated for by using larger samples. Often when we do not know the distribution of the variable, and have reason to suppose that it is not normal, we use non-parametric or distribution-free tests. Non-parametric methods are the only ones available for nominal and ordinal level data. Both methods are used for interval/ratio data, depending upon what we want to know.

Table 17.3, reproduced from Weinbach and Grinnell (2010), provides a useful guide to selecting the appropriate statistical test. Note that the use of computers in statistical analysis makes the task of nominating the most appropriate test based on your study conditions much simpler.

Table 17.3 Parametric and non-parametric statistical tests

Parametric statistical test			*Non-parametric statistical test*		
Test	*Dependent (criterion) variable*	*Independent (predictor) variable*	*Test*	*Dependent (criterion) variable*	*Independent (predictor) variable*
–	–	–	Chi-square	Nominal	Nominal
–	–	–	Fisher's exact	Nominal	Nominal (two categories)
–	–	–	McNamar's	Nominal (before)	Nominal (after)
One-sample t	Interval/ratio	Interval/ratio	Goodness of fit	Nominal	Nominal
Independent t	Interval/ratio	Interval/ratio	Mann-Whitney U	Ordinal/skewed interval	Nominal
Dependent t	Interval/ratio	Nominal	Kolmorogov-Smirnov	Ordinal/skewed interval	–
One-way ANOVA	Interval/ratio	Nominal	Wilcoxon Sign	Ordinal plus	(two repeated measures)

Parametric statistical test			Non-parametric statistical test		
			Kruskal-Wallis	Ordinal/ skewed interval	Nominal
Pearson's r	Interval/ ratio	Interval/ratio	Spearman rho	Ordinal/ skewed interval	Ordinal/ skewed interval
Simple linear regression	Interval/ ratio	Interval/ratio	Logistics regression	Nominal	Nominal

Source: Weinbach and Grinnell (2010).

Tests of significance

Chi-square

Chi-square is one of the most commonly used statistics in social work research because it measures the association between variables at the nominal or ordinal level. Like many other measures of association, chi-square can tell us whether two variables are related. It is a non-parametric test. We will begin our discussion of significance tests with this one.

Measuring association at nominal level

From Table 17.1, the cross-tabulation of raw scores from a survey to measure people's experience when they visit an income-support agency office, we would like to know whether there is a significant difference between the rural and urban experiences.

In order to find out whether there is a significant difference, we first form two hypotheses, as discussed in Chapter 3. These are the null hypothesis and the alternative hypothesis. Remember that in conducting tests of significance we are attempting to disprove the null rather than actually 'prove' the alternative:

- H_0: the null hypothesis—there is not a significant difference between the urban and the rural experience.
- H_1: the alternative hypothesis—there is a significant difference between the urban and the rural experience.

We first consider the case where H_0 is true.

If H_0 is true, we would expect the proportions of people having a good experience to be the same in both locations. What we look for is that the *observed frequencies* differ from the *expected frequencies*. If they do, then the null hypothesis does not ring true. To determine this, we firstly calculate the expected frequency using the following equation:

$$\text{Expected value} = \frac{\text{row total} \times \text{column total}}{\text{number of cases}}$$

There are 90 people overall with a good experience (row total). There are 150 people in the rural sample (column total). The total number of cases is 300. Calculating the expected frequency for the first cell:

$$150 \times 90/300 = 45$$

We would expect 45 rural people to have had a good experience. We can similarly calculate 'expected' values for the different levels of experience in the two locations (Table 17.4) using this formula.

Table 17.4 Experience at income-support agency offices by location— observed (and expected) frequencies

Experience at agency office	Location		
	Rural	City	Total
Good	33 (45)	57 (45)	90
Satisfactory	74 (67.5)	61 (67.5)	135
Bad	43 (37.5)	32 (37.5)	75
Total	150	150	300

We now look at a sample statistic, chi-square, that we will represent using the symbol χ^2.

To calculate chi-square, we sum the observed values minus the expected values squared and divide by the expected value:

$\chi^2 = \Sigma$ (observed value – expected value)^2/expected value

$$\chi^2 = \Sigma \frac{(O-E)^2}{E}$$

where:

χ^2 = chi-square value, O = observed frequency,
E = expected value and Σ = sum of (for all cells).

Table 17.5 illustrates the working out for each cell in our example.

Table 17.5 Example of calculation of chi-square value for income-support agency office experience by location

O	E	O − E	(O − E)	$\frac{(O-E)^2}{E}$
33	45.0	−12.0	144.00	3.20
74	67.5	6.5	42.25	0.63
43	37.5	5.5	30.25	0.81
57	45.0	12.0	144.00	3.20
61	67.5	−6.5	42.25	0.63
32	37.5	−5.5	30.25	0.81
				$\Sigma = 9.28$

In assessing the statistical significance of chi-square, we need to look up the result in a chi-square table. First, we need to note that our assessment is affected by the number of *degrees of freedom* (df). If you examine the data in the table of raw scores (Table 17.1), you will note that there are six cells. The value of chi-square is affected by the number of cells in our table, such that the larger the number of cells the more likely it is that the chi-square value will also be high. It is important that we do not jump to the conclusion that our results are significant before we consider the dimensions of our table. This is where the degrees of freedom come in. To calculate degrees of freedom, we multiply the number of rows (r) minus 1 by the number of columns (c) minus 1. Thus:

$$df = (r - 1)(c - 1)$$

From Table 17.1

$$df = (3 - 1)(2 - 1)$$
$$= 2 \times 1$$
$$= 2 \text{ degrees of freedom (df)}$$

We now look up our value in a chi-square table (Table 17.6). We need to be aware of our degrees of freedom and our level of significance, or −. If we take 0.05 as an acceptable level of significance, this suggests that we are willing to accept that our results are flawed in five out of 100 cases.

Table 17.6 Portion of a table showing the two-tailed area of a χ^2 distribution

Level of significance for a two-tailed test			
df	.20	.10	.05
1	1.64	2.71	3.84
2	3.22	4.60	5.99

To look up our result in the chi-square table we look down the left-hand side of the table under 2 degrees of freedom and then across to our accepted level of significance. In the table you will note that the result for chi-square at 2 degrees of freedom and a probability level of 0.05 is 5.99. If our result is greater than 5.99 we can be 95 per cent confident that a relationship exists. Since our result of 9.28 is greater than 5.99, we can be fairly confident that a relationship does exist (especially as this result is also significant at the 0.01 level).

Table 17.6 is a subsection of the χ^2 table supplied as Table 17.7 (a fuller table that will allow you to assess chi-square results in detail).

Table 17.7 Critical values of χ^2

Level of significance for a one-tailed test						
0	0.10	0.05	0.025	0.01	0.005	0.0005
Level of significance for a two-tailed test						
df	0.20	0.10	0.05	0.02	0.01	0.001
I	1.64	2.71	3.84	5.41	6.64	10.83
2	3.22	4.60	5.99	7.82	9.21	13.82
3	4.64	6.25	7.82	9.84	11.34	16.27
4	5.99	7.78	9.49	11.67	13.28	18.46
5	7.29	9.24	11.07	13.39	15.09	20.52
6	8.56	10.64	12.59	15.03	16.81	22.46
7	9.80	12.02	14.07	16.62	18.48	24.32
8	11.03	13.36	15.51	18.17	20.09	26.12
9	12.24	14.68	16.92	19.68	21.67	27.88
10	13.44	15.99	18.31	21.16	23.21	29.59
11	14.63	17.28	19.68	22.62	24.72	31.26
12	15.81	18.55	21.03	24.05	26.22	32.91
13	16.98	19.81	22.36	25.47	27.69	34.53
14	18.15	21.06	23.68	26.87	29.14	36.12
15	19.31	22.31	25.00	28.26	30.58	37.70
16	20.46	23.54	26.30	29.63	32.00	39.29
17	21.62	24.77	27.59	31.00	33.41	40.75
18	22.76	25.99	28.87	32.35	34.80	42.31
19	23.90	27.20	30.14	33.69	36.19	43.82
20	25.04	28.41	31.41	35.02	37.57	45.32
21	26.17	29.62	32.67	36.34	38.93	46.80
22	27.30	30.81	33.92	37.66	40.29	48.27

df	0.20	.10	0.05	0.02	0.01	0.001
23	28.43	32.01	35.17	38.97	41.64	49.73
24	29.55	33.20	36.42	40.27	42.98	51.18
25	30.68	34.38	37.65	41.57	44.31	52.62
26	31.80	35.56	38.88	42.86	45.64	54.05
27	32.91	36.74	40.11	44.14	46.94	55.48
28	34.03	37.92	41.34	45.42	48.28	56.89
29	35.14	39.09	42.69	46.69	49.59	58.30
30	36.25	40.26	43.77	47.96	50.89	59.70
32	38.47	42.59	46.19	50.49	53.49	62.49
34	40.68	44.90	48.60	53.00	56.06	65.25
36	42.88	47.21	51.00	55.49	58.62	67.99
38	45.08	49.51	53.38	57.97	61.16	70.70
40	47.27	51.81	55.76	60.44	63.99	73.40
44	51.64	56.37	60.48	65.34	68.71	78.75
48	55.99	60.91	65.17	70.20	73.68	84.04
52	60.33	65.42	69.83	75.02	78.62	89.27
56	64.66	69.92	74.47	79.82	83.51	94.46
60	68.97	74.40	79.08	84.58	88.38	99.61

Source: Weinbach and Grinnell (2010). This material was originally from Table IV of Fisher and Yates (1963).

Table 17.6 shows us that χ^2 for our sample is > 5.99, we say that we will reject hypothesis H_0 at the 0.05 level of significance and accept H_1. What does this mean?

> The significance of a test is the probability that we reject H_0 when H_0 is actually true (Type 1 error).

In this case, the probability that H_0 is true is 0.05. Another way of saying this is that there are five chances in 100 that we will conclude there is a relationship between the two variables when there is no relationship.

In our example, $\chi^2 = 9.28$. As 9.28 is much bigger than 5.99, we reject H_0 at the 0.05 level of significance and accept that there is a relationship between experience at the income-support agency and location. Usually, in social work or social science research, we say that 0.05 is an acceptable level of significance. If we wished to be more rigorous, we might choose a 0.01 level.

If we were to present our chi-square findings in a report of our work, we would list it in the following way:

$$\chi^2 = 9.28, df = 2, \rho < 0.05$$

That is, we list our chi-square result, the number of degrees of freedom and the probability that sampling error may have produced the result.

Chi-square is a non-parametric test. It can be used to test association between two variables at nominal or ordinal level when we don't know what their distribution is, or when samples have been drawn from different populations, or when sample size is small. Although less powerful than the parametric tests described below, this can sometimes be compensated for by using larger samples.

For more detail on how to measure association between variables measured at the nominal level, see de Vaus (2002, Chapter 14) and Weinbach and Grinnell (2010, Chapter 8).

Parametric tests for interval/ratio data

Parametrical statistical tests are more powerful tests than non-parametric tests. However, certain conditions must be met before these tests can be used. Parametric tests require that we know the distribution of the variables (usually normal) and that at least one variable is at the interval or ratio level of measurement.

Scattergrams

To get a good working hypothesis of the type of relationship (if any) between two interval/ratio variables that have been measured in pairs, we use a *scattergram*. We plot pairs of points on a graph, with one variable (usually the independent variable) being measured on the horizontal axis and the other (the dependent variable) on the vertical axis. We mark the point corresponding to each pair with a cross. The kinds of results to be expected are shown in Figure 17.1. There are various possibilities:

- There is a linear relationship between the two variables, and Y increases as X increases—the line has a positive gradient.
- There is a linear relationship between the two variables, and Y decreases as X increases—the line has a negative gradient.
- There is no relationship.
- There is a relationship—that is, the crosses do form a definite pattern, but it is not linear. It is a curvilinear relationship. Most of the tests we do will be concerned with linear relationships.

Figure 17.1 Scattergrams and corresponding values of r

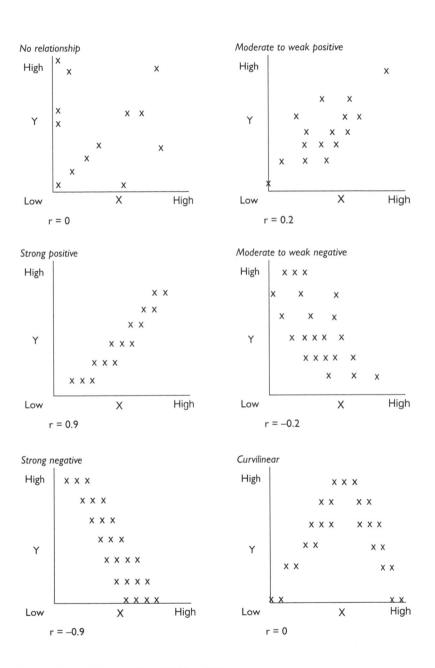

Source: Adapted from de Vaus (2002, p. 281).

Correlation co-efficients

The association between two variables can be summarised by a single figure known as the *correlation co-efficient*. There are many types of correlation co-efficients, which are used at different levels of measurement. Knowing what they mean, and which one is appropriate for your situation, is the most important thing to understand, as computers usually do the mathematics for you. The aspects of correlation co-efficients shown in the box are important factors.

Characteristics of correlation co-efficients

- Correlation co-efficients vary between −1 and 1. If the size of the correlation co-efficient is large (approaching 1 or −1), the relationship is strong; if the value is low (approaching 0), the relationship is weak. Correlations of 0 indicate that there is no correlation between the variables.
- Having a strong (high value) correlation co-efficient does not indicate causality. Correlation co-efficients only show whether two variables are associated (vary together), not that one caused the other.
- At ordinal and interval levels of measurement, correlation co-efficients also show the direction of a relationship using either a minus sign (indicating a negative relationship—variables change in different directions) or no sign (indicating a positive relationship—variables change in the same direction).
- Some co-efficients only indicate whether there is a linear relationship; some can also measure non-linear relationships.
- Different levels of measurement require different measures of association.

Source: De Vaus (2002).

Pearson's product-moment correlation co-efficient

If a scattergram seems to indicate a linear relationship between two variables, X and Y, then we may wish to investigate the relationship further. Pearson's product-moment correlation co-efficient is a useful measure to test whether there is an association between two variables at interval or ratio levels. It is easily calculated with the help of a computer (this is commonly called *the* correlation co-efficient or Pearson's r).

Pearson's r is calculated using the following formula:

$$r = \frac{N\Sigma XY - (\Sigma X)(\Sigma Y)}{\sqrt{[N\Sigma X^2 - (\Sigma X)^2]\ [N\Sigma Y^2 - (\Sigma Y)^2]}}$$

where:

r = Pearson's r

N = number of cases

ΣXY = sum of the XY column

ΣX = sum of the X column

ΣY = sum of the Y column

ΣX^2 = sum of the X^2 column

ΣY^2 = sum of the Y^2 column

Source: Weinbach and Grinnell (2011, p. 211)

This co-efficient always has a value between −1 and 1. A value of 1 means that there is a perfect positive linear relationship between the two variables; a value of −1 means that there is a perfect negative linear relationship between the two variables; while 0 means that there is no relation. (Note that we are talking about data that we have already ascertained is *not* curvilinear. The correlation co-efficient is not particularly meaningful in the case of a curvilinear relationship.)

It should be noted that very little reliance should be placed on correlation co-efficients for small samples.

We use as an example the data in Table 17.8 and Figure 17.2. Table 17.8 lists the results in two examinations of a class of 58 students. We are interested in whether there is a relationship between each student's two sets of marks.

Table 17.8 Class marks for two examinations

Exam 1	Exam 2
10 12 7 13 6 10 13 10 5 9 10 12 13 7	54 79 56 86 53 71 84 70 41 62 76 84
12 12 10 11 12 13 12 11 11 12 12 9 8 89	50 69 74 68 78 78 86 87 79 73 28
10 12 11 7 12 8 11 7 13 9 13 11 11 10	71 77 60 64 77 72 50 72 56 83 48 92
12 9 10 8 12 11 10 7 11 10 7 9 10 13	66 91 75 75 76 79 68 65 65 70 73 63
12 6 8	60 66 88 62 75 64 93 83 52 66

Figure 17.2 Scattergram showing relationship between two sets of examination marks

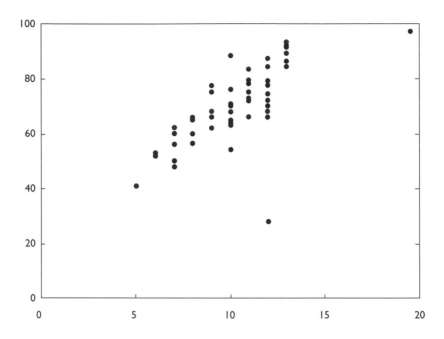

We first look at the scattergram (Figure 17.2). We note that there is a possible positive linear relationship between the two sets of marks. It is thus worth looking at the correlation co-efficient to verify this. If we calculate Pearson's correlation co-efficient using a computer, we find that r = 0.722005. A correlation co-efficient of .72 represents quite a strong linear relationship.

To determine an expression describing this relationship, we need to look at lines of regression.

Pearson's product-moment can be calculated in a number of different ways. For two clear and readable accounts refer to de Vaus (2002) or Weinbach and Grinnell (2010).

Regression

If we find that there is good reason to suppose that two variables (X, Y) are linearly related, we can use this fact to predict the value of the dependent variable based on the value of the independent variable. For example, r can tell us how likely it is that higher education will mean higher income, but regression analysis tells us how much the difference is likely to be. The regression co-efficient, or b, is the slope of the line and predicts how much a change in the independent variable (X) will cause a change in the dependent variable (Y). The regression co-efficient b is always expressed in the units of measurement of the dependent variable.

The equation of a straight line is given by:
$$Y = a + bX$$

where:

    $Y =$ the value we want to predict on the basis of a particular value of X

    $a =$ the point at which the regression line crosses the Y axis

    $b =$ the slope of the line or the regression co-efficient (it is always expressed in the units of measurement of the dependent variable)

    $X =$ the value of X on the X axis

Relationships between variables at the ordinal data level

Data at the ordinal, ratio and interval levels can be arranged in rank order, and can thus be associated with a set of ordinal numbers (1st, 2nd, 3rd, . . .). If we use cardinal numbers instead of ordinal numbers, we assign a number n to each rank. A common measure of association for random variables at these levels is Spearman's rank correlation co-efficient.

If R_x is the set of ranks for variable X, and R_y the set for Y, then the Spearman rank correlation co-efficient is given by:

$$S = 1 - 6\Sigma(R_x - R_y)^2 / (N(N^2 - 1))$$

This correlation co-efficient again has values between −1 and 1, and can be used in a similar way to Pearson's correlation co-efficient. It has the advantage that it can be used with ordinal level data and also with ratio and interval level data that may be related in some non-linear fashion.

Table 17.9 presents a sample of ten pairs of examination marks. (Note that 10 is not really a very realistic sample size for this kind of work, and has been used merely to demonstrate the method.)

Table 17.9 Sample of pairs of examination marks

Practical exam rank	Practical exam score	Theory exam rank	Theory exam score
10	74	1	22
9	70	2	35
8	68	3	41
1	15	4	48
7	60	5	60
6	59	6	62
2	22	7	63
5	48	8	76
4	47	9	77
3	38	10	79

The scattergram for the scores listed in Table 17.9 looks like Figure 17.3. The relationship is certainly not linear, but it looks as if there is a possibly curivilinear relationship. Spearman's rank correlation co-efficient for this data is –0.7, indicating quite a strong relationship.

Figure 17.3   Scattergram of relationship between pairs of scores

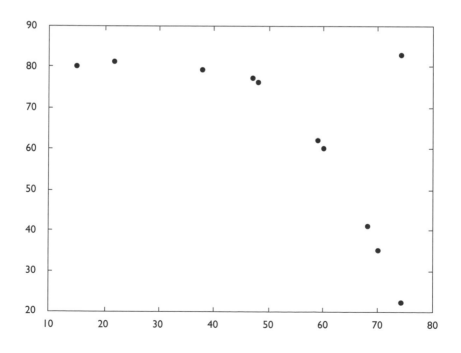

Other ways to measure bivariate relationships

There are other ways to test for statistical significance, but detailed discussion of them is beyond the scope of this book. You can go on to read for yourself about these other statistical tests, all of which use similar reasoning to these basic examples we have provided.

To conclude our overview of statistics for social workers, two of these other methods, t-tests and ANOVA, are described briefly, and examples of how these tests are used to interpret results is provided.

T-tests

The t-test, another parametric test that can be used in a number of ways, is an interval/ratio level test. We will briefly consider how to use it to test whether statistics of a sample can be compared to populations (a one-sample t-test), and how it can be used to test the differences between values of two populations (a two-sample t-test). While t-tests are designed to be used when the interval or ratio dependent variable is normally distributed, Weinbach and Grinnell (2010, p. 136) note that they can still be quite accurate even when the variables are a bit skewed.

One-sample t-test

T-tests can be used to test whether sample results can be generalised to the population—that is, to establish confidence intervals. The one-sample t-test is used to calculate whether there is a significant difference between the sample mean and the population mean. It can be used in situations where the population parameters are unknown. Similarly to the chi-square test, t-tests depend on the number of degrees of freedom. In the case of one-sample t-tests, the number of degrees of freedom is (n–1) where n is the sample size.

Originally, t-tests were used with small samples and Z-scores were used for large samples, but these days t-tests are used for both large and small samples. The t-test follows the same logic and uses tables in the same way as the Z-score described earlier in this chapter. Once you have the sample mean and standard deviation, you can calculate a t-score using a computer or a formula, then compare the t-score with the table value of t, using degrees of freedom (n–1) and the confidence level (usually 0.05) you wish to accept. If the value of t is equal to or greater than the value in the table, H_0 is rejected.

Two-sample t-test

T-tests can also be used to compare the means of two different populations. The logic for calculating the t-statistic and using degrees of freedom and a confidence level is the same, but the methods of calculating the t-statistic are different, depending on whether the samples you are comparing are independent (unrelated) or dependent (paired or matched).

T-tests are so popular in social work that Weinbach and Grinnell (2010, p. 136) report that sometimes they have been used in almost any situation where there is a nominal level dichotomous independent variable and an interval or ratio level dependent variable. They warn that if the interval or ratio level dependent variable is badly skewed within the population, then t-test results can be misleading. Another instance when t-tests are used inappropriately according to Weinbach and Grinnell (2010, pp. 136–7) is when researchers use a 'shotgun' approach, testing a single dependent variable against a long list of dichotomous independent variables to see whether there are any statistically significant relationships. While it is quite likely that some statistically significant relationships will turn up, these are likely to be spurious, or a Type 1 error. If there are reasons to believe that many independent variables are related to a single dependent variable, it is better to use multivariate statistical tests that have been designed specifically for this situation.

ANOVA

Analysis of variance (ANOVA) is a common and powerful test that is used when we want to make multi-group comparisons, or when there is more than one variable we wish to compare—a common occurrence in social work research. In such situations, we cannot use multiple t-tests, because by doing so we increase our likelihood of making Type 1 errors. Instead of having to make many calculations comparing different sets of means, ANOVA allows us to make an overall comparison of the difference of the means among various groups.

Most commonly, ANOVA (or analysis of variance) is used when there are three or more categories of the independent variable or when more than two variables are studied. While t-tests produce a t-value that can be checked in a table for statistical significance, ANOVA tests produce an F-ratio that is checked against its own table. ANOVA tests can be one-way (when there is one independent variable), two-way (when there are two independent variables) or N-ways (for N numbers of independent variables, also called factorial ANOVA).

ANOVA analyses the ratio of variance between groups (between-group variance or difference between the means) and the variation within groups (the within-group variance). If the between-group variance is large compared with the within-group variance, the F-ratio is large. As for t-tests and chi-square tests, degrees of freedom are important in calculating ANOVA results.

$$\text{F-ratio} = \frac{\text{between-group variance}}{\text{within-group variance}}$$

See Weinbach and Grinnell (2010, Chapter 7) for more detailed discussions of different types of t-tests and ANOVAs. Dudley (2010, Chapter 13) also has some good examples of social work research using t-tests and ANOVAs.

Example of use of statistical tests in social work research

Wendy Bowles (1995) studied the quality of life of adults with spina bifida in New South Wales (NSW) for her PhD research. From her experience as a social worker, she was concerned that people with spina bifida were often disadvantaged but did not protest about the conditions in which they were living.

As part of the reading she did to try to explain this, Bowles discovered a model of quality of life that proposed the lowest quality of life was defined by a condition termed 'adaptation', in which people were objectively disadvantaged, but reported no dissatisfaction with their circumstances because they had no hope that things would improve (Zapf 1986; Zapf et al. 1987). According to this model, people only report dissatisfaction when they have had some experience that things can be better—having objectively poor conditions and being dissatisfied (deprivation) is one step higher than adaptation because people in this category have some belief that it is possible for their situation to improve.

If this model could explain the situation Bowles (1995) had observed in the course of her work, she believed it also had important implications for the uncritical use of subjective-only measures of need in needs analyses. Indeed, it pointed to how dangerous it could be to use subjective measures of need without objective measures when dealing with severely disadvantaged groups of people.

Bowles conducted structured interviews with a stratified random sample of 117 adults with spina bifida, and compared these with the results from postal surveys from 180 Technical and Further Education students and with Census data.

People with spina bifida were found to be disadvantaged in every area of life studied, being in the 'adaptation' category for many domains. In this situation, the spina bifida group had significantly lower objective life conditions than the comparison group, yet were at least as satisfied with their circumstances, having adapted their expectations downwards. Qualitative results revealed that people with spina bifida suffered high levels of discrimination, social exclusion and isolation. They wanted jobs, leisure opportunities, relationships and to form their own families. Having little hope of attaining these, however, they had become resigned to their disadvantaged situations.

An example from this study of how t-tests and ANOVA were used comes from the domain of income.

People with spina bifida experienced significantly lower levels of income than the general population of New South Wales aged 15 years and over (see Table 17.10).

Table 17.10 Annual income of the spina bifida group, New South Wales population aged 15–44 years and comparison group

Annual income range $	Spina bifida group %	NSW population 15–44 years %	Comparison group %
0–14 999	70		23
0–12 000		38	
15 000–29 999	25		50
12 001–30 000		42	
30 000 +	5		
30 001 +		20	
Total	100	100	100
	(n = 113)	(n = 2 380 775)	(n = 171)

SB grp x NSW popn	Comp. grp x NSW popn
Chi-square = 50.44	Chi-square = 15.57
Significance: p < 0.001 (Sig)	Significance: p < 0.01 (Sig)

SB grp x Comp. grp
Chi-square = 63.089
Significance: p = 0.000 (Sig)
Strength: Cramer's V = 0.471

The median annual individual income for all people in the New South Wales population in 1991 was $12 001–$16 000 (Australian Bureau of Statistics, 1994); the annual median income for adults with spina bifida was $5000–$9999. The comparison group, on the other hand, had a higher median annual income than the overall population ($20 000 to $24 000).

When income levels were grouped into three categories, the proportion of people with spina bifida in the lowest income range was twice that of the general population of adults in New South Wales aged 15 to 44 years; the proportion in the middle income range was half the New South Wales figure, and less than a third of the New South Wales percentage was earning incomes in the highest bracket (Table 17.10). While the income levels of the comparison group were higher than those of the general population, they were not as different from the New South Wales population as the incomes of people with spina bifida.

The satisfaction scales for income level revealed results that were opposite to those that would intuitively be expected from the objective results. People with spina bifida, despite considerably lower average incomes than the New South Wales population and even lower incomes again compared with the comparison group, reported significantly greater satisfaction with level of income than did those in the comparison group (Table 17.11). People in both groups rated their present incomes as being a little under what they would have hoped for at this time in their lives (the 'expectation gap'). There was no difference in these expectation levels between the two groups.

Table 17.11 Subjective income scales: Spina bifida group by comparison group, t-test results

Variable	Group cases	Number of cases	Mean*	t-value	Two-tailed probability	Significance**
Income satisfaction	SB	115	3.2			
				2.76	0.006	**
	Comp.	179	2.8			
Expectation gap	SB	113	2.7			
				1.49	0.138	NS
	Comp.	178	2.5			

Mean represents the group mean on a scale of 1–5 where 1 = not at all satisfied, or low/worse than, and 5 = very satisfied, or high/better than
** NS = not significant, * = $p < 0.05$, ** = $p < 0.01$, *** = $p < 0.001$

Table 17.12 shows the highly significant differences in levels of satisfaction with income at all levels of actual income, between the spina bifida and comparison groups. Regardless of the amount of income received, people with spina bifida were more satisfied with their incomes than those in the comparison group. This is clearly a pattern of adaptation. However, satisfaction with income also increased with increasing income in both groups, demonstrating that people were more satisfied with increasing income whether or not they had spina bifida.

Despite their considerably lower incomes than the New South Wales population, and still lower incomes than the comparison group, people with spina bifida were more satisfied with their incomes than the comparison group. In response to further questions, the majority of people with spina bifida in the sample also reported that their incomes were sufficient, regardless of level of income or source of financial support. However, satisfaction did increase with level of income for both groups. Such results place the spina bifida group in Zapf et al.'s (1987) 'adaptation' category of quality of life for income. Clearly, people with spina bifida are objectively disadvantaged in this life domain, yet subjectively are highly satisfied with their incomes.

Table 17.12 Satisfaction with income by level of income and group: Spina bifida and comparison groups

Income range ($)	Spina bifida group		Comparison group	
	Mean	%	Mean	%
0–14 999	3.05	69	2.08	23
15 000–29 999	3.39	25	2.72	50
30 000 +	3.83	5	3.43	46
Total		100		100
		(n=111)		(n=171)
ANOVA				
Source of variation	F		Signif. of F	
Main effects	13.683		0.000***	
Income level	16.080		0.000***	
Group	25.131		0.000***	
Two-way interactions				
Income x group	0.752		0.473	
*p < 0.05	**p < 0.01		***p < 0.001	

Note: Mean represents the group mean on a scale of 1–5 where 1 = not at all satisfied, or low/worse than, and 5 = very satisfied, or high/better than

As Sen (1985, p. 29), cited in Travers and Richardson (1993, p. 16), has written:

> A poor, undernourished person, brought up in penury, may have learned to come to terms with a half-empty stomach, seizing joy in small comforts and desiring no more than what seems 'realistic'. But this mental attitude does not wipe out the fact of the person's deprivation.

Summary

In this chapter, we have examined how to present your data, and some of the statistics most commonly used by social workers when studying two variables with a brief reference to statistics for more than two variables. We have presented some of the fundamental methods used in statistical analysis and have covered descriptive and inferential statistics, organising our discussion according to the level of measurement. The aim has been to explain the logic of different tests and how to interpret the information provided by computer calculations. A detailed example of how these statistics are reported was also provided.

In particular, we have covered:

- some basic analytical concepts
- testing hypotheses—levels of significance
- relating two variables (correlation and regression).

Of course, bivariate analysis is only the beginning of the statistical calculations you can perform. Once you have explored the relationship between two variables, it is most likely that you will want to check on the effects of interfering variables, and how several variables relate or cluster together. To learn about this type of analysis, termed multivariate analysis, you need to consult advanced statistical texts and computer software manuals.

Discussion questions

17.1   What information should you include in a bivariate table?

17.2   What is the difference between Type 1 and Type 2 errors?

17.3   At what level of measurement do you use a chi-square test?

17.4   What can a scattergram tell you?

17.5   When would you use ANOVA?

17.6   A study has found that age and income have a correlation co-efficient of 0.65, whereas age and number of qualifications have a relationship of –0.85. What do these correlation co-efficients say about the relationships between age and income, and age and number of qualifications, respectively? Which relationship is strongest?

17.7   What is the difference between parametric and non-parametric statistics?

17.8   A social worker studying domestic violence in the outer suburbs finds that in a table cross-tabulating number of incidences of domestic violence by the type of couple relationship, the chi-square value is 4.23 in a table with four degrees of freedom. Is the relationship significant? What does this finding mean?

Exercise

Construct a cross-table for the variables APPEAL (information re appeal) and gender in Table 17.13. Calculate the chi-square value from the table. Is there a significant relationship between someone's gender and whether they were given information about their right to appeal?

Table 17.13 Summary information

Respondent (ID)	Type payment (PAY)	Location	Gender	Age	Staff respect (ATTIT3)	Info re appeal (APPEAL)	Staff behaviour (BEH1, BEH2)
J. Smith (001)	Sole parent	City	Female	18	3	No	Formal, rushed
P. Collins (002)	Disability support	City	Male	19	5	Yes	Friendly, took time for me
M. Chapman (003)	Young homeless	City	Male	16	1	No	Rude
A. Jones (004)	Unemployed	Country	Male	20	3	Yes	Okay, friendly
T. Black (005)	Sole parent	City	Male	25	2	Yes	In a hurry, didn't seem interested in my questions
006	Unemployed	City	Female	21	2	Yes	Rushed, rude
007	Aged pension	City	Male	85	5	No	Polite, busy
008	Unemployed	Country	Male	26	1	No	Not interested, accused me of not seeking work
009	Sole parent	City	Female	23	3	No	Okay, kids a nuisance
010	Sole parent	Country	Female	29	4	No	Just routine visit to ask if UB would be better, staff busy
011	Disability support	Country	Male	21	3	Yes	Staff kind, busy
012	Unemployed	City	Female	21	2	Yes	Rushed, formal
013	No payment	City	Female	53	4	Yes	Asking on behalf of my daughter, staff very nice

Respondent (ID)	Type payment (PAY)	Location	Gender	Age	Staff respect (ATTIT3)	Info re appeal (APPEAL)	Staff behaviour (BEH1, BEH2)
014	Aged pension	Country	Female	60	5	No	Very nice, very busy
015	Unemployed	City	Male	30	2	Yes	Formal, brusque
016	Unemployed	Country	Female	32	4	Yes	Formal but courteous
017	Sole parent	Country	Female	23	3	Can't remember	Okay
018	Unemployed	Country	Male	57	3	Yes	Very busy, no idea for jobs
019	Disability support	City	Female	40	3	Yes	Sympathetic but formal
020	Unemployed	City	Female	18	2	No	Okay

Further reading

De Vaus, D.A. 2002, *Surveys in Social Research*, 5th edn, Allen & Unwin, Sydney. Part IV, 'Analysing survey data', provides a clear and detailed account of the statistics in this chapter.

Pallant, J. 2011, *SPSS Survival Manual: A Step-by-step Guide to Data Analysis Using the SPSS Program*, 4th edn, Allen & Unwin, Sydney. Parts 3, 4 and 5 offer excellent explanations of the statistics covered in this chapter, with step-by-step guides to using SPSS for the data analysis.

Weinbach, R.W. and Grinnell, Richard M. 2010, *Statistics for Social Workers*, 8th edn, Allyn & Bacon, Boston. For a detailed discussion of the statistics in this chapter, see Chapters 5, 6, 7, 8 and 9.

PART V

Bringing it all together

18 Influencing policy and practice

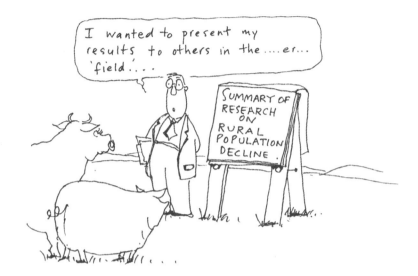

Having written your research proposal, received ethical approval and funding, designed your study, collected and analysed the data, you are finally ready to release your results. Thought the hard work was over? In many ways it has just begun.

This chapter covers two critical phases in the research process:

- making an impact, or influencing policy and practice
- writing up your research.

Planning for maximum impact of your results is just as important as planning the research itself. There are many good reasons why you should plan the dissemination of your results as carefully as you plan the research. These involve political, ethical and practical issues. *Ethically*, it is important to be accountable to those who were involved in the research, those who funded the research and other key stakeholders who will be affected by the research. *Politically*, it is important for the goodwill of the community that you plan some kind of report back to the people involved in the research process. Social work is a profession committed to goals of social justice. If research does not lead to action, it is hard to justify why social workers should be involved. Reporting results to the people who participated in the research is increasingly being acknowledged as an ethical and political imperative in social work research (D'Cruz and Jones 2004; Marlow 2010) and as contributing towards the social justice and empowerment agendas of social work research. *Pragmatically*, if you can demonstrate that the results of your research have led to specific outcomes in social work policy or practice, or have influenced decision-makers in some way, you are more likely to get funded for further research. Thus there are many good reasons why you should plan how to disseminate your results to a variety of audiences.

Most social work research projects have at least two audiences: the people who participated in the research and the funding body or sponsors. Usually a written report for sponsors is required by the research agreement.

We have discussed how reporting back to participants in a series of stages can be part of the research process itself. Whether or not it is built into earlier stages of your research design, it is important to plan some report-back mechanisms to your participants at the end of the process.

All the key stakeholders we identified in Chapter 1 are also potential audiences, as is the general community. Thus, when you are planning how to disseminate your findings, it is advisable to use several of the avenues discussed in this chapter in order to gain maximum impact.

In addition to reporting their results to research participants, sponsors and stakeholders, most social workers aim to report their results at conferences and publish them in journals whose readers are other professionals and colleagues. Your colleagues are another important audience. Reporting to them means you can contribute to the growing social work research culture and the knowledge base of our profession. The more we publish the results of our research in venues accessible to our colleagues, the more we will develop an evidence-based culture for our work and increase confidence in our profession.

In this chapter, we prepare you for disseminating your research so that it has maximum impact. First, we discuss how to develop an action plan. Then we outline several avenues for disseminating your results, some of which you might build into the action plan. Finally, we discuss writing up your report.

Planning for maximum impact

Planning the action you want to achieve as a result of your research is part of the research process. Ideally, you will have been developing a plan as you have been working through the findings and implications with your steering committee or whoever is working with you in the research project. Wadsworth (2011a) suggests writing an action plan once you know the results of your research. This is an important step in influencing policy and practice, and making sure that your results have an impact. If you have been working with an advisory group or steering committee through-out the research, writing an action plan and carrying it out are the final tasks that you will be undertaking with the group. If you did not have an advisory group, this is the time to form one. The advisory group consists of the key stakeholders in the research project: the people with an interest in the results (see Chapter 2). An advisory group can help you to brain-storm the implications of your research and what should happen as a result of your recommendations. At this stage in the research, several heads are generally better than one.

There are four steps in forming an action plan, according to Wadsworth (2011a, pp. 154–5). These are:

- *What* do you want to achieve as a result of the research?
- *Who* needs to know in order for these things to happen? Should you add people to an existing list?
- *Why* do we want to tell them? (How will these people contribute to the process of getting the action taken?)
- *How* should the findings be conveyed (and *when*)?

What needs to happen?

If they are specific enough, your findings and the recommendations will directly suggest what needs to happen as a result of your research. More general findings may require further discussion and brainstorming about what actions should follow.

In the income-support agency example in Chapter 5, if you uncover that there are problems in the way some people are treated when they visit an office, you may want to raise the awareness of staff and management about the problem. You may also want additional training for the staff and to institute ways of monitoring their improvement in this area. You might recommend that a working party be formed within the agency to decide the best ways in which the problem can be dealt with. If you are a researcher who is external to the agency, then your work with the steering committee/advisory group will be critical in achieving action.

Wadsworth (2011a) notes that recommendations may be short-, medium- or long-term. It is a good idea to structure your action plan according to these categories, to assist in developing a timeframe.

Who do we tell?

Understanding the formal and informal power structures of the key organisations relevant to your research topic (including organisations of 'the researched' as well as organisations controlling the funding, decision-making or other resources) is critical in making good decisions about 'who do we tell?' Wadsworth lists a series of questions to take into account, including: Who controls the resources you need to achieve your goals? Who makes the decisions? Who will be your supporters? Who is likely to try to block you? If your results are to have maximum impact, you must take into account the people who will both support and oppose you. You need to decide who they are and what will be the most effective way of making your results known to them. Plan which people are to be lobbied, depending on the results of your research.

Why we want to tell them

Part of deciding who you want to tell about your research involves thinking about what you want from these people. What do you want them to do? How do you want them to get involved? Researchers usually have few resources, so you need to target carefully which people you want to tell.

How to convey the findings

A written report is a requirement for most research projects. We will discuss the formal report later in this chapter. However, to achieve maximum impact, there are also other pieces of writing that will be required. People in the community, as well as policy-makers and decision-makers, may find a summary more accessible. For media interviews or news releases in local papers, you will need a succinct summary of key findings and recommendations.

When planning how to present your findings, work out where and how your target group is most likely to see them. Remember that written information will not be accessible to people in the community who don't read. There are many other ways to present your findings. A combination of methods will increase the potential impact of your research, and raise awareness about the next steps. Some of these methods are listed in the following section of the chapter.

When will we do this?

Timing is always important in developing your action plan. It is important to know when the key decisions are being made that will affect the issues you have researched, and to time your strategies accordingly. For example, just before an election can be an excellent time to ensure that politicians are interested in your results. Releasing your findings in time for key meetings, before budget decisions, or while key people are *not* on leave, is also an important consideration. The summer holiday period is not a good time to release your report!

Here is an example of an action plan, as devised by Wadsworth (2011a, p. 155) using the income-support agency example:

What we want	Who we tell	Why	How findings will be presented	What to get over	When
Better treatment for country clients	• Managers • Country staff	To improve services and ensure efficiency with better access	Meetings, article in departmental newsletter, focus groups of staff to discuss how to monitor changes	Experiences of country clients	April: article in newsletter. May–Oct: meet with all country offices. April next year: evaluate action plan

Planning for maximum impact

Develop a written action plan that includes

- *what* you want to achieve
- *who* needs to know
- *why* you want to tell them
- *how* the findings should be conveyed
- *when* this is to happen, timed for maximum impact.

We now consider some of the avenues that you could use under the 'how' of your action plan.

Avenues for publication and dissemination of results

Journal articles

There is a range of avenues through which you can publish the results of your research. The most prestigious journals are called refereed or peer-reviewed journals. The editors of journals such as international and national journals of social work send your article out to referees before they decide whether to publish your work. The referees, in turn, send in their comments and suggest changes needed before your paper will be published.

Monographs or stand-alone reports

Organisations that fund research may require a report or monograph that is published as a separate document in its own right. These stand-alone reports are longer than articles published in journals and usually involve more complex studies. They are often published on the internet, on the websites of the sponsoring organisation. The format for such reports follows the same general structure as outlined later in this chapter, although more detail is included than for journal articles. Usually an executive summary and a list of recommendations are included in these reports—though not in journal articles.

Conference presentations

Conferences are another important avenue for presenting research results. Unless you are a keynote speaker, usually no more than ten to fifteen minutes is allowed for presentation time. The discussion/question time that follows is a valuable opportunity to criticially review your work with colleagues before you submit it for publication. Many conferences also have the option of presenting your research in poster form or PowerPoint.

Newspapers, newsletters, e-newsletters

At the more informal end of the publication spectrum, your results could be published in newspapers or newsletters or in electronic media such as e-newsletters or websites with 'Events' pages. With this type of publication, it is particularly important that tables, graphs and other visual presentations of the results catch the readers' attention. Similarly, the title of your report should attract attention and make people want to find out more. Readers of informal or popular avenues for written research tend to be interested in the conclusions and recommendations of research rather than in the methodology or detailed results, so tailor your writing accordingly. Make sure your work is succinct. Always write in plain English and avoid jargon.

Media interviews

Media interviews are an important avenue for disseminating research results. You or your organisation may submit a news release to highlight major findings in the hope of being invited for an interview. Newspapers, radio and television reach a wide audience and can bring the results of your research to the notice of policy-makers and decision-makers. Local media such as community radio are also a useful means of communicating with various stakeholders about the research.

Meetings

Sometimes you or the organisation sponsoring the research will organise a seminar, public meeting or forum specifically to publicise your research results. Depending how the meeting is structured, this is an excellent opportunity to reach a wide range of people, including organisational staff, the people being researched (if they are different from the staff) and members of the wider stakeholder groups. We have seen how meetings to reflect on results can be an intrinsic part of action research and other research designs.

Whether speaking at a conference, writing a paper for a journal or newspaper or preparing for an interview on radio, it is imperative that you are succinct and present your ideas simply and within the word or time limit.

Avenues for disseminating your research findings

- Books or book chapters
- Academic and professional journals (refereed or not refereed)
- Stand-alone reports
- Conference papers, posters, PowerPoint
- Newsletters
- Newspapers, magazines
- Meetings
- Media interviews, articles, press releases
- Web-based publication and dissemination

Writing your research report

If you have followed the process that we have outlined throughout this book, writing up your report should be a relatively easy process. You will already have completed much of the work when you wrote your research proposal (see Chapter 19). Throughout the data-collection phases, you can be working on various parts of the report. It is better to start writing as you go, rather than leaving it to the end.

Writing the formal research report is an important part of ensuring that the findings from your research become public knowledge. It leaves a clear record of your work. It is also usually a requirement of the initial research agreement.

The following discussion covers the elements required for most research reports, distinguishing what is included in journal articles from other types of reports. Whatever the context, when reporting your research you need to provide a succinct summary of your project (abstract), outline your aims and the significance of the research in the broader context of the literature review (introduction/problem statement), describe your methodology and findings, discuss the limitations as well as the implications of your study and, finally, make conclusions and/or recommendations based on the evidence you have gathered.

Title
Your title should attract interest, and evoke the key issues in the research.

Table of contents
Longer or complex research reports (but not journal articles) begin with a table of contents (listing section headings and page numbers), which acts as a guide to various parts of the report. Highlight different levels of headings and sub-headings with indents and different fonts or font sizes.

Separate lists of tables, figures, maps or other important items in the report (for example, lists of abbreviations) may also follow the general table of contents and are placed before the introduction. Word processing packages usually include a Table of Contents function.

Acknowledgements
Acknowledgements often appear at the beginning of a report, either as a separate section, as part of the introduction, or as a footnote to the title. They are generally not used in journal articles. Acknowledgements thank others for their contribution to the research, and are often personal statements by the author/s about the support they received during the project.

Abstract
The abstract is written last and appears first. It is the brief summary that heads your report and is one of the most difficult parts of the report to write. In about 300–350 words, the aims of your study, the design and methodology, the key results and findings are summarised. Readers scanning journals or searching databases use the keywords and abstract to decide whether they will read the whole article. It is therefore imperative that the abstract is written in clear and concise terms that outline the important aspects of your study. Include the key words that you expect other researchers to use if they are doing research in your area.

The research report itself consists of five main elements, each of which includes several sub-sections. These are: introduction/statement of the problem; methodology; findings; discussion; and conclusion/recommendations. When you are drawing up the outline or structure for your own report, it is a good idea to divide the report into these five sections and write up sub-headings within each of them. Usually the largest sections will be the 'findings' and 'discussion' sections, so you will need to allow plenty of space for these. We now explore each of the five sections of a research report in more detail.

Introduction/statement of the problem

Most of the work for this section of the paper you have already completed in your original research proposal (see Chapter 19). If you have done this correctly, all you need to do for the first part of your research report is a cut-and-paste job from several sections of your research proposal.

Context of study

The major task of the introduction/statement of the problem is to explain the context of your research, showing why it is important and how it is relevant to social work practice, theory, policy or social issues. In the introduction, you set out the broad aims of the study as well as defining research questions and concepts (in quantitative studies), demonstrating through the literature search how and why you made the decisions that you did.

Auspices and assumptions

The auspices of the study are also clearly stated in the introduction, as well as the researcher's orientation, if this is appropriate. Some qualitative and feminist researchers are careful to state their own position in relation to the research—for example, how different or similar they are to the people they are researching, or what stake they have in the issues being examined, and what effects this might have on the research process. It is also important to make explicit any assumptions that underlie the approach you have chosen.

Literature review

In the introduction, the literature search is summarised and presented as an argument, which leads up to and justifies the approach that you have taken. You must demonstrate that you have read widely and understood the major debates in the literature, the research approaches that have been tried and the gaps that exist (hopefully some of which your research is addressing). All the important concepts that you have used in your research should be located in the wider context of the literature as well as the theoretical approach you have adopted. Most of this you have already completed in your research proposal. The only additions may be some more up-to-date literature about particular aspects of the research problem that have come to light after the research proposal was written.

The literature review is not an author-by-author account describing what you have read. Rather, divide the literature into themes or issues that are related to the issue and questions in your study, and use this structure to justify the approach you have taken. Be critical of what you have read, especially if you detect biases or flaws in other studies that influence the results and/or conclusions.

What to include in the introduction/problem statement

- Statement of topic, aims, research questions
- Significance of the research, its contribution to social work practice, theory, policy or knowledge
- Summary and critical discussion of literature review, justifying the broad design (qualitative, quantitative, feminist), theoretical approach of the study and the definition of major variables and research questions
- Researcher's own position in relation to the research
- Assumptions clearly stated
- Auspices of the study
- Quantitative studies: identify dependent and independent variables, state hypotheses

---

Methodology

The second major section of your research report is the methodology section. Again, much of this has been completed in your research proposal. There are several areas that you have to cover, and it is important to distinguish between them. Sub-headings in your report are an effective way to do this.

Design

This is a summary/overview of how your methodology addresses the research questions. Usually it begins broadly, indicating whether you have chosen qualitative, quantitative or a mix of approaches, and then narrows down to how you operationalised the variables (if quantitative), who you are going to research and what kind of research techniques you will use. Review Chapters 2, 3 and 4 for the sorts of information to include in your description of the design of your study.

Population and sample

Whether doing qualitative or quantitative research, it is important to report what population you are researching, how you drew your sample, what your unit of study is and on what basis (theoretical or statistical) you will be generalising your results. When describing who was in your sample, acknowledge any limitations in the sampling process that might lead to biases in the findings. Tables and graphs are an effective way of presenting data about your sample. Take care only to include information about the sample that relates to how it was selected. For example, if you stratified your sample for age, gender or region, you could provide tables showing the breakdown of the sample in terms of these variables. If you did not stratify your sample according to certain criteria then much of this information is left to the section on findings (see Chapter 5).

Instrumentation

Having spent so much time using your questionnaire, interview schedule or prompt sheet, it is an easy mistake to forget to describe it to the reader. In longer reports, it is expected that you will appendix the whole survey or list of questions as well as summarising the key aspects of it in the text of your report.

Describe how you developed the instrument, including sources from the literature, any pre-tests or pilot tests you performed, and major changes that were made as a result. Include some samples of the types of questions you asked, showing how they relate to the broader research questions. In quantitative studies, if you have not already provided the fine detail of how research questions and variables were operationalised, this is the place to do so. How you addressed questions of reliability and validity should also be included. In qualitative studies, it is more appropriate to discuss questions of rigour, rather than reliability and validity.

Data collection

Describe how the data were collected, where, how long it took and who collected them (for example, 'Interviews lasting from one to three hours were conducted by the researcher at locations convenient for the respondent, sometimes in the person's home, or at other places nominated by the respondent such as the local park, offices of the local X organisation or the respondent's workplace.'). Include in this description the measures taken to address scope and coverage (number of call-backs, how refusals were dealt with and so on—see Chapter 6).

Ethical issues and limitations of methodology

As part of the methodology section, you should include a brief discussion of any ethical issues you anticipated in the research process and how you dealt with them. Again, this will have been written up already in your documents for ethics committees and will be a matter of cutting and pasting. If other ethical issues arose that you did not anticipate, this is the place to discuss them, including how you dealt with them.

While the discussion section is most likely to include a discussion of the limitations of your study and areas for future research, it is also worth acknowledging any limitations in the methodology in this early part of the report. Being constructively critical of your own work is a strength. It assists future researchers who wish to replicate your methodology. It also forestalls other critics if you have shown that you are aware of the weaknesses or limitations in your work. Providing a critique of your work enables your results to be interpreted in a wider context.

Data analysis

Finishing the methodology section with a description of how you analysed your data is a good way to lead into the results or findings section of the report. In this last sub-section of the methodology section, you need to guide the reader through the steps you took to analyse your data. In quantitative studies, this could be an overview of which statistical techniques you used and how they were interpreted, mention of which computer software you used and an explanation of why these data analysis techniques were the most appropriate to address the research questions. In qualitative studies, you might discuss the theory driving the data analysis, how you coded your data, which software you used and how you developed themes. In this section of the report, you are providing the reader with a map of how to read the results you are about to present, and an explanation of how you arrived at them.

What to include in the methodology section of your report

- Design of the study
- Population and sample (including sampling techniques and sample description)
- Instrumentation (including how instrument was designed, pre-tests, pilot, reliability/validity or rigour. In quantitative reports, you would state how variables were operationalised and how this relates to the research questions.

- Data collection (including scope and coverage issues)
- Ethical issues, limitations of methodology
- Methods of data analysis

Findings

This section is usually one of the largest in the report. When planning how to present your results, it is a good idea to think of a series of sub-headings that relate to the major themes in your findings, or to the research questions themselves, or to some other logical sequence, so that as you describe your results, a story unfolds. Sometimes researchers follow the same sequence in reporting results that they followed in asking the questions, if the structure for the interview or questionnaire followed a logical sequence.

Before beginning the story emerging from the results, researchers usually present a description of the people in the research (the sample). In quantitative reports, simple, univariate results are then described, followed by the more complex results from bivariate and multivariate analyses addressing various research questions about relationships between variables. In qualitative reports, the results are presented according to the themes that have been identified, often also in increasing order of complexity.

Remember that you don't have to include all your results when you report your findings. Only include findings that directly focus on the relevant issues. Often many of your results will be discarded in the interests of concise and precise reporting.

Do not selectively weed out the data that invalidate your hypothesis or point of view! You must allow contradictory data to emerge in the interests of the development of knowledge.

As a general guideline, if the results can be more simply and clearly put in words, then use text and don't bother about tables or graphs. On the other hand, if it is more effective to summarise large amounts of detailed information in tables, then do so, remembering to comment on the tables in the text. Readers can use the tables to check whether your interpretations of the data are correct, or whether you have overlooked something important. When discussing tables, there is no need to state the obvious, but you should include an overview of the main points you want to emphasise and the meaning of key statistics. Generally, you do not have to explain the statistics you used. Simply list the results at the bottom of the table and comment on them in the text (see Chapters 16 and 17 for examples).

As a rule of thumb, in quantitative reports the findings are usually reported with little comment. This is saved for the discussion section, unless a decision has been made to combine the findings and discussion sections. Sometimes in qualitative research these two sections are combined in order to reduce duplication and to delineate the different themes more clearly. Similarly, in large, complex quantitative studies with many results to report, it is more sensible to combine the results and discussion sections according to particular themes or questions. Usually at the end of a complex results section, the results and issues arising from them are summarised briefly to provide the 'big picture' or overview, before the final conclusions and recommendations are made.

What to include when presenting findings

- Present a description of the sample of people involved in the research.
- Present all findings relevant to the research issues or questions, including contradictory or unexpected results.
- Not all the results have to be included.
- Arrange the findings in a sequence, using logic or the order of interview questions so that the results tell a story.
- In quantitative reports, start with simple descriptive findings and move on to the more complex explanatory results.
- In qualitative reports, structure the results according to the themes that emerged and the research questions.
- Use tables and graphs interspersed with text judiciously—choose between tables and text on the basis of the easiest, clearest and most accountable way of reporting findings.

Discussion

This is the section where results are summarised, explained and interpreted. Often the discussion is conducted in the light of the issues identified in the literature search at the beginning of the paper, highlighting the contribution your own results make to these debates. If your results are different from findings in previous studies, try to explain why this may be so (using theory, other research or your own data) and hypothesise about future research to explore these differences further. If previous studies support your findings, discuss this and the implications.

The discussion section is the place to comment on how your findings relate to theory development or specific issues, how the evidence you have gathered supports or does not support the hypotheses you made, and what implications arise from the findings. Reid (1993) notes that the discussion section is a balancing act between two negatives—not merely repeating the findings, and yet also not going off into flights of interpretation which are not supported by the evidence in your research. It is important that your discussion relates your findings back to the original research questions or issues that motivated the study in the first place.

Limitations

Usually the discussion includes a sub-section, or at least a few paragraphs, on the limitations of the study and areas for future research (which are sometimes suggested by the limitations).

Acknowledging the limitations of the study is very important when you discuss the meaning of the findings and how they can be used in practice. In quantitative reports, this will include a discussion about the overall soundness of your study (its internal validity) as well as the degree to which the findings can be generalised (external validity). In qualitative research, generalisability often relies on the theoretical strength of the work, as discussed in previous chapters.

As well as limitations in sampling, it is important to consider other methodological issues, including the design of the instrument (survey, interview), timing of interviews or impact of interviewers. In qualitative studies where 'objectivity' is not an issue, discussion of rigour and what makes the results credible is important.

The report is documentary evidence of your competence as a researcher, so you may be inclined in the interests of passing a subject or improving your career to over-emphasise the strength of your work and to downplay the weaknesses. You should guard against this and allow readers to assess the merit of your work. Similarly, you should be on the lookout for data that not only support your stance, but also negate it. Do not overlook alternative interpretations in the interests of supporting your argument.

Remember that in some studies the discussion and findings sections can be combined. When this is the case, it is important that the points raised in this section are included somewhere in the report.

Discussion section

- Summarise, explain and interpret your findings.
- Do not merely repeat findings and do not make interpretations that are not supported by the evidence in your study. Discuss findings in the light of issues raised in the literature review.

- Discuss implications of findings for current practice, policy and/or theory.
- Acknowledge the limitations of the study.
- Point to areas for future research.

Summary, conclusion and recommendations

In long or complex studies, the conclusion begins with a summary of the key findings. This includes all the important aspects of the study. Sometimes this summary is placed at the beginning of the discussion section. There can also be an 'executive summary'. Executive summaries are located at the beginning of government or stand-alone reports.

Executive summaries and recommendations are sometimes the only parts of a research report that busy workers and decision-makers read. This means that the main messages from your research have to stand out in these sections. In journal articles, there is no executive summary, and the conclusion and recommendations follow directly from the findings and discussion.

Conclusions must first refocus the issue (relate to the original research questions), second be justified in the light of your research design and the limitations of the study, and finally remind the reader about directions for future research.

Following the conclusions, many social work studies end with a list of recommendations. Recommendations may be about practice issues, policy matters, changes to existing services or advocating the need for new services. Often research recommendations are about changes in emphasis or priorities within existing services. Sometimes the sponsoring organisations that pay for the research specify that they have the right to approve, or at least to comment on, the recommendations made by researchers. Others consider this to be a breach of intellectual freedom and against the spirit of research. Wording recommendations is an important job for your advisory group. In action research designs, developing recommendations is an integral part of the research design.

Who has the final say over the recommendations of a research report is a political issue of ownership that should be understood by all parties from the beginning of the research process. If appropriate, negotiate this as part of the written contract with the sponsoring agency (see Chapter 1).

References

Research reports always include an alphabetical list of the references, books, articles and other sources of information (such as films and websites) that you cited in the report. Most journals and publishers have specific requirements regarding how you should present your references. There are several referencing systems and software packages available. If publishers do not prescribe a particular method, use one of the accepted means such as the Harvard system of referencing.

When listing your references, consistency and attention to detail is very important. Every source that you cite in the body of the report must be accurately referenced in this section.

Appendixes

Research reports such as stand-alone reports, books or longer book chapters often include appendixes. These are additional sections of the report and may include the original questionnaires or interview schedules, copies of letters, details about sampling and other procedural matters, and extra background data that support the arguments in the report. Journal articles usually do not include appendixes.

A structure for your research report

- Title page
- Table of contents*
- List of figures*
- List of tables*
- List of abbreviations*
- Abstract
- Introduction/problem statement
- Methodology
- Findings
- Discussion
- Conclusion/recommendations
- References
- Appendixes*

*Not generally included in journal articles

Summary

This chapter has discussed various ways to ensure that your research has maximum impact and leads to actions that make a positive difference in people's lives. Devising an action strategy is an important part of the research process, which needs the same careful planning as other stages in your project. With an action plan in place and good follow-up procedures to monitor its success, you will be in an excellent position to make sure that your research is effective and that all your hard work has been worthwhile.

Reporting back to the people involved in the research, as well as the sponsors and other stakeholders, and involving these groups in the action plan is an important aspect of social work research.

Write your research report with the target audiences and your purpose for the research in mind. Whether your report is at the formal or informal end of the spectrum, several elements will make it more effective: a catchy title, logical structure, clear layout with well-spaced headings, plain English, graphics and charts, and finally an eye-catching cover. Use the structure outlined in this chapter as a guide.

Discussion questions

18.1 What is the relative importance of the methodology versus the findings and conclusions sections of research reports in:
   (a) professional journals or conference presentations?
   (b) newspapers, newsletters, more informal sources of publication?
18.2 What is the purpose of the abstract?
18.3 List the main elements included in the introduction/statement of the problem section.
18.4 What are the six key aspects of the methodology section?
18.5 Should you discuss your findings as you present them?
18.6 What should be included in the discussion section?
18.7 What are the key elements to include in an action plan?

Exercises

18.1 Go to the library and select one quantitative and one qualitative research report in a journal, as well as one quantitative and one qualitative stand-alone report (either a book or a larger report):
   (a) List the structures of these four reports, noting similarities and differences.

(b) Compare the structures of these reports with the suggested structure for report writing in this chapter:
  (i) Are the research question/s and the background literature review clear? Do you understand the context of these studies?
  (ii) How is the methodology section set out? Is all the necessary information included?
  (iii) Are the findings related to the questions?
  (iv) Is the evidence sufficient to justify the conclusions?
  (v) Are the limitations of the studies acknowledged? How?
  (vi) Are the recommendations/conclusions related to the original research questions and relevant to social work practice or policy?

18.2 Scan news reports and newspapers for some examples of how research is being reported and used to make decisions or take action. Is there evidence of an action plan on the part of the researcher?

18.3 Interview some researchers about how they formulate action plans, or try to ensure that the results of their research are known about in the right places. What strategies do they use to get their message across? How effective have they been?

18.4 Write an action plan for a piece of research in which you have been involved. Alternatively, select a piece of research from earlier exercises and write an action plan for that. You may use Wadsworth's (2011a) framework or one of your own devising. Remember to include a timeframe and to nominate who will be responsible for which strategy.

Further reading

Babbie, E. 2010, *The Practice of Social Research*, 12th edn, Wadsworth, Belmont, CA. See Chapter 17, 'Reading and writing social research'.

D'Cruz, Heather and Jones, Martyn 2004, *Social Work Research: Ethical and Political Contexts*, Sage, London. Chapter 8, 'Reporting and disseminating research', provides a good discussion of the contextual issues surrounding report writing in social work.

Dudley, J. 2011, *Research Methods for Social Work: Being Producers and Consumers of Research (updated edition)*, 2nd edn, Allyn and Bacon, Boston, MA. Chapter 15, 'Preparing the report', contains a useful discussion on reporting to staff, the people who were researched, clients and empowerment.

Engel, R.J. and Schutt, R.K. 2010, *Fundamentals of Social Work Research*, Sage, Thousand Oaks, CA. See Chapter 12, 'Reporting research'—especially the distinctions between journal articles and other research reports, ethics of reporting, and sections on empirical methods to address literature reviews (similar to systematic reviews).

Hardwick, L. and Worsley, A. 2011, *Doing Social Work Research*. Sage, London. Chapter 9, 'Developing a research proposal and writing a research report', is an excellent account, aimed at students writing a thesis but useful for all social workers.

Marlow, C. 2011, *Research Methods for Generalist Social Work*, 5th edn, Brooks/Cole Cengage, Sydney. Chapter 13, 'Research writing', is a good introduction to research writing, including ethical issues.

O'Leary, Z. 2010, *The Essential Guide to Doing Your Research Project*, Sage, London. Chapter 15, 'The challenge of writing up', is especially good on constructing a story and finding your voice. See also Chapter 5, 'Crafting a research proposal'.

Wadsworth, Y. 2011, *Do It Yourself Social Research: The Bestselling Practical Guide to Doing Social Research Projects*, 3rd edn, Allen & Unwin, Sydney. Chapter 8, 'Getting your findings into action', is an excellent chapter on action planning.

19 *Developing a research proposal*

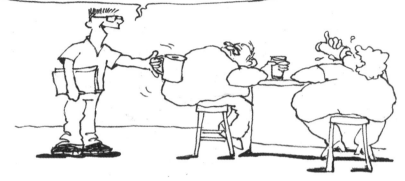

Chapters 2 and 3 introduced us to effective ways of transforming our problems into researchable questions. However, what *we* think is a good research idea may not be so apparent to our agency or to the funding source. Our good idea must be sold, and to do this we must demonstrate that we have the skills and knowledge to undertake a complex piece of research. The ability to construct a detailed research proposal is an extremely important skill in the current competitive environment. Chapter 19 discusses the funding sources and issues that affect our research, before outlining the steps that must be followed to develop a well-crafted research proposal. We also highlight the pitfalls to be avoided.

Before you begin to prepare a research proposal, think about forming the steering committee or advisory group to which we have referred throughout this book. This group will help you keep the proposal on track, including pointing out ethical issues, providing feedback on what is practical, and in some cases helping you demonstrate that you can access the people you wish to involve in the research. It is also important to seek the help of an experienced researcher—someone who can advise you about your proposal.

Funding your research

The first step in preparing a research proposal is to target an appropriate funding source. Sometimes this may be your own organisation. With the increasing pressure for evidence-based practice of various types, larger human service organisations have research sections that fund or approve research by their own employees, external organisations or partnerships between the two. Other employers encourage you to apply for external research grants, often as collaborative endeavours with other organisations. Federal and state governments fund research, as do philanthropic organisations.

Beginning researchers will often define their researchable problem before turning to the practical question of where to seek funds. Experienced researchers are more likely to develop their proposals in response to guidelines from funding bodies, and thus may be more likely to attract funding. Students would do well to begin collecting newspaper advertisements relating to funds available and, as an exercise, download funding guidelines so that they become aware of the types of external funding available and the current priority areas for research. This is an important part of your research training and will improve your skills in the long term. You may have a good idea for a piece of research on domestic violence, but you are unlikely to receive funds from a body that targets something else. Examine the objectives of the funding programs available and decide where you might find appropriate financial support.

You should also be aware of the budgetary limits of each funding program. Some bodies prefer to fund a number of small projects for less than, say, $20 000, while others invest their research funds in a few complex and more expensive proposals. We will examine budgetary issues later in this chapter. What is important to note here is that you should ensure that your budget matches the money available.

Don't be afraid to seek clarification from the funding body about its objectives and funding requirements. Most funding bodies welcome inquiries; it is better to ask before you submit your proposal than to receive a knockback because you misunderstood one of the questions. Most funding bodies are inundated with proposals for funding, however, so you should be aware that the success rate is low (often as low as 10 per cent). Don't be disheartened if you are unsuccessful with your first proposal. Many bodies provide feedback on and assessment of proposals, and you should use this feedback to improve your chances at a later date.

Seeking funding
- Establish your advisory group or steering committee. Include an experienced researcher who can advise you about the proposal.
- Be clear about your research question.
- Do your homework on funding bodies.
- Seek funds from appropriate funding bodies.
- Match your budget to available funds.
- Be aware that a minority of research proposals will be funded in any competitive round.
- If your proposal is knocked back, study the feedback and improve your proposal.

Developing your research proposal

As we have already noted, many granting bodies have guidelines or online application forms, which include the categories of information required from you. If so, you should follow these carefully. You should also note that some funding bodies require a preliminary summary of your proposal. These bodies then determine from the initial applications which applicants will be asked to submit full applications. All final applications for these organisations, and applications for other bodies, should include the categories to be discussed here. If funding guidelines do not include them, you need to address them in any case as part of good planning for your project. Your research proposal is the road map alerting you and the funding body to the way the research will unfold. It details your aims and outcomes, the research plan and your budget. The following sections outline the key aspects of a research proposal, and are included in most funding application guidelines.

Background
The background statement should contain a section introducing your research issue and succinctly describing why this issue is important. What is it you wish to study? You should demonstrate the depth of your knowledge about the research question, and indicate to the assessor that you have spent time researching the issue. If the issue has caused controversy lately, or proposed legislative reform is in the air, indicate that you are aware of this. Make the case for your proposed project and emphasise that you are the right person to undertake it, up front.

A literature review is an important part of your background statement. While this literature review will not necessarily be comprehensive, because of limited space, it should indicate that you are aware of the latest publications and reports. Additionally, if it is to be assessed by an academic committee, it should also include the current theoretical debate in the area you wish to address. You should also be cognisant of recent legislative reforms. If you are wishing to research aspects of domestic violence or child protection, for instance, you will need to indicate an understanding of the latest legislative and policy developments, and any proposed changes or problem areas.

Your background statement will provide information on existing knowledge in your topic area, and will clearly outline how your proposed research relates to the existing knowledge base. Will the research address theoretical development in the area? Will it challenge basic assumptions or treatment procedures? Will it explore a new area or gap in the literature where little information is available? Will it examine the effects of new legislation or policy development in unexplored areas—for example, in rural locations or among minority groups? Be clear about the value of your study and how it will contribute to our current understanding of the issues.

Aims and significance of the study

Following your background statement, you should list your aims in undertaking the study and the significance of the work. These should be concise and logical. Why are you proposing this study? Why is it so important at this particular point in time and who will directly benefit from your work? Note the importance of your work and how exciting it will be once the results are in. Remember you must sell the research, so do not be shy or hesitant in heralding its significance.

This section should also address the specific priorities of the funding body. Most will have three or four key areas—which may change from year to year—that are integral to the way the proposal will be assessed. If your funding body has specified that a priority for the current round is citizenship rights, and you are proposing to investigate child protection practices, then indicate how your research will contribute to enhanced rights for children. Addressing the funding organisation's current priorities is crucial to your ultimate success, so you should pay particular attention to the way you relate the significance of your work to these issues. Wherever possible, use the language of the application guidelines and demonstrate how your study relates to these ideas.

Outcomes

This section of your research proposal should detail the anticipated outcomes of your research. What will be the achievements of your work and how will these help the target group? What practice, policy or legislative implications will flow from your research? Note how these relate to the priorities of the funding body. In particular, you should detail how the results will be published, circulated or shared in order to achieve the proposed effects on practice, policy or legislation. Will this be in the form of a report, a conference paper, a journal article, a newspaper story or via a news conference? Be specific, because this is just as important a step as any other in the research proposal. You may conduct research that has the potential to markedly change society's thinking about an issue, but unless you disseminate the information appropriately, nothing will change.

Research plan

Having written a clear background statement and excited the reader with the potential significance of your work, your research will stand or fall on the detail provided in your research plan. A well-constructed and clear plan is critical to any research proposal, and it is in this section that you must demonstrate an understanding of the research process.

Methodology

Begin with a statement on the type of methodology you have chosen, why this is the most appropriate choice, and give a brief description of this methodology. We have outlined methodologies in Chapter 1. This chapter should assist you to determine the most appropriate methodology, or combination of approaches, for any study you are proposing. Your research plan will outline the steps in the research process, all of which are discussed more fully in Chapter 4. Should you choose a quantitative methodology, then you should outline the hypothesis you propose to test and your operational definitions. If you choose a qualitative methodology, you must outline your research problem.

Sampling

Your research plan will clearly define the population you wish to study and the sample to be drawn from that population (see Chapter 5). How will this sample be chosen, and how is this relevant to the study aims? Be precise about your sampling procedure and why it is the best possible choice for your study.

In outlining your sampling procedure, you should indicate how you propose to gain access to the specified population group. If you are studying survivors of domestic violence and your proposal suggests you will interview women entering refuges, your assessors will know that you have not done your homework. It is standard practice in women's refuges to protect women from everyone, including well-meaning researchers! Make sure you have checked on your proposed access to your sample. This may involve including a letter from your agency or another source such as the steering committee, indicating that you have access to the group in question.

In the case of violence, for instance, there may be a group for survivors of violence at the local health centre. You might seek permission from the group leader to interview consenting members and include a letter from this person indicating that this process is acceptable.

Method of data collection

Your research plan will include a discussion of the chosen method of data collection—that is, how you will be gathering the required information. Several chapters in this book have covered the types of method you might choose, including interviews, surveys, observations, secondary analysis and content analysis. You should indicate in your proposal which method or combination of methods you have chosen, and explain why it is the most appropriate and effective. In particular, you should note any ethical considerations arising from your chosen method. How will you ensure confidentiality? What strategies are in place should your interviewees become distressed?

Data analysis

Your research plan will detail the type of data analysis to be employed. What will you do with the data once you have collected it? What procedures and statistical analyses, if any, will you use to find answers to your research question, or patterns and themes in the data that relate to your research aims? You should always indicate any experience you may have had with the proposed methods and data analysis techniques.

In preparing this section, do not restrict it to one sentence. 'Data will be analysed using SPSS' is not sufficient to inspire the confidence of assessors in your knowledge of data analysis. Indicate in a few carefully crafted sentences that you actually understand the process of analysis and the way you intend to pursue it.

Limitations

The next section of your research plan will outline the limitations imposed by your proposed plan. The very nature of social research means that every study will have limitations, often due to factors that can never be entirely eliminated. For example, your sampling technique may limit your ability to generalise your findings. In the case of survivors of violence, you may only have been able to interview those women confident and articulate enough to join a group. This limitation should be noted in your proposal, as should any limitation evident in your data-collection method and data analysis. Do not ever try to hide limitations, but instead outline how you propose to minimise them.

Timetable

The final section of your research plan provides a timetable for the proposed project. This timetable should not only fit the funding guidelines (for example, some granting bodies require all research to be completed in one year), but should also fit your own schedule. Can you realistically meet the proposed timetable, given your other commitments? Can you achieve the proposed aims? Be realistic in setting targets for yourself.

Ethical considerations

Explicit acknowledgement of the ethical dimensions involved in your project is fundamental to demonstrating competence in a research proposal. You must be confident that your research meets the ethical aspirations and standards of social work. Your research proposal also has to demonstrate how you will meet the requirements of the research ethics bodies in your country.

In its *National Statement on Ethical Conduct in Human Research*, the Australian National Health and Medical Research Council (NHMRC 2007) sets out a framework of four fundamental values and principles to which all research with people must conform. These values are: respect for human beings; research merit and integrity; justice; and beneficence. In addition, the NHMRC lists values for specific research situations that you must address if your research is in one of these areas. The areas with specific ethical requirements include pregnant women, children and young people, people in dependent or unequal relationships, people highly dependent on medical care who may be unable to give consent, people with a cognitive impairment, intellectual disability or mental illness, people who may be involved in illegal activities, Aboriginal and Torres Strait Islanders and people in other countries.

For example, research proposals involving Aboriginal and Torres Strait Islander communities must show how they meet six core values: reciprocity, respect, equality, responsibility, survival and protection, spirit and integrity (NHMRC 2003). This set of mandatory ethical standards and guidelines was developed in consultation with Aboriginal and Torres Strait Islander groups and researchers. When planning such research, you would do well to consult the online booklet written for Aboriginal and Torres Strait Islander communities about how to manage researchers: *Keeping Research on Track: A Guide for Aboriginal and Torres Strait Islander Peoples About Health Research Ethics* (NHMRC 2006).

As part of the research proposal, you have to show that you have thought about how to minimise any ethical risks in your study and, further, show that these risks are worth taking in return for the knowledge that will be gained as a result. For example, in the proposed domestic violence study, is learning about the successful strategies people have used to leave a violent partnership worth the potential distress caused by asking them to tell you about their situation? In addition, your proposal must demonstrate that you have taken proper steps to protect the data you collect (for example, keeping personal details safe from being used for other purposes), to gain informed consent from participants, to protect their confidentiality and to ensure there will be no negative consequences, such as withdrawal of service due to 'speaking up'. You may also have to demonstrate how you will be inclusive, especially if your research includes the groups identified above.

Most agencies now have ethics committees as part of their organisational structure. The ethics committee will want to know how you propose to address these and other questions. Usually you will need to seek ethical clearance from this committee before your research proposal is funded. Sometimes you require ethical clearance from more than one organisation: the funding body and also the agency whose clients you are researching. Most funding agencies and ethics committees require consent protocols. Look over the example of the consent protocol in Chapter 7. Your proposal should indicate the procedure to be used to address ethical issues.

Administration of the research
In this section of the research proposal, you should outline the way the study will be organised, and what resources are needed to successfully complete the research. You should identify which group is managing the project, and any quality assurance or evaluation strategies in place, showing how this group is competent to oversee the research. You should also demonstrate

that your organisation manages finances responsibly, is accountable and otherwise meets any requirements to be able to accept funding, such as incorporation. This is also called an *organisational capability statement*.

You might indicate that your agency is allowing you to use your office and telephone, and to have computing, typing, printing and photocopying done at no cost to the research funding body. This is also included as part of your budget (see example below). Alternatively, if you are working independently, these costs will need to be factored into your budget. Note what staff are to be involved in the research. This may be agency personnel only, or you may need to employ a research assistant. If so, indicate what qualifications will be necessary and what their tasks and responsibilities will be. If you are the principal researcher, indicate this and list any consultants and others who will be contributing to the research.

Budget

Your budget is vital to the success or failure of your research project. If you have insufficient funds to complete the work, you will fail to achieve your aims and your research record may be damaged.

Precisely cost out all the items listed in your plan. Which of the listed activities will cost money? These will generally fall under categories of personnel, travel, equipment, maintenance and dissemination. Make sure these activities are accurately costed (seek quotes) and justified. Do not pad your budget with unnecessary items but at the same time do not skimp. Take care that all budget items are in line with the objectives and methods you have included in your proposal.

Note from the funding guidelines what items the sponsoring body will financially support, and make sure your requests are within reason. Finally, check and recheck your budget total to ensure you have not made a fundamental error in your adding up!

The following provides an example of a budget prepared for a small project to assess changes to domestic violence services in country towns. This application is for a regional research grant for small projects of between $20 000 and $30 000. Note that the principal researcher's time is costed as 'in-kind contribution'. If you have other partners, you would also include their 'in-kind contributions' in a separate column. Including the costs absorbed by your organisation is an important part of demonstrating value for money to the funding body. If you require additional funds for your own time, this should be added. Other personnel costs and travel costs should be computed on the current award rates. These may change periodically from what is listed in this proposal. You should also note that, depending on the size of the project, costs may include such items as lease of computers and other equipment items, and additional maintenance costs such as an office lease.

This example is indicative only, showing the kinds of costs that can be itemised. Many funding bodies have their own budget categories, usually in online forms, that you must complete. You should check the value of services in *your own currency at current prices*.

Budget justification

No matter what the size of your budget, you should provide a short justification for all budget items. Why is it necessary to employ a Level 6 research assistant? Why do you need 100 hours of transcription? Why do you need to travel? Why do you need a digital recorder? Assessors will expect each item to be justified with a brief statement. It may be that if this is not done well enough, your proposal could be funded at a lower rate than requested.

Budget items	Grant funds	In-kind contribution
Personnel		
Principal researchers, 2 x social workers, 1 day per week each (7 hours) x 40 weeks @ $31.50 per hour		$17640
Research Assistant, level 6, 1 day per week (7 hours) x 35 weeks @ $43.45 per hour	$10645	
Transcriber—100 hrs @ $31.23 per hour	$3123	
Project team members: 5 days' work each x 5 rural agency representatives @ $300.00 per day		$7500
On-costs 30%	$4130	$7540
Total personnel costs	**$17898**	**$32680**
Equipment		
Digital recorders x 2	$400	
Laptops, software		$10000
Maintenance		
Photocopying		$2000
Teleconferences for project team meetings: 4 meetings x 5 people @ $15.00 per hour per person (2 hrs per meeting)		$600
Telephone		$1500
Office space, meeting room, desks		$1500
Total equipment and maintenance	**$400**	**$15600**
Travel		
Sustenance rates x 4 overnight trips to rural towns A, B, C, D, 1 overnight trip to regional centre E, 2 researchers per trip, 4 x 2 @ $250 per day accomm plus meals	$2000	

Budget items	Grant funds	In-kind contribution
Sustenance rates for project team travelling to initial face-to-face meeting at regional centre: 4 members (1 is local)—4 × $250	$1 000	
Car rates		
Town A: 1000 km @ 30c km	$300	
Town B: 400 km @ 30c km	$120	
Town C: 700 km @ 30c km	$210	
Town D: 800 km @ 30c km	$240	
Car rates for project team members from towns A, B, C, D to attend initial project team meeting	$870	
Total travel	**$4 740**	0
Dissemination		
Report printing, distribution	$2 000	
Total dissemination	**$2 000**	
Totals	**$25 038**	**$48 280**

About you

You should include a section in your proposal that details your capability to conduct the research. Are you in a unique position to collect the data? For example, you may be a sexual assault counsellor in an area populated by people of diverse cultural backgrounds, and through your work have access to interviewees and case material that puts you in a unique position to study the effects of sexual assault in multicultural groups. Note the importance of your position. Have you conducted research before? If so, say so. If not, you might outline any research training and higher degree study you have undertaken. Outline your publishing record, particularly in the areas of the proposed research. If you have not published, note any staff seminars or student supervision you may have given in this area. What experience do you have that makes it important that you are the one to be funded for this particular piece of research? Don't sell yourself short. Nominate people as referees who know your work and appreciate your skills. Be confident of your ability to conduct the project and be convincing.

Sections of your research proposal

- Background
- Aims and significance of the study
- Research plan
- Ethical considerations

- Administration including organisational capability
- Budget
- Outcomes
- About you

Fine-tuning your proposal

Having reached this stage, you should now spend time going through and streamlining your proposal. Make sure you have not repeated yourself and that the proposal is clear, comprehensive and succinct. Make sure that there are no typing errors and that the proposal is well presented. Go back to the guidelines and check that you have kept within the page limits for the proposal. Some guidelines will indicate that they require nine (or six or 20) pages only. If this is the case, you can be sure that any additional pages will not be read. Keep within the limits! Note from the guidelines the expected font size, spacing and number of copies to be sent. Particularly note the submission date and whether faxed or emailed copies are accepted. You can be sure that deadlines will be strictly adhered to. Before sending in your proposal, ask colleagues to go through it and consider their advice on any modifications that should be made. Be sure you have done the best possible job you can.

Assessment of research proposals

Once your research proposal has been sent to your agency management committee or an outside funding body for assessment, you will have little to do but wait for feedback. The assessors will be focusing particularly on the merit of the proposed research and the ability of the researcher to conduct the work.

The merit of the proposed research will be judged by its potential outcomes. Will the research lead to a major advance in our understanding of the proposed issue, to an important advance in practice strategies, to the solution of a problem, or to policy development or legislative reform? If the answer to any of these questions is yes, then the assessment committee will be interested to read on.

The merit of the research will be judged further by the ability of the agency to provide the infrastructure to support the proposal and by the capacity of the researcher to devote the time and resources required to the project. If those points are soundly addressed in the proposal, the assessors will examine carefully the research plan for thoroughness and detail.

If the plan meets with approval, the assessors will finally examine the researcher's potential to successfully complete the project. Particularly relevant will be research experience, publishing record, work history and experience in the proposed areas. If you have covered all these sections effectively, your proposal has a very high chance of funding success. If so, it is now time to begin the hard work!

Summary

Chapter 19, the final chapter in our book, has, first, examined the issues to be considered when developing a research proposal and, second, illustrated how to develop a competitive proposal. There is a great deal of time and effort between a 'good idea' and an adequate proposal for funding support. You must address the agency, professional, personal and practical issues before developing a proposal for funding that will meet with approval.

We have outlined the sections to be included in a proposal. You should bear in mind that only a limited number of proposals will be successful in any given funding round. You should therefore see the research proposal as a very important step in your research project, and as worth a great deal of your time and energy. You must convince the funding body that you and your project are worthy of investment!

This brings *Research for Social Workers* to an end. We hope that you are ready to include research as one of the fundamental tools in your professional toolkit, and that you are inspired to contribute to the growing social work research culture and knowledge base. With the increasing pace of change in our globalised world, the importance of research as a means to influence change and to include the voices of those not usually heard is growing. Now is the time for you to take up the challenge to join the social work research culture, to work towards an equitable and just society.

Discussion questions

19.1 How should you investigate possible sources of funding for a proposed research project?

19.2 What are the constraints your agency might impose on your proposed research?

19.3 What professional issues will affect your proposal?

19.4 Outline the personal issues to be assessed before you begin developing your proposal.

19.5   What practical issues must be addressed before you submit your proposal?

19.6   Outline the sections to be included in your research proposal.

19.7   How might these differ depending on your methodology?

19.8   Why is an accurate budget so important to your research?

19.9   Given your current position, how might you go about gaining research experience?

19.10 What issues will guide the assessors of your research proposal?

Exercises

19.1   Find an advertisement for research funding in the newspaper or online. Send for or download funding guidelines. Note the priorities of the funding body, the timeline for completion of the project and the funding limits.

19.2   Begin a file of advertisements as outlined in Exercise 1. Collect funding guidelines for three different grant programs. Note how they differ.

19.3   Ask your agency supervisor or the management committee for a copy of any successful research proposals. Note how these are constructed. Why do you think they were successful?

19.4   Seek copies of unsuccessful research proposals. Why do you think they were unsuccessful? Here you may need to consult funding guidelines.

19.5   In your work situation, you may have noticed that there are some issues that warrant further investigation. Make a list of these and determine how you might improve the situation through research.

Further reading

There is a wealth of information about proposal writing on the internet and also in most research texts. Most universities and many large human service organisations have guidelines for how to write proposals. There are also some excellent web links—for example:

Research Proposal Guide: How to Write a Research Proposal, <http://researchproposalguide.com>. This site has links to many proposal-writing sites from various universities.

Geron, S.M. and Steketee, G.S. 2010, 'Applying for research grants', in B. Thyer (ed.), *The Handbook of Social Work Research Methods*, Sage, Thousand Oaks, CA, pp. 619–30. Contains useful general guidance on proposal writing, as well as providing links for North American social work research.

Hardwick, L. and Worsley, A. 2011, *Doing Social Work Research*, Sage, London. Chapter 9, 'Developing a Research Proposal and Writing a Research Report', offers many good pointers to writing proposals, from a UK social work perspective.

References

Abrami, P.C., Borokhovski, E., Bernard, R.M., Wade, C., Tamim, R., Persson, T. and Surkes, M.A. 2010, 'Issues in conducting and disseminating brief reviews of evidence', *Evidence & Policy: A journal of research, debate & practice*, vol. 6, no. 3, pp. 371–89.

Ackerly, B.A. and True, J. 2010, *Doing Feminist Research in Political and Social Science*, Palgrave Macmillan, Basingstoke.

Alhabib, S., Nur, U. and Jones, R. 2010, 'Domestic violence against women: Systematic review of prevalence studies', *Journal of Family Violence*, vol. 25, no. 4, pp. 369–82.

Alston, M. 1995, *Women on the Land: The hidden heart of rural Australia*, UNSW Press, Sydney.

——1996, *Goals for Women: Improving media representation of women's sport*, Centre for Rural Social Research, Charles Sturt University, Wagga Wagga, NSW.

Annandale, E., Harvey, J., Cavers, D. and Dixon-Woods, M. 2007, 'Gender and access to healthcare in the UK: A critical interpretive synthesis of the literature', *Evidence & Policy: A journal of research, debate & practice*, vol. 3, no. 4, pp. 463–86.

Australian Association of Social Workers (AASW) 2010, *Code of Ethics*, AASW, Canberra, <www.aasw.asn.au/document/item/740>. Accessed 12 July 2011.

Australian Bureau of Statistics 1994, *1991 Census of Population and Housing: Basic community profile*, Cat. No. 2722.1, ABS, Canberra.

Australian Institute of Community Practice and Government (AICPG), n.d. *Help Sheets: Conducting a community needs assessment*, <http://www.ourcommunity.com.au/manage ment/view_help_sheet.do?articleid=10>. Accessed 12 August 2011.

——n.d. *Help sheet: Auditing your community assets*, <http://www.ourcommunity.com.au/management/view_help_sheet.do?articleid=9>. Accessed 12 August 2011.

Babbie, E. 2010, *The Practice of Social Research*, 12th edn, Wadsworth, Belmont, CA.

——2011, *The Basics of Social Research*, Wadsworth, Belmont, CA.

Barusch, A., Gringeri, C. and George, M. 2011, 'Rigor in qualitative social work research: A review of strategies used in published articles', *Social Work Research*, vol. 35, no. 1, pp. 11–19.

Basile, K., Lang, K., Bartenfeld, T. and Clinton-Sherrod, M. 2005, 'Report from the CDC: Evaluability assessment of the Rape Prevention and Education Program—Summary of findings and recommendations', *Journal of Women's Health*, vol. 14, no. 3, pp. 201–7.

Begg, P. and Thompson, S. 2011, 'Tackling solastalgia: Improving pathways to care for farming families', in R. Giles, I. Epstein and A. Vertigan (eds), *Clinical Data Mining in an Allied Health Organization: A real world experience*, Sydney University Press, Sydney, pp. 83–100.

Bennett, B. and Zubrzycki, J. 2001, 'Indigenous social workers: Putting stories into practice', conference paper, AASW National Conference, Melbourne.

Berg, B.L. 2007, *Qualitative Methods for the Social Sciences*, 7th edn, Pearson, New York.

Blum, E., Heinonen, T. and White, J. 2010, 'Participatory action research studies', in B. Thyer (ed), *The Handbook of Social Work Research Methods*, Sage, Thousand Oaks, CA.

Boaz, A. and Pawson, R. 2005, 'The perilous road from evidence to policy: Five journeys compared', *Journal of Social Policy*, vol. 34, no. 2, pp. 175–94.

Bowles, W. 1995, 'Quality of life of adults with spina bifida: An issue of equality', unpublished PhD thesis, University of New South Wales, Sydney.

Bowles, W., Collingridge, M., McKinnon, J., Agllias, K., Dawood, A., Irwin, J., Maywald, S., Noble, C., O'Sullivan, J. and Zubrzycki, J. 2011, *Online Student Supervision Training: Accessible and cooperative learning in social work,* Australian Learning and Teaching Council, <www.altc. edu.au/resource-online-studentsupervision-csu–2011>. Accessed 15 October 2011.

Bradshaw, J. 1977, 'The concept of social need', in N. Gilbert and H. Specht (eds), *Planning for Social Welfare: Issues, models and tasks,* Prentice-Hall, Englewood Cliffs, NJ, pp. 29–96.

British Association of Social Workers (BASW) 2002, *The Code of Ethics for Social Work,* <http:// cdn.basw.co.uk/membership/coe.pdf>. Accessed 12 August 2011.

Brown, T. and Hampson, R. 2009, *An Evaluation of Interventions with Domestic Violence Perpetrators,* Family Violence Prevention Foundation of Australia, Canberra, <www. violencefreefamilies.com.au/Intervention%20Domestic%20Violence%20Perps%20Web. pdf>. Accessed 19 November 2011.

Brueggemann, W.G. 2006, *The Practice of Macro Social Work,* 3rd edn, Thomson Brooks/Cole, Belmont, CA.

Campbell, N. and Fonow, M. 2009, 'Introduction', *Frontiers: A journal of women studies,* vol. 30, no. 1, p. 1.

Cardoso, J. and Thompson, S.J. 2010, 'Common themes of resilience among Latino immigrant families: A systematic review of the literature', *Families in Society,* vol. 91, no. 3, pp. 257–65.

Carson, E., Chung, D. and Day, A. 2009, 'Evaluating domestic violence programs, standardisation and organisational culture', *Evaluation Journal of Australasia,* vol. 9, no. 1, pp. 10–19.

Central Coast Community Congress Working Party 2003, *Making Headway: Building your community. How to get started—an asset based community development toolkit,* <www. communitybuilders.nsw.gov.au/Making_Headway_ToolKit.pdf>. Accessed 20 November 2011.

Clark, A. 2005, *Situational Analysis: Grounded theory after the postmodern turn.* Sage, Thousand Oaks, CA.

Corbin, J.M. and Strauss, A.L. 2008, *Basics of Qualitative Research: Techniques and procedures for developing grounded theory,* 3rd edn, Sage, Thousand Oaks, CA.

Curran, C., Burchardt, T., Knapp, M., McDaid, D. and Bingqin, L. 2007, 'Challenges in multidisciplinary systematic reviewing: A study on social exclusion and mental health policy', *Social Policy & Administration,* vol. 41, no. 3, pp. 289–312.

Daniel, B., Taylor, J. and Scott, J. 2010, 'Recognition of neglect and early response: Overview of a systematic review of the literature', *Child and Family Social Work,* vol. 15, no. 2, May, pp. 248–57.

David, M. and Sutton, C. 2011, *Social Research: An introduction,* 2nd edn, Sage, Thousand Oaks, CA.

Davis, K. 2008, 'Intersectionality as a buzzword: A sociology of science perspective on what makes a feminist theory successful', *Feminist Theory,* vol. 9, pp. 67–85.

D'Cruz, H. and Jones, M. 2004, *Social Work Research: Ethical and political contexts,* Sage, London.

de Vaus, D. 2002, *Surveys in Social Research,* 5th edn, Allen & Unwin, Sydney.

Denzin, N.K. and Lincoln, Y.S. (eds) 2005, *Strategies of Qualitative Inquiry,* 2nd edn, Sage, Thousand Oaks, CA.

——2011, *The Sage Handbook of Qualitative Research,* 2nd edn, Sage Publications, Thousand Oaks, CA.

Dillman, D.A., Smyth, J.D. and Christian, L.M. 2009, *Internet, Mail and Mixed-Mode Surveys: The tailored design method,* John Wiley & Sons, Hoboken, NJ.

Dixon-Woods, M., Cavers, D., Agarwal, S., Annandale, E., Arthur, A., Harvey, J. and Sutton, A.J. 2006, 'Conducting a critical interpretive synthesis of the literature on access to healthcare by vulnerable groups', *BMC Medical Research Methodology,* vol. 6, p. 35.

Domestic Violence Crisis Service 2011, *What is Domestic Violence?* Domestic Violence Crisis Service, Canberra, <www.dvcs.org.au/domesticviolence.html>.

Dominelli, L. 2005, 'Social work research: Contested knowledge for practice', in L. Dominelli, M. Payne and R. Adams (eds), *Social Work Futures: Crossing boundaries, transforming practice*, Palgrave Macmillan, Basingstoke, pp. 223–36.

Dudley, J.R. 2010, *Research Methods for Social Work*, 2nd edn, Pearson, Boston, MA.

——2011, *Research Methods for Social Work: Being producers and consumers of research (Updated Edition)*, 2nd edn, Pearson, USA.

Dullea, K. and Mullender, A. 1999, 'Evaluation and empowerment', in I. Shaw and J. Lishman (eds), *Evaluation and Social Work Practice*, Sage, London.

Engel, R.J. and Schutt, R.K. 2009, *The Practice of Research in Social Work*, 2nd edn, Sage, Thousand Oaks, CA.

——2010a, 'Survey research', in R.M. Grinnell and Y.A. Unrau (eds), *Social Work Research and Evaluation*, 9th edn, Oxford University Press, New York, pp. 326–65.

——2010b, *Fundamentals of Social Work Research*, Sage, Thousand Oaks, CA.

Fisher, R.A. and Yates, F. 1963, *Statistical Tables for Biological, Agricultural and Medical Research*, Longman, London.

Fook, J. (ed.) 1996, *The Reflective Researcher*, Allen & Unwin, Sydney.

——2000, 'Deconstructing and reconstructing professional expertise' in B. Fawcett, B. Featherstone, J. Fook and A. Rossiter (eds), *Practice and Research in Social Work: Postmodern feminist perspectives*, Routledge, New York, pp. 104–19.

——2002, *Social Work Critical Theory and Practice*, Sage, London.

Fook, J. and Gardner, F. 2007, *Practising Critical Reflection: A resource handbook*, Open University Press, Maidenhead.

Freire, P. 1970, *Pedagogy of the Oppressed*, Herder & Herder, New York.

Garton, L., Fenton, J. and Paton, A. 1992, *Review of Sexual Assault Services: Report on X Sexual Assault Service*, NSW Department of Health, Sydney.

Geron, S.M. and Steketee, G.S. 2010, 'Applying for research grants', in B. Thyer (ed.), *The Handbook of Social Work Research Methods*, Sage, Thousand Oaks, CA, pp. 619–30.

Giles, R., Vertigan, A.E., Epstein, I. and Rhodes, D. 2011, 'Introduction', in R. Giles, I. Epstein and A. Vertigan (eds), *Clinical Data Mining in an Allied Health Organization: A real world experience*, Sydney University Press, Sydney, pp. 1–26.

Glaser, B.G. 1978, *Theoretical Sensitivity: Advances in the methodology of grounded theory, vol. 2*, Sociology Press, Mill Valley, CA.

——1992, *Basics of Grounded Theory Analysis*, Sociology Press, Mill Valley, CA.

Glaser, B. and Strauss, A. 1967, *The Discovery of Grounded Theory*, Aldine, Chicago.

Gochros, H. 2010, 'Qualitative interviewing', in R.M. Grinnell and Y.A. Unrau (eds), *Social Work Research and Evaluation*, 9th edn, Oxford University Press, New York, pp. 301–25.

Gray, M. 1995, 'The ethical implications of current theoretical development in social work', *British Journal of Social Work*, vol. 25, pp. 55–70.

Gray, M. and Schubert, L. 2010, 'Turning base metal into gold: Transmuting art, practice, research and experience into knowledge', *British Journal of Social Work*, vol. 40, pp. 2308–25.

Greenwood, D. and Levin, M. 2007, *Introduction to Action Research: Social research for social change*, 2nd edn, Sage, Thousand Oaks, CA.

Grinnell, R.M. and Unrau, Y.A. (eds), 2010, *Social Work Research and Evaluation*, 9th edn, Oxford University Press, New York.

Gunnarsson, L. 2011, 'A defence of the category "women"', *Feminist Theory*, vol. 12, no. 1, pp. 23–37.

Haene, L. 2010, 'Beyond division: Convergences between postmodern qualitative research and family therapy', *Journal of Marital and Family Therapy*, vol. 36, no. 1, pp. 1–12.

Hall, R. 2008, *Applied Social Research: Planning, designing and conducting real world research*, Palgrave Macmillan, Melbourne.

Hallberg, L.R. 2006, 'The "core category" of grounded theory: Making constant comparisons', *International Journal of Qualitative Studies on Health and Wellbeing*, vol. 1, pp. 141–8.

Hannes, K. and Claes, L. 2007, 'Learn to read and write systematic reviews: The Belgian Campbell Group', *Research on Social Work Practice*, vol. 17, no. 6, pp. 748–53.

Hardwick, L. and Worsley A. 2011, *Doing Social Work Research*, Sage, London.

Healy, K. 2006, 'Asset-based community development: Recognising and building on community strengths', in A. O'Hara and Z. Weber (eds), *Skills for Human Service Practice: Working with individuals, groups and communities*, Oxford University Press, Melbourne.

Hemingway, P. and Brereton, N. 2009, *What is a Systematic Review?*, Haywood Medical Communications, <www.whatisseries.co.uk/whatis/pdfs/What_is_syst_rev.pdf>. Accessed 20 November 2011.

Heron, J. and Reason, P. 2006, 'The practice of co-operative inquiry: Research "with" rather than "on" people', in P. Reason and H. Bradbury (eds), *Handbook of Action Research*, Sage, London, pp. 144–54.

Homan, M.S. 2008, *Promoting Community Change: Making it happen in the real world*, Thomson Brooks Cole, Sydney.

Hopp, F., Thornton, N. and Martin, L. 2010, 'The lived experience of heart failure at the end of life: A systematic literature review', *Health & Social Work*, vol. 35, no. 2, pp. 109–17.

Howe, D. 1994, 'Modernity, postmodernity and social work', *British Journal of Social Work*, vol. 24, pp. 513–32.

Huberman, A.M. and Miles, M.B. 2002, *The Qualitative Researcher's Companion*, Sage, Thousand Oaks, CA.

Humphries, B. 2008, *Social Work Research for Social Justice*, Palgrave Macmillan, Basingstoke.

Humphries, B. and Truman, C. 1994, *Re-thinking Social Research*, Avebury, Aldershot.

Ife, J. 2010, *Human Rights from Below: Achieving rights through community development*, Cambridge University Press, Melbourne.

Johnson, C.V., Bartgis, J., Worley, J.A., Hellman, C.M. and Burkhart, R. 2010, 'Urban Indian voices: A community-based participatory research health and needs assessment', *American Indian & Alaska Native Mental Health Research: The journal of the National Center*, vol. 17, no. 1, pp. 49–70.

Kaufmann, W. 1973, *Without Guilt & Justice: From decidophobia to autonomy*, Dell, New York.

Kerlinger, F. 1973, *Foundations of Behavioural Research*, 2nd edn, Holt, Rinehart and Winston, London.

Kretzmann, J. and McKnight, J. 1993, *Building Communities from the Inside Out: A path towards finding and mobilizing community asset*, Center for Urban Affairs and Policy Research, Chicago.

Lesley, C. 2002, Discussion re culturally sensitive interviewing, Northwest Regional Advocate, Disability Service Aboriginal Corporation, personal communication.

Lindquist, E.L. 1938, *A First Course in Statistics*, rev. edn, Houghton Mifflin, Boston, MA.

Logan, T.K. and Royse, D. 2010, 'Program evaluation studies', in B. Thyer (ed.), *The Handbook of Social Work Research Methods*, 2nd edn, Sage, Thousand Oaks, CA, pp. 221–40.

McArdle, J. 1998, *Resource Manual for Facilitators in Community Development*, 2nd edn, Vista, Melbourne.

McNiff, J. and Whitehead, J. 2006, *All You Need to Know About Action Research*, Sage, London.

McTaggart, R. (ed.) 1997, *Participatory Action Research: International contexts and consequences*, State University of New York Press, New York.

Maddern, G. 2011, 'New surgical technologies: When can they be introduced?', paper presented at *2011 Quality and Scientific Program 'Clinical Effectiveness: Rethinking Treatment and Technology'*, Hunter New England Local Health District, 2011.

Marlow, C.R. 2010, *Research Methods for Generalist Social Work*, 5th edn, Brooks/Cole Cengage, Sydney.

Mathias, K.R., Mathias J.M.P. and Hill, P.C. 2011, 'An asset-focused health needs assessment in a rural community in North India', *Asia Pacific Journal of Public Health*, vol. 20, no. 10, pp. 1–12.

Merriam, S. 2009, *Qualitative Research*, Jossey-Bass, San Francisco.

Moore, P. 2009, *Community Needs Assessment Toolkit*, Missouri Association for Community Action, <http://scholar.googleusercontent.com/scholar?q=cache:jnBKDEsvLoIJ:scholar google.com/+community+needs+assessment+toolkit&hl=en&as_sdt=0,5>. Accessed 20 September 2011.

Morris, T. 2006, *Social Work Research Methods: Four alternative paradigms*, Sage, Thousand Oaks, CA.

Naples, N. 2003, *Feminism and Method*, Routledge, New York.

National Association of Social Workers (NASW) 2008, *Code of Ethics of the National Association of Social Workers*, <http://www.socialworkers.org/pubs/code/code.asp>.

National Health and Medical Research Council (NHMRC) 2003, *Values and Ethics: Guidelines for ethical conduct in Aboriginal and Torres Strait Islander Health Research*, Commonwealth of Australia, Canberra, <www.nhmrc.gov.au/_files_nhmrc/publications/attachments/e52.pdf>. Accessed 20 November 2011.

——2006, *Keeping Research on Track: A guide for Aboriginal and Torres Strait Islander peoples about health research ethics*, Commonwealth of Australia, Canberra, <www.nhmrc.gov.au/_files_nhmrc/publications/attachments/e65.pdf>. Accessed 20 November 2011.

——2007, *National Statement on Ethical Conduct in Human Research*, Commonwealth of Australia, Canberra, <www.nhmrc.gov.au/_files_nhmrc/publications/attachments/e72.pdf>, Accessed 20 November 2011.

Norton, M. 2008, 'Systematic reviews: Can qualitative social work research live up to the zeitgeist?' *Qualitative Social Work*, vol. 7, no. 3, pp. 381–6.

Oakley, A. 1985, *The Sociology of Housework*, Basil Blackwell, London.

O'Leary, Z. 2010, *The Essential Guide to Doing Your Research Project*, Sage, Thousand Oaks, CA.

Owen, John M. 1993, *Program Evaluation: Forms and approaches*, Allen & Unwin, Sydney.

Padgett, D. 2008, *Qualitative Methods in Social Work Research*, 2nd edn, Sage, Thousand Oaks, CA.

Pallant, J. 2011, *SPSS Survival Manual*, 4th edn, Allen & Unwin, Sydney.

Payne, M. 2008, *Modern Social Work Theory*, 3rd edn, Palgrave Macmillan, Basingstoke.

Payne, M. and Askeland, G.A. 2008, *Globalisation and International Social Work: Postmodern change and challenge,* Ashgate, Aldershot.

Pearson, K. (ed.) 1930, *Tables for Statisticians and Biometricians*, Imperial College of Science and Technology, London.

Pearson, M. and Coomber, R. 2010, 'The challenge of external validity in policy-relevant systematic reviews: A case study from the field of substance misuse', *Addiction*, vol. 105, no. 1, pp. 136–45.

Petticrew, M. and Roberts, H. 2005, *Systematic Reviews in the Social Sciences: A practical guide*, Blackwell, Oxford.

Pyke, S.W. and Agnew, N.M. 1991, *The Science Game: An introduction to research in the social sciences*, Prentice-Hall, Englewood Cliffs, NJ.

Reason, P. and Bradbury, H. 2006, *Handbook of Action Research Participative Inquiry and Practice*, Sage, London.

Reid, W.J. 1993, 'Writing research reports', in R.M. Grinnell Jr (ed.), *Social Work Research and Evaluation*, 4th edn, Peacock Publishers, Itasca, IL.

Reinharz, S. 1992, *Feminist Methods in Social Research*, Oxford University Press, New York.

Reissman, C.K. 2008, *Narrative Methods for the Human Sciences*, Sage, Thousand Oaks, CA.

Richards, L. and Richards, T. 1990, 'Critiquing qualitative computing: Grounded theory method versus code and retrieve technique', paper presented to Social Research Conference, Brisbane, December.

Roberts, H. (ed.) 1981, *Doing Feminist Research*, Routledge & Kegan Paul, London.

Rossiter, A. 2000, 'The postmodern feminist condition: New conditions for social work', in B. Fawcett, B. Featherstone, J. Fook and A. Rossiter (eds), *Practice and Research in Social Work*, Routledge, London, pp. 24–38.

Rothery, M. 1993, 'The positivistic research approach', in R.M. Grinnell Jr (ed.), *Social Work Research and Evaluation*, 4th edn, Peacock Publishers, Itasca, IL, pp. 38–56.

Rowntree, M. 2010, '"Living my life with grace is my revenge": Situating survivor knowledge about sexual violence', *Qualitative Social Work*, vol. 9, 447–60.

Royse, D. 2009, *Research Methods in Social Work*, 5th edn, Thomson Higher Education, Belmont, CA.

Rubin, A. and Babbie, E. 2010, *Essential Research Methods for Social Work*, 2nd edn, Brooks/Cole, Cengage Learning, Belmont, CA.

——2011, *Research Methods for Social Workers*, 7th edn, Brooks/Cole, Belmont, CA.

Saks, M. and Allsop, J. 2007, *Researching Health: Qualitative, quantitative and mixed methods*, Sage, London.

Sands, R.G. 2004, 'Narrative analysis: A feminist approach', in D.K. Padgett (ed.), *The Qualitative Research Experience*, Wadsworth/Thomson Learning, Belmont, CA, pp. 48–78.

Sarantakos, S. 2005, *Social Research*, 3rd edn, Palgrave Macmillan, Melbourne.

Seccombe, K. 2011, *'So You Think You Can Drive a Cadillac?': Welfare recipients' perspectives on the system and its reform*, 3rd edn, Allyn & Bacon, Boston.

Seigel, L.W., Attkisson, C.C. and Carson, L.G. 1987, 'Need identification and program planning in the community context', in F. Cox et al. (eds), *Strategies of Community Organisation Practice*, Peacock, Itasca, IL.

Slone, D.J. 2009, 'Visualising qualitative information', *The Qualitative Report*, vol. 14, no. 3, pp. 489–97.

Smith, R. 2009, *Doing Social Work Research*, McGraw Hill/Open University Press, Berkshire.

Smith, V., Devane, D., Begley, C.M., and Clarke, M. 2011, 'Methodology in conducting a systematic review of systematic reviews of healthcare interventions', *BMC Medical Research Methodology*, vol. 11, no. 1, pp. 15–20.

Stanley, L. and Wise, S. 1990, 'Method, methodology and epistemology in feminist research process', in L. Stanley (ed.), *Feminist Praxis: Research, theory and epistemology in feminist sociology*, Routledge, London.

Strauss, A. 1990, *Qualitative Analysis for Social Scientists*, Cambridge University Press, Melbourne.

Strauss, A.L. and Corbin, J.M. 1990, *Basics of Qualitative Research: Grounded theory procedures and techniques*, Sage, Newbury Park, CA.

——(eds) 1997, *Grounded Theory in Practice*, Sage, Thousand Oaks, CA.

——1998, *Basics of Qualitative Research: Techniques and procedures for developing grounded theory*, 2nd edn, Sage, Thousand Oaks, CA.

——2008, *Basics of Qualitative Research: Techniques and procedures for developing grounded theory*, 3rd edn, Sage, Thousand Oaks, CA.

Strier, R. 2007, 'Anti-oppressive research in social work: A preliminary definition', *British Journal of Social Work*, vol. 37, no. 5, pp. 857–71.

Sullivan, C.M. 2011, 'Evaluating domestic violence support service programs: Waste of time, necessary evil or opportunity for growth?', *Aggression and Violent Behaviour*, vol. 16, pp. 354–60.

Sullivan, W.P. and Rapp, C.A. 2009, 'Honoring philosophical traditions: The strengths model and the social environment', in D. Saleebey (ed.), *The Strengths Perspective in Social Work Practice*, 5th edn, Pearson, Boston, MA, pp. 220–39.

Taylor, J.B. 1993, 'The naturalistic research approach', in R.M. Grinnell Jr (ed.), *Social Work Research and Evaluation*, 4th edn, Peacock, Itasca, IL, Chapter 4.

The Cochrane Library, <http://onlinelibrary.wiley.com/o/cochrane/cochrane_search_fs.html?newSearch=true>. Accessed 20 November 2011.

Thompson, N. 2009, *Practising Social Work: Meeting the professional challenge*, Palgrave Macmillan, Basingstoke.

Thompson, N. and Thompson, S. 2008, *The Social Work Companion*, Palgrave Macmillan, Basingstoke.

Travers, P. and Richardson, S. 1993, *Living Decently: Material well-being in Australia*, Oxford University Press, Melbourne.

Trinder, L. 2000, 'Reading the texts: Postmodern feminism and the "doing" of research', in B. Fawcett, B. Featherstone, J. Fook and A. Rossiter (eds), *Practice and Research in Social Work: Postmodern feminist perspectives*, Routledge, New York, pp. 39–61.

Tutty, L.M. and Rothery, M. 2010, 'Needs assessments', in B. Thyer (ed.), *The Handbook of Social Work Research Methods*, Sage, Thousand Oaks, CA, pp. 149–62.

Victor, L. 2008, 'Systematic reviewing', *Social Research Update*, vol. 54, pp. 1–4.

Wadsworth, Y. 2011a, *Do It Yourself Social Research: The bestselling practical guide to doing social research projects*, 3rd edn, Allen & Unwin, Sydney.

Wadsworth, Y. 2011b, *Everyday Evaluation on the Run*, 3rd edn, Allen & Unwin, Sydney.

Weinbach, R.W. and Grinnell, R.M. Jr 2010, *Statistics for Social Workers*, 8th edn, Allyn & Bacon, Boston, MA.

Whyte, William F. 1955, *Street Corner Society*, University of Chicago Press, Chicago.

Winokur, M., Holtan, A. and Valentine, D. 2009, 'Kinship care for the safety, permanency, and well-being of children removed from the home for maltreatment', The Cochrane Library, no. 3, <http://onlinelibrary.wiley.com/doi/10.1002/14651858.CD006546.pub2/pdf/standard>. Accessed 20 November 2011.

Yegidis, B.L. and Weinbach, R.W. 2009, *Research Methods for Social Workers*, 6th edn, Allyn & Bacon, Boston, MA.

Yegidis, B.L., Weinbach, R.W. and Myers, L.L. 2012, *Research Methods for Social Workers*, 7th edn, Pearson, Boston, MA.

Zapf, W. 1986, 'Development, structure and prospects for the German social state', in R. Rose and R. Shiartori (eds), *The Welfare State, East and West*, Oxford University Press, Oxford.

Zapf, W., Glatzer, W., Noll, H.H., Habich, R., Berger-Schmitt, R., Brever, S., Diewald, M., Kerber, U., Mohr, H.M. and Wiegand, E. 1987, 'German social report: Living conditions and subjective well-being, 1978–1984', *Social Indicators Research*, vol. 19, no. 1, pp. 5–171.

Zwijsen, S.A., Niemeijer, A.R. and Hertogh, C.M. 2011, 'Ethics of using assistive technology in the care for community-dwelling elderly people: An overview of the literature', *Aging & Mental Health*, vol. 15, no. 4, pp. 419–27.

Author index

Subject index